The CRAFT Treatment Manual for Substance Use Problems

Also Available

Clinical Guide to Alcohol Treatment:
The Community Reinforcement Approach
Robert J. Meyers and Jane Ellen Smith

The CRAFT Treatment Manual for Substance Use Problems

WORKING WITH FAMILY MEMBERS

Jane Ellen Smith
Robert J. Meyers

Foreword by William R. Miller

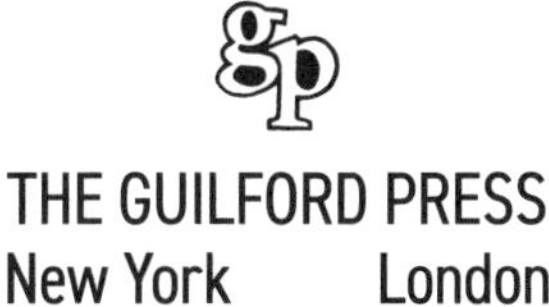

THE GUILFORD PRESS
New York London

A Division of Guilford Publications, Inc.
370 Seventh Avenue, Suite 1200, New York, NY 10001
www.guilford.com

Printed in the United States of America

This book is printed on acid-free paper.

Last digit is print number: 9 8 7 6 5 4 3 2 1

Library of Congress Cataloging-in-Publication Data is available from the publisher.

ISBN 978-1-4625-5110-1 (paperback) — ISBN 978-1-4625-5111-8 (hardcover)

To my sisters, Susan Paradise, Kathryn Constantine, Judith Hakim, and Maria Ricci. You are each unique in terms of your rich personality, chosen life path, playful pursuits, and creative spirit, but you share our family's overwhelming capacity for compassion and devotion to each other. I couldn't love you more.

—J. E. S.

To my two sons, Nicholas Andrew Meyers and Oliver Joseph Meyers, whom I love with all my heart.

—R. J. M.

About the Authors

Jane Ellen Smith, PhD, is Professor of Psychology at the University of New Mexico (UNM). She was the first woman to be tenured in the Psychology Department, to become Director of Clinical Training, and to become Chair of the Department, a role she filled for 12 years. Specializing in both alcohol treatment and eating disorders, Dr. Smith has published over 120 scientific articles and chapters and eight books, and was lead author of the first CRAFT manual in 2004. She is a recipient of the Presidential Teaching Fellowship, UNM's highest teaching award, as well as the UNM Alumni Association's Erna S. Fergusson Award for exceptional accomplishments and/or distinguished service to the university. Dr. Smith, with her colleagues, is responsible for a $15.6 million National Institutes of Health grant focused on hiring diverse biomedical faculty to enhance inclusive excellence efforts at UNM.

Robert J. Meyers, PhD, is Director of Robert J. Meyers, PhD, and Associates, and is Emeritus Research Associate Professor of Psychology at UNM, where his primary affiliation is with the Center on Alcohol, Substance use, And Addictions (CASAA). An internationally sought speaker who has delivered trainings throughout the world, Dr. Meyers is the developer of CRAFT. He is a recipient of the Dan Anderson Research Award from the Hazelden Betty Ford Foundation and the Early Career Investigator Award from the Research Society on Alcoholism. He has published nearly 100 scientific articles or chapters and 10 books, including the CRAFT self-help book *Get Your Loved One Sober.*

Foreword

The impetus to rejuvenate and refine an early version of the Community Reinforcement and Family Training (CRAFT) approach and fully test it actually came from the front-desk staff of our large public addiction treatment program. "Almost every day we receive these desperate calls from family members who are worried about a loved one's drinking or drug use. They don't want to kick the person out, but it's gotten really bad and they don't know what to do. What should we tell them?"

Back in the 1980s there were three main responses. The first was "I'm sorry, but there is nothing we can do until the person contacts us to ask for help." Indeed, while insurers might pay to treat the drinker or drug user, there was no coverage to help their distressed family members directly. Having to say that to distraught family members also distressed our staff.

A second option was to refer the family members to Al-Anon, a 12-step program where they could receive compassionate support from peers with similar experience. The Al-Anon program encourages family members to detach and accept that they are helpless to influence their loved one. People who attend Al-Anon often do benefit themselves, but for their primary concern the message was the same: "There's nothing you can do until the person is ready to ask for help." They didn't feel detached, nor did they want to wait passively for their loved one to "hit bottom."

Then there was "the Intervention," originally developed by the Johnson Institute, a kind of surprise party where the person is confronted by a roomful of people concerned about his or her substance use. A specially trained facilitator would work with the family, usually for a fee, preparing them for the eventual confrontation. This normally required weeks or months while they identified and trained the Concerned Significant Others (CSOs) who were willing to participate, and found a treatment program ready to admit the person on the designated date. Usually there would be a vehicle waiting outside to take the person off to treatment, and often some negative consequences would be announced if the person refused to go. About 70% of families ultimately decided not to go through with the Intervention, often for fear of damage to family relationships.

And that was it: Wait for the person to suffer enough to be "ready," go to Al-Anon, or plan an Intervention. Were there no other possibilities?

Based on his successful experience with using a community reinforcement method to treat people suffering from substance use disorders, Bob Meyers developed CRAFT as a very different approach. Invite the CSOs to come in themselves, even if their loved one was unwilling. The message was not one of helplessness but quite the opposite: that "there *are* things you can do." Always conscious of safety first, the CRAFT team taught family members how to use positive reinforcement rather than punishment to help their loved one make better choices and hopefully accept help. Families learned how to positively encourage *the right stuff* and not inadvertently make it any easier for the person to continue using. The clinical procedures described in this manual are clear and doable, and I had the further privilege of witnessing *how* people were treated: with warmth, encouragement, empathy and, yes, positive reinforcement for every step in the right direction.

It sounds good, but the proof was in the outcome. In a definitive clinical trial, CSOs were randomly assigned to receive, without fee, one of three professional treatment methods, each provided by therapists trained and believing in their approach. Some received Al-Anon facilitation therapy, helping them to get engaged in the fellowship and to work the Al-Anon program. Others received an intervention facilitated by therapists trained in the Johnson Institute approach, and a third set of participants were offered CRAFT. Families in all three conditions personally benefited: Their depression, anxiety, and physical symptoms decreased. The major difference was in what happened with their loved ones. In the Al-Anon condition, few CSOs got their loved one into treatment, which is fair enough because influencing the substance user is not a goal in Al-Anon. As usual, 70% of families in the Intervention group decided not to go through with it. In the CRAFT condition, however, two-thirds of families succeeded in getting their loved one into treatment within about 6 weeks on average. CSOs observed that even before beginning treatment, their loved one's drinking had decreased to about half its previous level. Two subsequent randomized trials found that CRAFT families engaged at least two-thirds of drug users in treatment, and this finding has been replicated by research teams in several other nations. CRAFT works.

What you have in this manual from Bob Meyers and Jane Ellen Smith is seasoned professional advice from the very psychologists who have grown and tested the CRAFT approach, based on their decades of clinical experience and research. CRAFT has been successfully delivered in individual, group, and even self-directed formats. The procedures are specific and learnable, offering hope and change for distressed families that are wondering what to do. It is also rewarding work, with some of the most motivated clients you will ever see: the CSOs themselves. We who go into helping professions hope that we can contribute to the alleviation of suffering in the world, and here is a practical and effective way to do it.

WILLIAM R. MILLER, PHD
Emeritus Distinguished Professor of Psychology and Psychiatry, University of New Mexico

Preface

In all probability you know someone with a serious substance use problem who absolutely refuses to get help. Or if you don't find *yourself* in this situation, it is likely you have a friend, or a client, who does. The Concerned Significant Others (CSOs) of treatment-refusing individuals (Identified Patients; IPs) suffer tremendously. This distress stems from day-to-day anxiety regarding the IP's well-being, but also from the chronic fallout associated with the IP's substance use: the CSO's social embarrassment or isolation, financial uncertainty, depression, chaotic home environment, or domestic abuse. What options do these CSOs have? Although many CSOs have found comfort and support over the years through mutual-help groups like Al-Anon and Nar-Anon, CSOs have wanted more.

Community Reinforcement and Family Training (CRAFT) is a scientifically supported behavioral treatment that works directly with the *family members or friends* (the CSOs) of treatment-refusing individuals with substance use problems (the IPs). "Community reinforcement" represents CRAFT's belief that IPs must learn how to find healthy rewards (reinforcement) in their communities (e.g., at home, work, school, or place of worship, or through hobbies and their social life) that do not revolve around substance use. CRAFT accomplishes this objective by inviting the typically eager *CSO* to attend therapy—without the IP. During CRAFT sessions, the CSO is taught how to modify her or his own behavior at home in order to reward *non-using* IP behavior and to withdraw rewards when the IP uses. The CSO also learns to communicate in a positive manner with the IP and to use the array of new skills ultimately to invite the IP to begin treatment. Throughout, the CSO is *never* blamed for an IP's drinking or drug use. And of central importance: CRAFT offers each CSO the opportunity to enhance her or his overall well-being, regardless of the outcome for the IP.

Empirical studies going back as far as the 1980s show that CRAFT-trained CSOs are successful at getting their treatment-refusing IPs into treatment two-thirds of the time, on average. This success is evidenced regardless of the CSOs' ethnicity or race and no matter what their relationship is to the IP (e.g., spouse, partner, sibling, parent, friend). CRAFT's success also is not dependent upon the IP's drug of choice.

This clinician-friendly treatment manual describes CRAFT's objectives and walks therapists step-by-step through each CRAFT procedure while incorporating illustrative cases complete with clinician–CSO dialogue. Uniquely, each procedure-oriented chapter is built around a checklist that is an outline of the main components of the procedure.

The checklists are intended to serve as handy guides that new CRAFT therapists bring into sessions. This manual also contains all of the necessary forms for conducting CRAFT and includes examples of how these forms would have been completed by the individuals represented in the case examples. Drawing on our years of experience training and supervising CRAFT clinicians, the chapters also offer specific tips for enhancing the delivery of each procedure and for avoiding common pitfalls.

All of the components contained in this treatment manual are critical, as CRAFT therapists must strategize with their clients (the CSOs) how to facilitate behavior change in a person who is not even in the therapy room (the IP). Despite this complexity, CRAFT appeals to many clinicians because it relies on a motivational (nonconfrontational) style, solid clinical judgment, and a creative approach to problem solving. And since they are working with CSOs as opposed to individuals with substance use problems, CRAFT therapists do not have to be experts in substance use treatment to be effective.

This manual offers a complete description of CRAFT and a guide to doing it. And yet, research on therapy outcomes shows that reading a treatment manual (or even attending a multiday workshop) should be supplemented by individualized performance feedback (e.g., having one's recorded therapy sessions reviewed) if possible, and preferably by an expert in the particular treatment (Miller & Moyers, 2021; Miller & Rollnick, 2014). To learn about CRAFT-based supervision that includes an explicit program for becoming a certified CRAFT therapist, visit Dr. Meyers's website at *www.robertjmeyersphd.com*. Although this certification is *not* required for clinicians to practice CRAFT, it is strongly encouraged.

Foundational material for this CRAFT treatment manual is drawn from Smith and Meyers (2004, 2010) and Meyers and Smith (1995).

A word about pronouns: To minimize confusion, we have opted to use "she or he" and "he or she" when singular pronouns are needed to discuss CSOs and IPs. We put she/her/hers first when referring to CSOs (e.g., "she or he") and he/him/his first when writing about IPs (e.g., "he or she"). We have made this choice for simplicity of language and do not mean to exclude those who use gender-neutral pronouns.

Contents

Purchasers of this book can download and print enlarged versions of the forms and handouts at *www.guilford.com/smith9-forms* for personal use or use with clients (see copyright page for details).

Chapter 1

What Is CRAFT?

Gloria is desperate. She is riddled with anxiety and sadness. The stress is almost unbearable. She has tried *everything* to get her husband to stop drinking and using drugs, ranging from begging him to screaming at him. She also has threatened to leave him on more than one occasion, but she knows she never will. She does *not* want to simply detach from him. Gloria just wants her "old husband" back. Occasionally he *does* dramatically reduce his substance use, and for a short period of time she catches a glimpse of the loving man she married years ago. But these changes never last. Gloria is desperate.

TREATMENT-REFUSING INDIVIDUALS WITH SUBSTANCE USE PROBLEMS

According to a 2018 national survey, approximately 20.3 million U.S. adults had a substance use disorder (SUD) during the previous year, but only 3.7 million people received any type of substance use treatment (Substance Abuse and Mental Health Services Administration, 2019). The major reasons given by these individuals for *not* seeking treatment included believing they did not need treatment, or not being ready to stop using (McKetin, Voce, Burns, & Quinn, 2020; Substance Abuse and Mental Health Services Administration, 2019). Notably, the loved ones of these treatment-refusing individuals reported that approximately five family members or friends were impacted directly by the treatment-refusing individual's substance use problem, such as through social embarrassment, financial concerns, domestic mistreatment, chaotic family environments, and anxiety-related emotional or physical problems (Hussaarts, Roozen, Meyers, van de Wetering, & McCrady, 2011).

COMMUNITY REINFORCEMENT AND FAMILY TRAINING

Community Reinforcement and Family Training (CRAFT) is a research-supported treatment for the family members (e.g., spouses, partners, siblings, adult children) or friends of individuals with substance use problems who *absolutely refuse* to seek therapy. The family members or friends are called Concerned Significant Others (CSOs), and the individuals with substance use problems who *should* be in treatment (but who refuse to attend) are called Identified Patients (IPs). CRAFT was developed to support CSOs who did not know where to turn to get help for their loved one. These CSOs did not want to "detach" from their IPs, and they were unwilling to use a confrontational approach to force them into a program. Without other options, CSOs returned to unsuccessful methods for getting IPs into treatment: threatening, pleading, arguing, and resorting to the "silent treatment."

CRAFT is an outgrowth of the Community Reinforcement Approach (CRA), a scientifically supported behavioral treatment for individuals with SUDs that originated in the 1970s (Azrin, 1976; Azrin, Sisson, Meyers, & Godley, 1982; Hunt & Azrin, 1973). The early CRA researchers realized that the wives of the alcohol-abusing men in their studies could be highly influential in bringing about positive change (Sisson & Azrin, 1986), as evidenced by their active roles in CRA's relationship therapy sessions (see Chapter 12). Recent research has made it even *more* apparent that individuals such as these (CSOs) should begin treatment *themselves* if their loved one with a substance use problem (IP) refuses to enter treatment. The two major reasons are as follows:

1. CSOs receiving CRAFT can play a valuable role in getting their IPs to enter treatment (Archer, Harwood, Stevelink, Rafferty, & Greenberg, 2019; Roozen, de Waart, & van der Kroft, 2010). This appears to be based on the findings that:

- CSOs have a tremendous amount of valuable information about their IPs that can be extremely helpful when preparing a detailed, well-conceived plan to get an IP to enter treatment.
- CSOs have extensive contact with their IPs, and consequently have many opportunities to influence an IP's behavior in a direction that supports treatment engagement and reduced substance use.
- IPs who eventually begin treatment often have reported that one of the major reasons for their decision to do so was their family's influence (Cunningham, Sobell, Sobell, & Kapur, 1995; Meyers, Roozen, Smith, & Evans, 2014; Perumbilly, Melendez-Rhodes, & Anderson, 2019).

2. CSOs frequently suffer both emotionally and physically due to their ongoing involvement with an individual with a substance use problem who refuses help (Lander, Howsare, & Byrne, 2013). Not surprisingly, these CSOs report a lower quality of life than the general population (Birkeland et al., 2018; Dawson, Grant, Chou, & Stinson, 2007; Kaur, Mahajan, Sunder Deepti, & Singh, 2018). Examples of the common types of problems CSOs experience and that CRAFT addresses (Roozen et al., 2010) include[1]:

- Social withdrawal/isolation
- Depression
- Anxiety/stress
- Relationship problems
- Physical/health problems
- Domestic violence
- Financial uncertainty/loss

CRAFT therapists work with CSOs to accomplish three main goals:

1. To help the substance-using individual (IP) reduce alcohol/drug use, preferably prior to entering treatment.
2. To influence the IP to enter treatment.
3. To enhance the CSO's happiness and functioning overall, regardless of whether the IP enters treatment.

How are these goals accomplished? Essentially, the CSOs focus on moving their IPs toward a path promoted by CRA: one in which their IP's life is rewarding *without* it revolving around alcohol and drugs. Importantly, since working with CSOs is one (large) step removed from having the IPs sitting in the therapy room themselves, CRAFT therapists must be highly creative when they develop strategies for CSOs to start rewarding the IP's *non-using* behavior and to stop rewarding the IP's using behavior. In this book, we review these strategies and present the CRAFT program, describe how it works, and explain why this type of therapy can be a valuable way to treat those closest to the IP. We do *not* present a detailed discussion of an intake assessment, since most agencies and clinicians have their own preferred (or mandated) assessment process. We do, however, suggest several assessment instruments that might be appropriate for a CRAFT CSO (see Box 1.1).

CRAFT's Scientific Support

CRAFT has an excellent research record (see Chapter 13; see also Archer et al., 2019; Roozen et al., 2010, for reviews). Studies show that, through work with CSOs, CRAFT is successful at getting treatment-refusing substance-abusing individuals (IPs) to seek treatment about two-thirds of the time (with multiple studies showing even higher rates). This success has been found across a variety of CSO–IP relationships (romantic partners, parents/children, siblings, friends) and drug or alcohol choices (Archer et al., 2019). Importantly, in addition to the research demonstrating high treatment-engagement rates, CRAFT has also shown very good outcomes as far as improvements in CSOs' anxiety, depression, family cohesion, and relationship happiness *regardless* of whether their IP started treatment (Roozen et al., 2010).

Therapists Who Are Drawn to CRAFT

Therapists who tend to embrace CRAFT are ones who have good clinical skills overall, such as being empathic, nonjudgmental, genuine, and warm. They also believe in the importance of a strong therapeutic alliance, and readily support clients with encouragement and praise as needed. For example, these therapists are willing to work with CSOs to give up the self-blame they feel for their IP's substance use, and to discuss CSOs' acts of courage—namely, their sacrifices and determination to keep the family going. Clinicians who are drawn to CRAFT tend to rely on a motivational style as opposed to a confrontational one. Additionally, they have a cognitive-behavioral or a behavioral theoretical orientation or are open to new therapeutic approaches. Last, these clinicians recognize the importance of ongoing supervision when first implementing a new treatment.

BOX 1.1

Measures Commonly Used with CSOs

Measures to Assess CSO Functioning

Overall functioning:

- Outcome Questionnaire–45 (Lambert et al., 2004)
- Significant Other Survey—Self-Administered (Benishek et al., 2012)

Depression:

- Beck Depression Inventory–II (Beck, Steer, & Brown, 1996)

Anxiety/stress:

- Beck Anxiety Inventory (Beck & Steer, 1993)
- State–Trait Anxiety Inventory—State Version (Spielberger, Gorsuch, Lushene, Vagg, & Jacobs, 1983)

Anger:

- State–Trait Anger Expression Inventory–2 (Spielberger, 1999)

Self-esteem:

- Rosenberg Self-Esteem Scale (Rosenberg, 1965)

Perceived impact of IP's substance use:

- Family Member Impact (Orford, Templeton, Velleman, & Copello, 2005)

Social support:

- Multidimensional Scale of Perceived Social Support (Zimet, Dahlem, Zimet, & Farley, 1988)
- Perceived Support Scale (Krause & Borawski-Clark, 1995)
- Social Support Questionnaire—Short Form Revised (Sarason, Sarason, Shearin, & Pierce, 1987)

Support of IP's sober or using behaviors:

- Sobriety Support subscale of the Spouse Sobriety Influence Inventory (Yoshioka, Thomas, & Ager, 1992)
- Enabling Behaviors subscale of the Behavior Enabling Scale (Rotunda, West, & O'Farrell, 2004)

Measures to Assess the CSO–IP Relationship

- Relationship Happiness Scale (Azrin, Naster, & Jones, 1973; Smith & Meyers, 2004, Chapter 12, Figure 12.6). *Note*: This version is for romantic partners. The categories can be modified to fit other types of CSO–IP relationships.
- Dyadic Adjustment Scale (Busby, Crane, Larson, & Christensen, 1995)
- Revised Conflict Tactics Scale (Straus, Hamby, Boney-McCoy, & Sugarman, 1996)
- Conflict Tactics Scale—Short Form (Straus & Douglas, 2004)
- Areas of Change Questionnaire (Margolin, Talovic, & Weinstein, 1983)

Measures to Assess CSO Report of IP Substance Use and Treatment

- Form-90—Collateral (Miller, 1996)
- Treatment Services Review–6 (Cacciola et al., 2008)

We have heard clinicians report many reasons why they find CRAFT so appealing. Some of the more common ones include:

- It works! CRAFT is highly effective at getting treatment-refusing individuals into treatment.
- They recognize the need for a science-supported program that does *not* tell desperate CSOs that nothing can be done and does *not* say they must confront the substance-abusing individual.
- CRAFT is effective with CSOs (and IPs) who represent many different cultures, ages, and CSO–IP relationships (e.g., romantic partners, parents/children, siblings).
- CRAFT can be used for IPs who have alcohol problems *and* for IPs experiencing problems with illicit drugs.
- This "menu-driven" program relies on clinicians to use their clinical skills, such as determining *which* procedures should be introduced and *when* with different clients.
- Therapists are not expected to pressure CSOs to engage in procedures or tasks that CSOs are uncomfortable attempting.
- Therapists enjoy working with CSOs due to their high level of motivation.
- CRAFT allows therapists to contribute to the substance use field without necessarily being a substance use expert.

CRAFT PROCEDURES

CRAFT was designed to be approximately a 12-session program with the 50-minute sessions occurring weekly, but of course flexibility is acceptable depending on client needs. This treatment comprises a set of procedures—nine primary ones in all (see below)—that you use to teach CSOs new behaviors and strategies geared toward influencing the treatment-refusing loved one to reduce substance use and enter treatment. Each procedure begins with you offering a cogent rationale and outlining the components of the procedure. You then work collaboratively with the CSO to personalize the material such that it suits the particular CSO and IP. Each procedure ends with precise instruction regarding how to implement the procedure outside of the session and how to address any obstacles that might surface in the process. An overview of each of the main CRAFT procedures follows, along with brief case illustrations.[2]

1. Informing and Motivating the CSO

A significant part of the first CRAFT session is devoted to reassuring CSOs that although they will be part of the solution to their IP's problem, it does *not* mean that CSOs are responsible for the substance use. The session also offers factual details about the CRAFT program (see Chapter 2) and instills hope that their loved ones will get better.

> Catalina (CSO) had debated with herself for about 6 months as to whether there was anything she could do to help her drug-abusing close friend get into treatment. At the

conclusion of Catalina's first CRAFT session, she is convinced she has come to the right place. She feels more motivated than ever to actively work to help her friend, and she knows she will be given the best tools and guidance to accomplish this task.

2. Functional Analysis ("Road Map") of a Loved One's Drinking or Using Behavior

CRAFT's functional analysis (FA) is the CSO's depiction of the context for the IP's substance use. This "road map" includes the IP's triggers for using substances, as well as the consequences (both positive and negative). Such a depiction allows you and the CSO to start developing a strategy for intervening (see Chapter 3).

Tori (CSO) realizes upon doing a road map of her husband's heavy Friday night drinking that his primary positive consequences (rewards) include receiving his coworkers' admiration for being entertaining, and being able to unwind/relax after a stressful week of work. With the help of her CRAFT therapist, Tori plans a pleasurable activity to compete with the Friday night high-risk time. The event is dinner at home with a fun, high-energy married couple that do not drink. Importantly, the couple and Tori's husband greatly enjoy each other's company.

3. Improving CSOs' Communication Skills

When helping CSOs establish plans for new ways of interacting with their IPs, preparatory skills training is needed (see Chapter 4). The most important of these skills is positive communication, as it plays a role in each of the other CRAFT procedures. Communication training entails practicing socially skilled options for handling important conversations with IPs that then typically result in an increased willingness of IPs to listen.

Jeremiah (CSO) and his 18-year-old daughter (IP) find themselves in yelling matches whenever the topic of her marijuana-smoking boyfriend comes up. The daughter has been grappling with her own marijuana problem, and so Jeremiah is trying to limit her exposure to marijuana cues (and get her into treatment). After practicing communication skills in CRAFT, Jeremiah might say something like the following to his daughter:

> "I know you and your boyfriend are really tight; I actually know what that's like [*understanding statement*]. And I probably should have spoken up earlier and tried to help when I realized that both of you were struggling [*partial responsibility statement*]. Anyway, I worry about you [*feelings statement*], so now I'm just doing my best to try to keep you safe [*positive statement*]. I'm happy to do whatever I can to help [*offer to help statement*], but I don't know all the answers, and so I need your help, too, when it comes to making sure you are safe and happy [*positive, specific statement*]."

4. Rewarding Non-Using Behavior

The critical strategy of Rewarding Non-Using Behavior (see Chapters 5 and 6) teaches CSOs how to give rewards only when their IPs are *not* using substances, thereby increasing the frequency of the non-using behavior.

Hayley (CSO) reminds her sister (IP) that they used to enjoy taking a walk after work each day in order to de-stress and to have some hearty laughs. Hayley tells her sister she would love to start taking walks with her again, but only if the sister has refrained from using pills that day. When the sister shows up for their walk the next day, she is substance-free, and so the two sisters head out to the trail already laughing.

5. Withdrawing Rewards for Using Behavior

The related strategy of Withdrawing Rewards for Using Behavior, often used in conjunction with the previous one (Rewarding Non-Using Behavior), teaches CSOs how to withdraw rewards consistently when their IPs are using substances, thereby decreasing the frequency of the using behavior (see Chapter 7).

Kirsten (CSO) tells her husband (IP) she misses their Saturday morning countryside drives that involved stopping at various farmers' markets along the way. Kirsten says she would like to go on these excursions again and has mapped out a few new routes if they decide to do so. She tells her husband she is interested in going only if he has not been drinking the night before. Kirsten's husband expresses interest in the Saturday excursion, but he drinks Friday night anyway. After breakfast Saturday morning he asks Kirsten whether she is ready to hit the road. Kirsten reminds him that the plan was to go if he did not drink the night before. She tells him that although the trip is off, she is looking forward to trying again the next weekend.

6. Allowing for Natural, Negative Consequences of Use

A structured plan of allowing for natural, negative consequences of use (see Chapter 8) assists CSOs in refraining from engaging in certain behavior with their inebriated/high IPs that inadvertently may be *supporting* continued substance use.

Katie (CSO) is asked to think about her pattern of routinely preparing a warm meal for her son (IP) when he returns home late in the evening after using drugs with his friends. Upon reflection, Katie admits that ever since she started doing this for her son, he seems to be coming home later, and more "out of it." The CRAFT therapist acknowledges that Katie is simply trying to make sure her son gets a healthy dinner, but wonders whether she might be making it a little easier for her son to keep getting high (and for using increased amounts of drugs) when she takes care of him in this manner. Katie decides to cease this behavior and to let her son know in advance about her plan and its rationale.

7. Problem Solving

In CRAFT, CSOs learn a structured approach for breaking down problems into manageable pieces and generating specific plans (and backup plans) for resolving them (see Chapter 9).

Jamie (CSO) is struggling to come up with possible coping strategies to suggest to a partner (IP) for those evenings when he reports strong cravings. The therapist teaches Jamie how to use CRAFT's problem-solving skills to narrow down the problem, generate multiple solutions, select a reasonable solution, address potential obstacles, and establish a backup plan. Jamie plans to present the suggested solution to her partner the next day.

8. Helping CSOs Enrich Their Own Lives

In the procedure Helping CSOs Enrich Their Own Lives, the Happiness Scale and the Goal Setting exercise (see Chapter 10) are used to explore CSOs' happiness in various areas of their lives and to develop successful strategies to work toward new goals.

Marta (CSO) wants to set a physical activity goal for herself in the "Health and Wellness" category from the CRAFT Happiness Scale (see Form 10.2 at the end of Chapter 10). She knows from experience that she will be more likely to accomplish her goal (strength training for 30 minutes three times a week) if she exercises with another person. A good friend has hinted about having Marta join her when she works out, but Marta has never taken the friend up on the offer. Marta commits to asking her friend that evening if she could join her for some strength training starting the upcoming Saturday afternoon.

9. Inviting the IP to Enter Treatment

The next set of procedures, which are introduced after considerable groundwork has been laid, revolves around preparing and practicing the invitation for the IP to attend treatment (which includes motivational "hooks"), and lining up an appropriate therapist (see Chapter 11).

Kamilla (CSO) is ready to invite her partner Elizabeth (IP) to enter treatment. She has rehearsed the positive conversation multiple times with the CRAFT therapist. The invitation to her partner would sound something like this:

> "Elizabeth, you mean the world to me [*feelings statement*]. And I can understand why you get upset when I try to talk with you about your weekend drinking and smoking, because you said it seems like I'm trying to change who you are as a person [*understanding statement*] That's not what I'm trying to do; I'm just worried about you [*feelings statement*]. I know it doesn't help that I'm working weekend nights and so I'm not available to do stuff [*partial responsibility statement*]. Anyway, I've been in therapy for a few weeks now to try to figure out how to deal with my stress over your weekend substance use [*specific behavior statement*]. I'm actually hoping that you'll join me for one session, just to see what it's like. Then if you decide you're willing to try it yourself, you'd have your own therapist. And I've been told that your therapist would let you be in charge of what you decide to work on and when. Of course, I'd be hoping that you'd look at your marijuana use, but that would be up to you. You've talked about wanting to get reconnected with your family. Maybe that's something you could focus on in therapy, too?"

When to Present the Various CRAFT Procedures

How are these nine primary CRAFT procedures distributed across the (approximately) 12 sessions? A reasonable starting point would be to assume that each procedure occurs in its own separate session, yet there are common exceptions to this. Most of the variations revolve around outcomes either anticipated or associated with the all-important "homework": those between-session assignments that CSOs complete that are based on the skills learned in the CRAFT procedure that week (see Chapter 2, Box 2.5; Chapter 3, Box 3.1). For example, you could decide that a second procedure (e.g., Problem Solving) should be added to a session to equip the CSO to successfully complete the homework assignment. Alternatively, it would be reasonable to spend more than one session on a specific procedure if, for instance, the CSO had difficulty carrying out the homework that was based on the previous week's CRAFT procedure. In this situation, you might decide to review the procedure again before developing a modified homework assignment. Also, occasionally there is insufficient time to complete a procedure during the session. In these cases, you would determine whether enough of the procedure had been covered such that the CSO could attempt to finish it for homework. Of course, the outcome would be reviewed at the start of the next session.

In what order should the different CRAFT procedures be introduced? The order in which the CRAFT procedures are presented in this book is not necessarily the exact order in which they need to be conducted with every CSO, and yet we describe them in an order that would be considered reasonable for many CSOs. Importantly, there are clear recommendations for the timing of those procedures that form the foundation for other procedures. For example, it is imperative that Improving CSOs' Communication Skills (Chapter 4) is taught in one of the earliest CRAFT sessions so that these skills can be incorporated into procedures that require positive communication skills (e.g., Rewarding Non-Using Behavior, Chapter 5; Withdrawing Rewards, Chapter 7). Some of the other procedures, such as Problem Solving (Chapter 9), are introduced when clinically indicated. The section at the beginning of each chapter that describes a CRAFT procedure (Chapters 2–11) entitled "Procedure Timing" should be helpful as you make your decision as to when the procedures in question should be conducted.

USING THE CHECKLISTS AS GUIDES

The chapters that present CRAFT procedures each contain a checklist that provides a detailed outline of the main components of the CRAFT procedure being covered. The expectation is that new CRAFT therapists will refer to these checklists as treatment guides during their sessions with CSOs. Importantly, the format of these chapters is organized in line with the checklists, thereby facilitating movement back-and-forth between the checklist and both the relevant instructions for each component of a procedure *and* an illustrative clinician–CSO dialogue.

DECIDING WHETHER CRAFT IS RIGHT FOR A CSO

CRAFT has received widespread support across many types of individuals and scenarios, but you still must use your own expert clinical judgment in deciding whether a *specific* CSO might safely benefit from CRAFT. Particular caution is advised, for example, for CSOs who report that domestic violence is a concern. Safety considerations must be a top priority, given the link between substance use and domestic violence (Cafferky, Mendez,

Anderson, & Stith, 2018) *and* the fact that several CRAFT procedures are *designed* to be unpleasant for IPs when they are using substances (see Chapter 2). Since many of the CRAFT studies excluded CSOs who reported that their IPs had engaged in domestic violence in recent years or had exhibited severe violent behavior at any point in the past, their outcomes (and safety) in CRAFT were not tested. Again, caution is advised.

CSOs who themselves had an SUD or a serious mental health condition were not routinely included in most CRAFT studies, but that does not necessarily suggest they should be excluded from CRAFT treatment. In fact, a study by Dutcher et al. (2009) allowed CSOs with their own substance use problems to participate, and reasonable results were obtained (see Chapter 13). The main consideration would be whether you believe that the CSO would be able to carry out the CRAFT-related tasks.

A few additional CSO presentations merit enhanced scrutiny in terms of their suitability for CRAFT, given that the CRAFT studies either did not test them, or issues became apparent in the course of conducting the studies. CSOs in the CRAFT studies were at least 18 years old. It is unknown whether a younger individual would be an appropriate CSO candidate—likely it would depend on the maturity of the person and the type of CSO–IP relationship. In terms of the extent of the CSO's contact with the IP, many CRAFT studies required contact on an average of at least 3 days a week. The belief was that CSOs who had limited contact with their IPs would not have sufficient opportunities to influence the IPs' behavior to any meaningful extent. Although one can surmise that there is nothing magical about the 3-day criterion, nonetheless you should keep in mind that it is critical for CSOs to interact with their IPs in order to promote and support behavior change. Finally, during the CRAFT studies it occasionally became apparent that a CSO was unwilling to participate fully in the program and instead expected the CRAFT therapist to somehow *make* the IP enter treatment. This is not a workable arrangement since CRAFT entails teaching CSOs skills and then having them go home and implement the procedures with their IPs.

THE BIG PICTURE: WORKING TOGETHER TOWARD A COMPREHENSIVE PLAN

It would be a mistake to assume the CRAFT program is merely a package containing odds and ends of therapy procedures. Instead, CRAFT is a comprehensive treatment that begins with an investigation of the factors that are driving or maintaining each IP's substance-using behavior, and then proceeds to devising a plan for CSOs to intervene. However, CSOs must learn specific skills and practice them in session before the plans (i.e., the homework assignments) can be enacted at home. Once the plans are in play, CRAFT therapists check on their progress regularly, and troubleshoot any problems that arise. Throughout the CRAFT treatment process, the need for CSOs to follow through with contingencies (such as rewarding their IPs only when they are *not* using) is stressed. Additionally, CSOs are reminded that each new procedure and homework assignment is but one step in the overall CRAFT program, and that the various steps work together to achieve treatment engagement. In Chapter 2, we discuss the first procedure: Informing and Motivating the CSO.

NOTES

1. Research documentation of these various CSO problems can be found in Benishek, Kirby, and Dugosh (2011); Dawson et al. (2007); Haugland (2005); Hussaarts et al. (2011); Kaur et al. (2018); Mancheri, Alavi, Sabzi, and Maghsoudi (2019); Nadkarni et al. (2019); Orford (2017); Orford, Velleman, Copello, Templeton, and Ibanga (2010); and Tsuji, Aoki, Irie, and Sakano (2020).
2. The cases throughout this book are fictionalized composites of cases.

Chapter 2

Informing and Motivating the Concerned Significant Other

The first CRAFT procedure is called Informing and Motivating the CSO. In addition to offering the opportunity for engaging a CSO and building an alliance, the procedure provides an overview of the CRAFT program, a description of its elements, and a basic explanation of the theory upon which it is based. It also begins the task of determining the best strategies for a CSO to change her or his behavior toward the substance-abusing loved one (IP) in a manner that ultimately should influence the IP to enter treatment.

This first meeting provides CSOs with much more than factual details about the CRAFT program; it offers hope that their loved ones will get better. Importantly, it makes CSOs aware of their own critical role in this recovery process, which includes learning new skills and modifying how they interact with their IP. CSOs react to this news with a variety of emotions, such as surprise, optimism, annoyance, anxiety, determination, or discouragement. It is not unusual for CSOs to ask whether they are at fault for the IP's substance use, since CSOs are the individuals being asked to make changes. Consequently, a significant part of your job in this first session is to reassure CSOs that although they will be part of the solution to their IP's problem, it absolutely does *not* mean that CSOs are responsible for the substance use. Furthermore, you frame the CSOs' prior efforts to get their IPs to stop abusing substances as herculean acts of courage and devotion that were based on the CSOs' best knowledge at the time.

THE BASICS

General Description

Informing and Motivating the CSO begins with an invitation for CSOs to share their IP's story; the ways in which the IP's substance use has created difficulties for the CSO and others, and the many attempts CSOs have made to address the problem. After conveying empathy and support, you review relevant assessment findings, and then shift the focus to the CRAFT program's offerings. You then present an overview of CRAFT's goals, principles, and procedures, linking them to the CSO's own unique situation. The need for CSOs to play a significant role in CRAFT is highlighted, and examples of typical CSO tasks and assignments are given. Positive expectations are enhanced by reviewing the scientific support for CRAFT.

Throughout the session, you watch for opportunities both to remind CSOs that the IP's substance use is *not* the CSO's fault, and to gain insight into possible CSO motivators in addition to the primary one of getting their IP into treatment. The importance of CSOs' safety is assessed and stressed throughout.

Procedure Timing

The first CRAFT procedure, Informing and Motivating the CSO, is conducted in the first CRAFT session. We assume that prior to this session the CSO's intake assessment will have been conducted already, either by you, your agency's intake worker, or a referring therapist. However, it is unlikely that the results of the testing, the "feedback," will have been communicated to the CSO yet. Thus, the testing feedback is incorporated into the first CRAFT procedure.

Form

- Informing and Motivating the CSO: Checklist (Form 2.1)

CLINICIAN GUIDANCE AND SAMPLE DIALOGUE

To illustrate the CRAFT procedures in this book, each chapter contains a sample case that highlights a representative clinician–CSO dialogue for the particular procedure. The components for the first CRAFT procedure, Informing and Motivating the CSO, are presented below and outlined in Form 2.1, Informing and Motivating the CSO: Checklist, found at the end of this chapter. Note that both the numbered and the italicized subheadings used in this chapter correspond to items on the checklist, thereby allowing you to easily cross-reference between the checklist items and the detailed chapter instructions for the matching CRAFT components. As stated earlier, the expectation is that new CRAFT therapists will have these checklists readily available to resort to as guides during sessions.

The order in which we introduce the topics in this chapter (i.e., the various components/steps of the procedure) does not need to be adhered to strictly, but this order seems reasonable for most CSOs. Clinical issues that arise during the session may dictate a different course, however. As mentioned, this procedure makes the assumption that some type of assessment was already conducted, the content of which will have been determined by factors such as agency and clinician preference, available length of time for assessments, and instrument copyright issues (see Chapter 1, Box 1.1, for several options for suggested instruments). We also assume you will have read through the assessment results prior to starting this session. Periodically the assessment does not contain information about the CSO's perception of which substance is being used by the IP, as well as how much or how often (see Box 1.1, Form-90—Collateral). In such a case, if the CSO does not offer this information automatically near the start of this CRAFT session, it would be useful to ask for it. Although these details will be collected in the next procedure, during the functional analysis (FA; see Chapter 3), this basic information could help frame the remaining topics in the first CRAFT session.

Case Description

The CSO (Kelsey) is the non-Hispanic white 46-year-old younger sister of the 50-year-old IP (Riley). Kelsey lives with her husband and two children. Recently her brother (IP) moved into her basement apartment after losing his job and apartment due to drug use. Kelsey and her brother have maintained a reasonably close relationship over the years despite the many family problems his substance use has created. Although Riley's illicit drug use has decreased somewhat in his new living situation, his drinking has increased considerably. Both Kelsey and her 75-year-old parents have not known where to turn for help.

1. Invite the CSO to describe the IP's substance use and the problems created by it.

Have the CSO describe some of the problems created by the substance use.

A CSO's description of the problems created by the IP's substance use provides insight into the CSO's own valued objects or feelings that have been lost as a result of the IP's use. Examples include no longer feeling financially secure as a result of the IP getting fired, being too embarrassed to attend social events with an IP who is inebriated or high, and worrying about the children witnessing too much arguing between their parents. It is helpful to later remind CSOs that they are moving toward regaining these lost "valuables" (financial stability, social activities, family harmony) as a way to keep them motivated to work hard in treatment.

Allow the CSO time to express frustration about the IP's use and offer empathy in response.

CSOs need time to express their strong feelings about their IP's use, and you must be responsive by conveying compassion and warmth so that rapport building is enhanced from the onset of the session.

Explore the CSO's underlying positive feelings for the IP.

Getting in touch with positive feelings toward the IP can help CSOs transition away from a conversation that dwells on the problems of the past and creates movement toward the part of the session that is focused on actively making changes. Yet some CSOs are consumed by their anger over the problems created by the IP's substance use, and thus have difficulty identifying any underlying positive feelings. It might help to ask these CSOs a question along the lines of "Besides feeling angry as you think about your loved one, what else do you feel?"

THERAPIST: Kelsey, it's clear from what you've shared about your brother that his substance use has been extremely hard on pretty much everyone in your family. He's responsible for a lot of painful memories. At the same time, I'm guessing that you care deeply for Riley, or you wouldn't have come in.

Let the CSO know it is time to move forward so that the problem can be tackled.

THERAPIST: The information you've shared about your brother's substance use will be very helpful in planning our work together. And now it's time to take that big step: to at least temporarily set aside the pain Riley has caused so that we can focus on making changes that will influence his future *and* your entire family in a healthy way. What do you think: Are you ready to take the leap?

2. Explore the CSO's past attempts to stop the IP's substance use and explain how CRAFT is different.

Explore the CSO's past attempts to get the IP to stop using.

THERAPIST: Kelsey, in preparation for moving forward, it is often helpful for me to hear about what's already been done. Can you tell me some of the specific things you or your parents have done in an attempt to get Riley to stop using?

CSO: Sure. We've all tried to talk with him about his drug use, but it gets us nowhere. And I won't let him hang out with my kids when he's messed up. My parents regularly threaten to stop lending him money because they know he spends it on drugs and never pays them back.

THERAPIST: Thanks. That's very helpful. As far as talking to him about his use, do you have those conversations when he's under the influence or when he hasn't been using?

CSO: Probably mostly while he's still high, because that's when he upsets us.

THERAPIST: OK. And when you say you don't let him hang out with your kids when he's messed up, what does that look like? What do you do?

CSO: If he comes up out of the basement and he's been drinking, I tell him he can't be around the kids. But I've made some exceptions, like on my daughter's birthday. He didn't seem that bad, so I told him he could be part of the birthday party as long as he was quiet.

THERAPIST: And what about when your parents threaten to stop loaning him money? *Do* they stop?

Note: See the next section (below) to understand why the therapist is inquiring about the timing of conversations and the consistency of the CSO's (and her family's) behavior toward the IP.

CSO: Not for long. When he was living in his own apartment, they worried that he might be out of food, so they caved a few times.

Explain that CRAFT will be different from the CSO's past attempts, both in terms of how CRAFT procedures are executed and the consistency required.

As far as the execution of CRAFT procedures, one of the main issues to highlight is the *timing* of conversations with the IP. CSOs routinely attempt serious conversations with IPs when the CSOs themselves are upset and the IPs are under the influence. The result is that these conversations are not delivered in a positive manner, and an already compromised IP is even less likely to listen (see Chapter 4). Having CSOs consistently following through with contingencies is stressed as well.

THERAPIST: The CRAFT program entails asking you, and probably your parents, to act in a way that's totally in line with what you've already tried to do, but with a few important differences. For example, instead of talking with your brother about his substance use when he's high, we'll focus on talking to him when he's definitely *not* high. And CRAFT involves learning specific skills, so I'll teach you how to best communicate with your brother about difficult topics. Also, in terms of refusing to let Riley see your kids when he's been drinking, we'll still focus on behaviors like that, but we'll make sure you're willing to follow through with them *consistently*, regardless of the circumstances. It will be important for you to let your parents know our basic plan, so they can be consistent in their messages to him, too.

Note: In describing her attempts to get her brother to stop using, this CSO had made it clear that she and her parents were not consistently following through with their contingencies. If the CSO had not readily divulged this information, the therapist would have asked specifically about it.

Explain how CSOs get "stuck" trying to fix their IP's problem by doing the same thing again and again, even though it is not working.

THERAPIST: It sounds like you've been working really hard to get your brother to stop using. But I bet you've felt stuck at times—maybe like you're spinning your wheels? For instance, it sounds like you've been trying to talk to him about the reasons why he should stop using. And when that hasn't worked, have you found yourself redoubling your efforts and talking to him even more?

CSO: Yes. More and *louder*! And you're right—it's not working.

THERAPIST: And that's why you're here. I'm hoping that you'll be willing to experiment with some of the procedures that this program has to offer; that you'll be open to trying new techniques.

3. Present and discuss the intake assessment results.

Regardless of who conducts the intake assessment (see Chapter 1, Box 1.1, for questionnaire suggestions), you should review the results at least briefly with CSOs during their first CRAFT sessions. This is done so that you can (a) acknowledge the effort the CSOs put into completing the questionnaires; (b) let the CSOs know they are not alone, that many others experience similar problems; (c) give some indication of how CRAFT can address the CSOs' identified problems; (d) explain how progress will be assessed over time with some of these measures; and (e) point out the CSOs' strengths. The amount of feedback you provide will depend on several factors, such as how interested the CSO appears to be in hearing the results, and whether the findings are helpful in supporting and motivating the CSO.

Although the assessment feedback does not need to be done at any particular time during the session, it tends to fit better in the earlier part. Therapists sometimes start the session with the feedback, especially if the CSO is quite anxious to hear the findings. Other clinicians wait until the CSO has had a chance to express frustration with the IP and to describe the unsuccessful treatment engagement attempts. Delaying the feedback presentation until CSOs have shared information about themselves and their IP enables you to link the assessment findings with this new information, and thus possibly make it more meaningful to CSOs. Regardless, it is important not to run short on session time before providing the feedback.

Present the findings from the CSO's assessment.

THERAPIST: I can't thank you enough for carefully completing all of those questionnaires. I know it was a *lot* of questions, but the information will be very helpful for our work together. And as I mentioned when you started them, about half of the questionnaires focused on how *you* are doing right now and the other half were about your relationship with Riley. I'm just going to go over the main findings now, but if you're left with any questions once I'm done, please let me know.

CSO: I'm kind of curious, so I'm glad you're going over these.

THERAPIST: Of course! OK. I'll start with the results about you specifically. As I'm sure you noticed, those questionnaires primarily were about your mood and the amount of social support you felt you had. As far as your mood, it looks like you're experiencing a moderate amount of anxiety and a mild amount of depression. In terms of support, it sounds like you feel as if you're getting a decent amount of social support.

Discuss the CSO's reaction to the findings.

THERAPIST: What do you make of this information?

CSO: I'm not surprised about the anxiety, because I know I'm a pretty nervous person to begin with. And this stuff with my brother has made it even worse, because I keep worrying about the poor role model he's being for my kids and the toll it's all taking on my parents. I don't think I'm usually depressed, but maybe I *have* been a bit down the last few weeks. It's probably because I haven't been able to get Riley into treatment.

THERAPIST: That's totally understandable. Other people in your situation often feel anxious and depressed. I think the fact that you have good social support is certainly helping though, and your healthy self-esteem level is probably enhancing your resilience.

Give an example of how an identified CSO problem can be addressed by CRAFT.

THERAPIST: As you'll see in a minute, one of the goals of CRAFT is to help the family members, like you, feel better themselves. For now, I'll just say that we can work on some of your own issues if you'd like, such as your day-to-day anxiety. It will be up to you, of course. And since I'll be readministering some of these measures again in a few weeks, we can see whether your anxiety and depression are improving.

Note: The therapist would repeat this feedback process with the results of the CSO–IP relationship questionnaires (see Chapter 1, Box 1.1, for sample questionnaires).

4. Outline CRAFT's three major goals.

The three main goals of CRAFT are to (a) reduce the IP's substance use, (b) get the IP to enter treatment, and (c) enhance the CSO's happiness and functioning. A comprehensive list of points to emphasize when presenting these goals is found below. It is not necessary to cover each point—simply focus on the ones that appear most applicable to your CSO.

Present CRAFT Goal 1: Reduce the IP's substance use.

The points to emphasize when introducing this first CRAFT goal include:

- Decreased use should make it more likely that the IP will be open to seeking treatment.
- If the IP does not seek treatment, decreased use will be particularly important.
- Some IPs temporarily *increase* their use when they realize their CSOs are changing their own behavior, but this usually reverses if CSOs remain consistent.
- CSOs should stay in treatment even if their IPs significantly reduce use, since:
  - *Any* ongoing use leads many CSOs to fear that it will escalate again.
  - The problems associated with the use likely will remain to some degree.
  - The use of illicit drugs is subject to legal consequences.

Present CRAFT Goal 2: Get the IP to enter treatment.

The important points to stress for the second CRAFT goal are:

- Preliminary steps must be in place (e.g., communication training) before the treatment invitation is extended.
- The safety of CSOs is the number one concern when preparing to extend this invitation and to deal with the consequences.
- If IPs successfully reduce their use considerably on their own (without formal treatment), attempts to engage the IP in treatment should *not* be abandoned because:
  - CSOs tend to feel less stressed/burdened if their IP is in treatment.
  - IPs can learn valuable skills in a treatment program that can help with relapse prevention or further reductions in use.

Present CRAFT Goal 3: Enhance the CSO's happiness and functioning.

Finally, the main points to emphasize for CRAFT's third goal include:

- CRAFT helps CSOs find happiness in life regardless of whether their IP enters treatment.
- Healthy and happy CSOs who are functioning well are good for the entire family.
- As CSOs become more engaged in enjoyable, substance-free activities, their IPs often want to participate in these healthy activities, too.

Provide examples of how these goals will be addressed.

THERAPIST: How are we going to tackle these three CRAFT goals? As I mentioned, there are basic skills that I will teach you first, such as positive communication. This is a very handy skill, not only because it will prepare you to eventually invite Riley to begin treatment but it will also provide you with a tool for other difficult conversations that have nothing to do with Riley, such as with friends or coworkers. I'll also teach you how to increase the chance that Riley selects *non-using* activities over using ones.

5. Explain why CSOs are crucial to CRAFT and describe their roles.

Explain why CSOs are crucial to CRAFT.

You should tell CSOs that they are crucial to CRAFT because:

- CSOs have valuable knowledge about their IPs' using patterns that is helpful when planning how to intervene.
- CSOs have a lot of contact with their IPs, and thus have many opportunities to influence their behavior.
- IPs often report that their family's influence is what prompted them to seek treatment.
- CSOs often need help themselves due to problems resulting from their IPs' use.

THERAPIST: Kelsey, I'd like to explain why you're considered a crucial player in this treatment for your brother. We've learned from studies that people like you, who seek our services for a resistant loved one, typically know a lot about the individual's substance use patterns, *and* they tend to have a fair amount of contact with the person, so they're in a great position to influence the substance use behavior.

CSO: I hope I can help. Riley has been sort of avoiding me lately by barely leaving his room.

THERAPIST: Don't worry. Together we'll come up with ways to draw him out of his room so you can interact with him more. Also, you mentioned earlier that you've noticed he drinks more on the weekends, even though he's home all week. So that's an important substance use pattern of his that you've recognized already. We'll explore that more in our next session. I also want to mention that despite their outright resistance, people with substance use problems commonly report that they ended up seeking treatment specifically *because of their family member's influence.*

CSO: Really? That makes me feel more hopeful.

THERAPIST: Good! The final reason why we encourage people like you to participate in CRAFT has to do with our third goal: We want to help the loving family members with some of their *own* issues, or with problems that have resulted from the substance user's behavior. The bottom line is that we want to help make *your* life happier. As an example, you've already said that your brother's drinking and drug use has been stressful for you and your parents, and I'm guessing it's been stressful for your husband and kids, too.

CSO: You're right, it's been stressful for all of us. I guess I try to pretend it hasn't been, but it has.

THERAPIST: Then we'll definitely want to find ways to help decrease the stress in your life *before* Riley gets into treatment. I've got some ideas that we can sort out together. Maybe they'll help with your anxiety that we spoke about earlier, too.

Describe several CSO roles in CRAFT.

It is also important to explain CSOs' roles in CRAFT and exactly what will be expected of them. Their responsibilities include (a) learning new skills for interacting with their IPs (e.g., positive communication, the rewarding of *substance-free* behavior, the withdrawal of rewards at times of use), (b) completing assignments during the week (trying out the new skills at home), (c) taking care of their own safety at all costs, (d) learning to make their own happiness and well-being a priority, and (e) continuing to support their IPs once they are in treatment (such as by attending therapy with the IPs).

6. Explain CRAFT's principles.

Mention CRAFT's two basic principles of reinforcement.

The CRAFT program is built on two principles of reinforcement or reward: (a) eliminating positive reinforcement (rewards) for substance-using behavior, and (b) enhancing positive reinforcement (rewards) for non-substance-using behavior.

Give an example of these principles of reinforcement.

THERAPIST: As far as the first principle, eliminating rewards for your brother's substance use, CRAFT will show you that you can have some control over making sure rewards *aren't* associated with Riley's drug use. For example, maybe you've been going out of your way to keep the kids quiet so as not to disturb their uncle when he comes home high or intoxicated and is sleeping in. Since this actually would be considered a type of reward for being high or inebriated, we might consider changing this and having your family go about their normal business, including the noise, so that it's not so easy for him to sleep in when he's under the influence.

CSO: It's funny you mention that, because I *have* been trying to keep the noise down!

THERAPIST: That's not surprising, because on the surface it seems like the normal, polite thing to do. But it might not be helping in the long run. And as far as the second principle, enhancing rewards for your brother's *non-substance* use behavior, we'll sort this out together once I know more about your brother. For example, maybe we can find something fun that you, or you and your family, can do with your brother that doesn't involve any alcohol or drugs.

CSO (*laughs*): We used to all love doing jigsaw puzzles together, but I don't know if he'd enjoy that anymore.

THERAPIST: Kelsey, you're showing a great understanding of these principles, because knowing whether Riley *enjoys* a non-using activity will be very important. If he doesn't enjoy it anymore, it definitely won't serve as a reward. But we've got time to sort that out.

Note: The therapist takes advantage of an opportunity to compliment the CSO for "getting" CRAFT principles.

7. Give an overview of the CRAFT program and procedures.

Provide an overview of the CRAFT program.

It is helpful to lay out the "nuts and bolts" of the CRAFT program since it is probably quite different from other treatments with which the CSO is familiar. This overview should also convey the message that the CSO's involvement is critical and that the program will be tailored to her or his specific situation.

- CRAFT is different from other programs (e.g., Al-Anon) because it entails getting CSOs to work actively toward getting their IPs to enter treatment, but without using confrontation (e.g., Johnson Institute Intervention [JII]).
- CRAFT is built around showing CSOs how to reward their IPs' *non-using* behavior and to withdraw rewards when their IPs are using substances.
- CRAFT is menu driven inasmuch as only the procedures that are relevant to a CSO's case are used.
- CRAFT relies on CSOs to attempt the agreed-upon homework assignments.
- CRAFT offers skills training that can be used in other areas of CSOs' lives (e.g., communication, goal setting, problem solving).
- CRAFT does not pressure CSOs to do anything that they do not want to do.

Mention several of the CRAFT procedures.

In addition to this program overview, you should describe a few of the CRAFT procedures (all of which are discussed in detail in subsequent chapters). But prior to doing this with a CSO, you should prepare yourself for possible pushback (see Box 2.1). Also keep in mind that it is neither necessary nor advisable to present all of the CRAFT procedures to the CSO. Instead, present several that appear most relevant to the particular case. The CRAFT procedures are as follows:

- *FA ("Road Map") of a Loved One's Drinking or Using Behavior*: A procedure that outlines the context (triggers, positive and negative consequences) for both substance-using and substance-free IP behaviors so that CSOs can develop a plan for influencing them (see Chapters 3 and 6).
- *Improving CSOs' Communication Skills*: A step-by-step approach to building positive communication that relies heavily on role plays (see Chapter 4).
- *Rewarding Non-Using Behavior*: A strategy for teaching CSOs how to provide rewards only when their IP is *not* using substances, thereby increasing the frequency of non-using behavior (see Chapter 5).
- *Withdrawing Rewards for Using Behavior*: A strategy for teaching CSOs how to withdraw rewards consistently when their IP is using substances, thereby decreasing the frequency of the using behavior (see Chapter 7).
- *Allowing for Natural, Negative Consequences of Use*: A structured plan to help CSOs refrain from engaging in "helpful" behaviors with an inebriated/high IP that inadvertently facilitate substance use (see Chapter 8).
- *Problem Solving*: A structured approach to breaking down problems into manageable pieces and developing specific plans for resolving them (see Chapter 9).
- *Helping CSOs Enrich Their Own Lives*: Tools that explore CSOs' happiness in various areas of their lives and then help them develop strategies to work toward new goals (see Chapter 10).
- *Inviting the IP to Enter Treatment*: Guidelines for crafting the IP treatment invitation, for lining up an appropriate therapist, and for preparing CSOs for a variety of possible IP reactions (see Chapter 11).

BOX 2.1

"I Already Tried That and It Didn't Work"

In the process of describing the CRAFT procedures and the type of CSO activities they require, CSOs sometimes insist they have "already tried that and it didn't work." Upon investigating, CRAFT therapists commonly discover either that:

- The CSOs have *not* actually learned and used a similar procedure.
- The CSOs *have* learned a procedure that was quite similar to the CRAFT procedure in question, but they did not implement the procedure correctly or did so inconsistently.

As a CRAFT therapist, your response might be:

> "It sounds like the communication skills training you learned from your earlier therapy *does* overlap somewhat with CRAFT's communication skills procedure. And I hear you saying that it didn't work. Still, I'm hoping you'll keep an open mind, because usually we find that there's something different about the CRAFT procedure and the version of it that people have already tried. Sometimes the difference can be pretty subtle, and sometimes it's just a matter of being more consistent in how you follow through with it. Importantly, communication skills are just one part of the larger CRAFT program. So what do you think: Are you willing to hang in there and give it a shot?"

Link at least one of the procedures to the CSO's particular situation.

THERAPIST: You mentioned that there might be some fun alcohol-free family activities that you could invite your brother to participate in. In order to sort this out, we'd use CRAFT's procedure for "Rewarding Non-Using Behavior." This would help us figure out whether it's a good activity and how you'd set it up. But we'd also use CRAFT's procedure for "Withdrawing Rewards for Using Behavior" in case Riley showed up to the activity intoxicated or high. Finally, we'd practice "Improving CSOs' Communication Skills" so you'd have a chance to learn an effective and comfortable way to invite him.

8. Build positive expectations on the basis of scientific support.

Present the four main outcomes showing evidence of CRAFT's success.

Research shows that CRAFT:

1. Is successful at getting resistant substance-using loved ones into treatment about two-thirds of the time (see Box 2.2).
2. Has been successful across a variety of CSO–IP relationships (spouses/partners, parents/children, siblings, friends).

BOX 2.2

Reassuring CSOs That They Can Be Successful

CSOs sometimes ask about the one-third of the CSOs who were *un*successful at getting their IPs into treatment. You might respond to these inquiries with reassurance and by offering several case-specific reasons why you are optimistic. You could also explain that, in the majority of the cases with an unengaged IP, the CSOs never actually invited their IP to attend treatment. Unsuccessful outcomes are commonly the result of the CSO losing contact with their IP, being solely interested in therapy for themselves from the start, or being afraid to mention therapy to their IP.

3. Works for many different types of drug use (e.g., alcohol, marijuana, methamphetamine).
4. Helps CSOs feel better themselves (i.e., less depression, anxiety) regardless of whether their IP enters treatment.

Discuss the CSO's reaction to the four main CRAFT outcomes.

THERAPIST: What do you make of what I'm telling you about the CRAFT research and how well it works?

CSO: I want to be optimistic, but part of me wonders if I'm going to end up with the one-third who *aren't* successful. It could happen.

THERAPIST: Well, there are no absolute guarantees, but based on what I already know about you and your brother, I think we've got a good shot at it. He lives in the same house as you right now—that's actually quite helpful because it gives you lots of opportunities to try out new behaviors with him. And it sounds like the two of you have a good relationship, so I'm guessing that although you might not change his mind about treatment right away, eventually he'll listen. Plus, I bet we can rely on the help of your parents, and maybe even your husband, too. There will be lots of people working together toward one goal.

9. Place responsibility for the substance use on the IP.

Explain that while CRAFT helps CSOs change their behavior toward the IP, it does not suggest that CSOs are responsible for their IP's substance use.

THERAPIST: One of the points I really want to drive home today is that although we are talking about ways I can work with you to change *your* behavior toward your brother, it absolutely does not mean you're responsible for his drinking or drug use. And as you know, the reason why we have to look at your behavior in the first place is because Riley won't come in himself—yet.

CSO: I know. But maybe I should have recognized the struggle he was having and done something earlier.

Offer supportive statements as needed to reemphasize the point.

THERAPIST: Kelsey, siblings aren't raised to know how to deal with a substance use problem that one of them develops later in life—right? You took your brother into your own home when he had no place to go because he lost his job and his apartment. And now you've even come into therapy to try to help *him*. That sure sounds to me like you're doing whatever you can to take good care of him.

10. Discuss confidentiality and safety.

Inquire about the best and safest way to contact the CSO, including whether any identifying information can be left in a message or with another person at the time of such a contact.

Common options include calling or texting the CSO's cell phone, and calling a friend or family member of the CSO. Be sure to determine whether information about the caller (e.g., therapist's or agency's name) can be shared with anyone who answers the phone, or whether it can be left as a text or voice message.

Ask whether the IP knows that the CSO is in treatment, and if not, whether there are safety concerns.

THERAPIST: You mentioned that Riley doesn't know you've begun therapy, but you wouldn't be concerned if he accidentally found out by taking a phone message at your house if someone from this office called. I guess I mostly want to make sure you'd really be OK, including being safe, if he finds out accidentally.

CSO: It's funny, but in some ways it would almost be easier if he found out accidentally; I wouldn't have to figure out how to tell him. No, I don't have any safety concerns whatsoever when it comes to my brother.

Determine whether additional precautions need to be taken due to the threat of domestic violence.

The CRAFT studies excluded CSOs who reported at intake that their IPs had engaged in domestic violence or criminal assault in the previous 2 years, or had demonstrated severe violent behavior (e.g., used a weapon, inflicted injuries that required hospitalization) at any point. Therefore, no claims can be made about whether it is safe to treat CSOs using CRAFT if they have experienced violence at the hand of their IP. Being particularly cautious is important, given that several CRAFT procedures (see Chapters 7 and 8) are designed specifically to be unpleasant for IPs (if they are using substances). For more information on assessing the potential for domestic violence, see Box 2.3, and for information on developing a protection plan, see Box 2.4. You should be mindful of the strong link between substance use and domestic violence regardless of whether you are considering offering CRAFT or another treatment for a CSO (see Cafferky et al., 2018).

11. Review a healthy IP reinforcer and identify the CSO's own rewards.

Discuss at least one reinforcer that the IP could gain/regain with treatment.

BOX 2.3

Domestic Violence Precautions: Assessment

Agencies typically have their own standard protocols for assessing the threat of domestic violence. These protocols might contain one or more of the measures outlined in Chapter 1, Box 1.1, under the section "Measures to Assess the CSO–IP Relationship." The topics generally covered include:

Assess the potential for violence and its severity.

- Assess the potential for the IP to become violent (e.g., Is there a history of violence?).
- Evaluate the *severity* of the potential violence in cases where there appears to be a threat (e.g., Did past threats/violence require medical attention? Were police called? Were weapons used?).

Determine the level of social support.

- Ask whether social support is available in the event of a violence threat:
  - If a support person is available: Get details regarding access to that person.
  - If a support person is not available: Help identify one.

Identify any triggers or "red flags" for violence.

- Identify triggers for IP violence (precipitants for the outbreak).
- Identify "red flags" for IP violence (reliable signals that violence is about to occur).

Note: This material is drawn from Smith and Meyers (2010). Additional information can be found in Smith and Meyers (2004).

BOX 2.4

Safer CSO Responses and a Protection Plan

Agencies generally have a standard process for working with CSOs if domestic violence is a threat. Common topics include:

Develop safer CSO responses.

- Talk about the need to develop safer CSO responses and help develop a plan for them.
- Discuss the importance of responding (e.g., leaving) at the earliest signs of possible violence.

Discuss self-protection (escape, safe houses, restraining orders).

- Address the three categories of protection:
  - Be prepared to exit quickly (e.g., small bag packed, closest exit known).
  - Be familiar with local temporary refuges (e.g., safe houses/domestic violence shelters, a friend's home).
  - Be aware of available legal interventions (e.g., calling 911, getting a restraining order).
- Determine which of these types of protection (if any) would be best suited to the CSO's situation and examine the steps to implementing them.

Note: This material is drawn from Smith and Meyers (2010). Additional information can be found in Smith and Meyers (2004).

THERAPIST: I want to be sure we finish on a high note today given how intense much of our discussion has been. I know we've already talked about this indirectly: What is something major that Riley stands to gain by stopping his alcohol and drug use?

CSO: Oh, that's easy. He'll be in a better position to get a new job and to eventually have enough money to get his own place again.

Discuss at least one way the <u>CSO</u> would benefit directly if the IP stopped using substances.

THERAPIST: And what about yourself? How will *you* benefit from Riley stopping his substance use?

CSO: The first thing that comes to mind is that I won't have to worry so much about him *and* the effect he's having on our parents. That would be major.

THERAPIST: Excellent. Can you think of anything else?

CSO: I'm not concerned about getting my basement apartment back once he leaves; that's honestly not an issue. I'd feel really good for *him* though if he gets his life back on track. And I guess I've been embarrassed at family functions when he's shown up drunk or high. Not only would it be great not to have to worry about that happening anymore but he'd be fun to hang out with again, too.

THERAPIST: I bet you also wouldn't have to worry about him being a bad influence on your kids then.

CSO: True. And he used to have fun babysitting for them when they were really small. If he gets better, I'd think about letting him do that again if he wants to. That would free me up for other things, which would be a bonus for sure.

Raise the issue of what the CSO might like to get out of therapy explicitly for her- or himself.

Some CSOs are ready to start working on goals for themselves early in treatment, whereas others prefer to wait until they have spent time addressing their IP's problems first. Regardless, you should introduce the topic of CSO rewards early on, because some CSOs need relief from the constant focus on their IP's problems and find the thought of attending to their own needs comforting. The procedure that specifically helps CSOs establish and work toward personal goals is described in Chapter 10.

THERAPIST: Now let's think for a minute about what else you might get out of therapy for yourself—things that will be separate from what you'll get as a result of Riley reducing or stopping his use. After all, remember that the third goal of CRAFT is to increase the functioning and happiness of the loved one, which is *you* in this case. In an upcoming session I'll be asking you to set some goals for yourself.

CSO: I've never been in therapy before, so I'm not sure what to say. But it's kind of exciting to think about focusing on myself. There *are* a few things I'd like to work on—things that I haven't let myself make a priority. Maybe with new communication skills I'll get the courage to get involved in the school board. I've always played around with that idea.

THERAPIST: Armed with new communication skills and a clear strategy for getting you active with the school board, I think you'll have a good chance of making that happen.

Note: Before the session concludes, the therapist would collaborate with the CSO to develop a homework assignment for the week (see Box 2.5).

COMMON PROBLEMS TO AVOID

The initial CRAFT session has several overall goals and contains many components, which can sometimes be daunting to new CRAFT therapists. Common problems and safeguards against them are outlined below.

Problem: You should be mindful of the tendency to go down the lengthy session checklist (Form 2.1) point by point in an effort to cover every element. This can result in losing sight of the importance of establishing rapport with the often anxious and depressed CSO.

Safeguards:

- Remind yourself that it is better to carry over some of the checklist items to the second session than to lose the emotional connection with the CSO.
- If you catch yourself frantically crossing off items on the checklist while repeatedly glancing at the clock, tell yourself to pause and "breathe." This is probably a good time to stop and ask the CSO about any questions she or he might have.
- Each time you complete an item on the checklist, ask yourself whether you took the time to make the material personally relevant to the CSO.

Problem: While it is important for CSOs to use therapy time to share their IP "horror stories" and to express their own feelings (anger, frustration, fear, sadness), some therapists

BOX 2.5

The First "Homework" Assignment

It is important to *assign* homework in each session and to *start* each session by reviewing homework. The Homework Assignment Guidelines (see Chapter 3, Box 3.1) provide the details regarding how to best do this, and they include determining whether your CSO prefers a more neutral term for this between-session activity, such as "assignment," "exercise," "task," or "experiment." With that said, there are many examples of specific assignments made throughout this manual. During the first session with a CSO, you will have discussed homework assignments and their importance when you gave the CRAFT overview and when you described CSO roles in CRAFT. When making the first assignment (in collaboration with the CSO) at the conclusion of the first CRAFT session, it is acceptable to start off slowly: many CSOs appear rather overwhelmed at the end of this session *and* you will not have had a chance to cover the homework assignment guidelines yet. Thus, a reasonable first assignment might be asking the CSO to jot down any questions or concerns about CRAFT that arise during the week. Of course, other assignments would be reasonable as well, particularly if additional CRAFT procedures were started in this first session. As will become apparent throughout this manual, relatively standard homework assignments are linked to the various CRAFT procedures.

have difficulty redirecting the conversation into a future-focused "problem-solving" mode. The result is a session that *overemphasizes* the negative aspects of the IP and the CSO–IP relationship, as opposed to one that highlights all the ways in which CRAFT can help make changes.

Safeguards:

- In preparation for the session, estimate the amount of time you would like to devote to the CSO describing the problems created by the IP's substance use (5 minutes? 10?). Prepare and rehearse a statement that allows you to interrupt and redirect the CSO when the allocated time is up. Role-play with colleagues if appropriate.
- You might find it more comfortable to inform CSOs at the start of the session that there is a lot of material to cover, and ask for their understanding in the event that you jump in and move them on to the next topic.

Problem: Some clinicians report that they are caught off guard when CSOs respond with defensiveness, anger, despair, or self-blame when the topic of the CSO's inadvertent support of their IP's substance use arises in the context of hearing about certain CRAFT procedures (e.g., Allowing for Natural, Negative Consequences of Use; see Chapter 8).

Safeguards:

- Assume CSOs *will* be upset when this topic is raised, and plan a response that both shows empathy and explains how the procedure fits within the larger CRAFT program.
- You might prefer starting this potentially difficult conversation by asking CSOs for "permission" to discuss an important and possibly upsetting topic.
- Be sure to raise this topic only when there is ample time to process it fully during the session.

SUMMARY

This chapter describes the first CRAFT session with CSOs. This introductory session serves many purposes: providing information about the goals of CRAFT and insight into the various procedures, conveying the expected role of CSOs as they participate in CRAFT while at the same time instilling confidence that they are up to the task, reassuring CSOs that an IP's substance use problem is not the CSO's fault, and beginning the process of identifying reasons for the IP's substance use and reinforcers for changing this behavior. Of course, one of the most important objectives of the session is to offer CSOs hope that is rooted in the science that underlies CRAFT.

FORM 2.1

Informing and Motivating the CSO: Checklist

1. Invite the CSO to describe the IP's substance use and the problems created by it.

- ☐ a. Have the CSO describe some of the problems created by the substance use.
- ☐ b. Allow the CSO time to express frustration about the IP's use and offer empathy in response.
- ☐ c. Explore the CSO's underlying positive feelings for the IP.
- ☐ d. Let the CSO know it is time to move forward so that the problem can be tackled.

2. Explore the CSO's past attempts to stop the IP's substance use and explain how CRAFT is different.

- ☐ a. Explore the CSO's past attempts to get the IP to stop using.
- ☐ b. Explain that CRAFT will be different from the CSO's past attempts, both in terms of how CRAFT procedures are executed and the consistency required.
- ☐ c. Explain how CSOs get "stuck" trying to fix their IP's problem by doing the same thing again and again, even though it is not working.

3. Present and discuss the intake assessment results.

- ☐ a. Present the findings from the CSO's assessment.
- ☐ b. Discuss the CSO's reaction to the findings.
- ☐ c. Give an example of how an identified CSO problem can be addressed by CRAFT.

4. Outline CRAFT's three major goals.

- ☐ a. Present CRAFT Goal 1: Reduce the IP's substance use.
- ☐ b. Present CRAFT Goal 2: Get the IP to enter treatment.
- ☐ c. Present CRAFT Goal 3: Enhance the CSO's happiness and functioning.
- ☐ d. Provide examples of how these goals will be addressed.

5. Explain why CSOs are crucial to CRAFT and describe their roles.

- ☐ a. Explain why CSOs are crucial to CRAFT.
- ☐ b. Describe several CSO roles in CRAFT.

(continued)

6. Explain CRAFT's principles.

- ☐ a. Mention CRAFT's two basic principles of reinforcement.
- ☐ b. Give an example of these principles of reinforcement.

7. Give an overview of the CRAFT program and procedures.

- ☐ a. Provide an overview of the CRAFT program.
- ☐ b. Mention several of the CRAFT procedures.
- ☐ c. Link at least one of the procedures to the CSO's particular situation.

8. Build positive expectations on the basis of scientific support.

- ☐ a. Present the four main outcomes showing evidence of CRAFT's success.
- ☐ b. Discuss the CSO's reaction to the four main CRAFT outcomes.

9. Place responsibility for the substance use on the IP.

- ☐ a. Explain that while CRAFT helps CSOs change their behavior toward the IP, it does *not* suggest that CSOs are responsible for their IP's substance use.
- ☐ b. Offer supportive statements as needed to reemphasize the point.

10. Discuss confidentiality and safety.

- ☐ a. Inquire about the best and safest way to contact the CSO, including whether any identifying information can be left in a message or with another person at the time of such a contact.
- ☐ b. Ask whether the IP knows that the CSO is in treatment, and if not, whether there are safety concerns.
- ☐ c. Determine whether additional precautions need to be taken due to the threat of domestic violence.

11. Review a healthy IP reinforcer and identify the CSO's own rewards.

- ☐ a. Discuss at least one reinforcer that the *IP* could gain/regain with treatment.
- ☐ b. Discuss at least one way the *CSO* would benefit directly if the IP stopped using substances.
- ☐ c. Raise the issue of what the CSO might like to get out of therapy explicitly for her- or himself.

Chapter 3

Functional Analysis of a Loved One's Drinking or Using Behavior

One of the major goals of the CRAFT program is to teach CSOs to change their behavior toward the IP (treatment-refusing substance user), so that, in turn, the IP alters his or her behavior in response. In order to position yourself to guide the CSO's behavior change, you first need a complete picture of the context in which the IP's substance-using behavior occurs. A "functional analysis" (FA) is a procedure that can do just that, as it outlines the antecedents or "triggers" of the behavior, as well as its short- and long-term consequences. FAs, which are sometimes called "road maps," are an integral part of the overall CRA program (see Chapter 12; see also Meyers & Smith, 1995, Chapter 2). A modified version of the CRA FA is needed for CRAFT, since it is the *CSO* who actually completes the FA of the IP's behavior.

CRAFT actually uses two types of FAs. This chapter focuses on the FA that targets a *problem* behavior, such as substance use. This type of FA works toward decreasing or eliminating that problematic behavior. Once the factors that are promoting and maintaining an IP's substance use are understood, a plan can be developed with the CSO for changing her or his own behavior in an effort to influence the IP. The second type of FA focuses on a *healthy* IP behavior, and its goal is to create a plan that ultimately increases this particular behavior. This second type of FA is covered in Chapter 6.

THE BASICS

General Description

The CRAFT FA for a problem behavior consists of a semistructured interview that gathers information from the CSO about a common/typical IP substance use episode. As with all CRAFT procedures, a checklist specific to the procedure is provided to guide the process (see Form 3.1, found at the end of this chapter). The CRAFT Functional Analysis of a Loved One's Drinking or Using Behavior (Form 3.2 or "the FA form," also found at the end of this chapter) is the form that is used to record the CSO's responses (see Figure 3.1 later in the chapter for a completed sample version). As evident from the FA form, you gather information about the triggers that set the stage for the substance use. These triggers are both external (in the IP's environment) and internal (within the IP). The details of the consequences of the substance use, both positive and negative, are collected as well. The positive consequences are the "rewards" the IP experiences for using the alcohol or drugs—basically, the reasons he or she continues to use. The negative consequences are the "downside" to the substance use: the negative things that have happened to the IP and loved ones as a result of the alcohol or drugs. The specific questions about the substance use itself (e.g., amounts) are intentionally placed in the middle of this first type of FA so that the link from triggers to use to consequences is more obvious. Once you obtain all of this information, you explain its clinical utility and generate a homework assignment with the CSO.

Typically, you would jot down on the FA (Form 3.2) the details being collected during the interview while the CSO is positioned such that she or he can watch what you are doing. Alternatives to this include (1) having the CSO write the information on the form instead of you, (2) having either you or the CSO write the information on a whiteboard or paper easel that is set up (lined and labeled) to look like an FA form (in this case, a picture should be taken of the completed FA so that it can be saved and printed), and (3) using the whiteboard function while conducting the session remotely. Regardless, the CSO should have a copy of the completed form, and a copy should be placed in the CSO's file for future reference.

Procedure Timing

The FA for a substance use problem is usually administered in the first or second CRAFT session with the CSO, and is referred back to at various points in treatment as plans are being developed.

Forms

- Functional Analysis of a Loved One's Drinking or Using Behavior: Checklist (Form 3.1)
- CRAFT Functional Analysis of a Loved One's Drinking or Using Behavior (Form 3.2)

CLINICIAN GUIDANCE AND SAMPLE DIALOGUE

The components for the FA that are described in this chapter correspond to the items on the checklist in Form 3.1. As noted, each checklist in this book is intended to be used by therapists as a guide during sessions. The checklists can also be utilized by clinical supervisors when reviewing recorded sessions of their clinicians. Once again, the chapter presents a representative case with a sample clinician–CSO dialogue for illustration purposes.

Case Description

We illustrate the administration of the FA with the case of Samantha, a non-Hispanic white single mom (CSO) who is seeking treatment for her 25-year-old son's drinking problem. Samantha reports that her son Jeff (the IP) also uses various illicit drugs at times, but only after he has already been drinking. Jeff is living at home again since he has insufficient funds to continue paying rent for his apartment. He works part-time as a salesperson at a cell phone store, but he is in danger of losing that job due to absences. Jeff's limited social life is with his coworkers. He has never been married and has no children.

1. Introduce the FA and explain its purpose.

Link the FA with two CRAFT goals (to decrease the IP's use and get the IP into treatment) and with the CSO's general role.

THERAPIST: Samantha, this procedure today is aimed at getting a good picture of your son's drinking. This procedure is called a "functional analysis," because it analyzes the function, or the purpose, of a behavior. But I like to call it a "road map" because it lays out the path leading up to and following someone's substance use. Anyway, once we have this picture of Jeff's drinking, we can start working toward getting him to decrease his drinking, and eventually to get into treatment—two of CRAFT's main goals. And as a reminder, *you* will play a critical role in influencing your son to change his own behavior by changing some of the ways you interact with him.

Explain how the CSO's knowledge of and contact with the IP makes her or him well suited for doing the FA.

THERAPIST: As we're going through this exercise, you'll probably be thinking that it would be much easier if Jeff were sitting here in front of me so that *he* could answer all these questions. We're both hoping he will decide to enter treatment soon. Still, we've found that family members like you are extremely helpful at sharing important information about their loved one's substance-using behavior, because they know so much about the person's daily routines and habits. And family members also tend to have a lot of contact with the drinker—which is going to be very useful as we move into other CRAFT procedures.

Describe some of the specific information that will be collected (external/internal triggers, positive/negative consequences) and explain how it will be used.

Triggers are the IP's high-risk situations for using substances, both the environmental factors (external triggers) and thoughts or feelings (internal triggers). The CSO will help the IP learn to respond differently to triggers, either by avoiding them altogether or by using healthy coping strategies instead. *Consequences* are the immediate "rewards" (reinforcers) the IP experiences from using substances (positive consequences), as well as the longer-term negative outcomes (negative consequences). The CSO will also help the IP find healthier ways to get some of those desired rewards, and will assist if the IP is willing to work on reversing some of the negative outcomes of the substance use. Examples of the therapist explaining the collection of information about both triggers and consequences are provided here:

THERAPIST: This procedure involves me asking questions about your son's *triggers* for drinking, such as who he drinks with and where this typically occurs. This will help us figure out Jeff's high-risk situations—ones that we'll probably need to help him find other ways to deal with or to avoid. I'll also be asking about Jeff's thoughts and feelings right before he drinks, which will give us an idea of what he hopes to get out of the drinking right when he's making the decision to drink.

CSO: I can tell already that this is going to be interesting.

THERAPIST: I'm glad you think so! Let me tell you a little more about this exercise. It also looks at the consequences of your son's drinking—both the positive and the negative. By discussing the things Jeff likes about drinking we'll be able to help your son find *healthy* ways to get some of those same things he likes. And by looking at the negative things that have happened to him because of his drinking we should be able to see the important things he's lost and might be willing to work to get back.

Give the CSO a copy of the FA form and point out the column headings so that she or he can follow along.

2. Settle on a common using episode for the IP and begin to collect information.

Ask the CSO to describe a common/typical substance use episode of the IP's—a pattern that happens fairly often.

Infrequently occurring episodes provide fewer opportunities for the CSO to step in and influence the IP's behavior and are usually less urgent to address. Furthermore, the findings from these episodes are less likely to generalize to other episodes in the IP's life. In terms of precisely how you should ask about a common using episode, you should use your own personal style. Two examples of different ways to ask the same basic question include:

THERAPIST: Can you describe a common drinking episode of your son's? This should be a particular pattern that takes place fairly regularly in terms of when and where it happens.

THERAPIST: Tell me a story about your son's typical drinking episode. Include as many details as you can, such as where it happens and why he seems to be doing it.

Before the CSO spends too much time describing an episode, check to make sure the type of episode occurs regularly.

Sometimes a CSO offers an episode and the therapist proceeds with using it for the FA, only to later determine that the episode is not actually a commonly occurring one.

THERAPIST: Correct me if I'm wrong, but based on what you've told me, it sounds like your son drinks a fair amount just about every day of the week—right? As far as the drug use that follows his drinking at some parties, how often does Jeff go to these parties? If he attends them most Friday nights, for example, we'd consider that a common pattern. But if he only goes once in a while, we'd want to focus on some other more frequent drinking pattern first. The frequent episodes will give you more chances to step in—once you've learned new ways to try to influence his behavior.

Focus on one common episode; do not jump around between multiple episodes describing different drugs and/or occasions.

In the case of an IP using multiple substances, part of settling upon an episode for the FA requires that you and the CSO decide which substance(s) should be focused on first. As noted in the case description, the IP's illicit drug use only occurs *after* the IP already has been drinking, and thus alcohol will be the selected substance use target here.

THERAPIST: It sounds like your son's pattern of drinking on Friday nights with friends from work is quite different from his weekday pattern where he mostly drinks at home on his own. Not only is the setting different, but as you said, he also goes on to use drugs after he drinks at those parties. Since different things probably influence his drinking at those two different times, we should pick just one to focus on right now. What are your thoughts about where you'd like to start—his weekday or his Friday night drinking?

Often the decision regarding which type of episode to choose is clear. Yet for the current case an argument could be made for either type of common episode:

- Friday night drinking:
  - The use of illicit drugs routinely follows the drinking, and the drinking/use occurs outside the home, potentially making the episode more serious, but . . .
  - The CSO may be less successful trying to influence this type of episode, as it appears to be associated with a social reward and she is not in the vicinity of where the episode occurs.
- Weekday drinking:
  - The frequency of the weekday drinking is high, raising concerns about its seriousness as well, but . . .
  - The CSO is less concerned about the IP's safety since the drinking is occurring at home and there are no illicit drugs involved.

Note: Assume the CSO's anxiety over the illicit drug use results in her selecting the Friday night drinking episode. Although social rewards (drinking at a party with coworkers) can be quite pleasurable, and the CSO is not near the IP when this activity occurs, she can still be successful in generating ideas for other enjoyable social rewards *and* in developing a method for getting her son to sample them.

Complete the FA form as much as possible once the CSO begins to describe the episode.

Filling in the form while the CSO is first telling the story of the IP's substance use behavior eliminates the need to later ask questions that already have been addressed, thereby avoiding CSO frustration. Being familiar with the layout of the questions on the FA form (Form 3.2) is helpful, because the CSO will be sharing information in no particular order at this point and you will be jumping around the form to jot down responses.

When next proceeding to clarify and fill in gaps in the FA form, use a conversational style whenever possible and do not feel compelled to fill in every blank.

You should avoid mechanically going down question after question in each column on the FA form, as this may interfere with building rapport with the CSO. And every question does *not* need to be addressed in order for the FA to contain sufficient information. This is fortunate, because CSOs will not know the answers to some of the specific questions about their IP's use, and they might be unable to even venture a guess at times. With that said, the case dialogue we use in this chapter covers all of the items on the worksheet as a way of illustrating how the questions might be posed and answered.

3. Outline external triggers.

Explain the concept of a high-risk situation—how it is important to look at the IP's environment (external triggers) at the time of the episode because triggers "set the stage" for the IP's substance use.

CRAFT's discussion of external triggers will likely resonate with CSOs who are familiar with Alcoholics Anonymous (AA) or Narcotics Anonymous (NA), because these triggers sound quite similar to AA's/NA's notion of the "people, places, and things" that threaten sobriety.

THERAPIST: Now I'd like to go back and fill in some of the remaining details about your son's Friday night drinking on this worksheet. Let's start with the first column on the left: "external triggers" (*points to the first column on the FA* [see Figure 3.1]). External triggers are things in your son's environment that are often associated with his drinking, like the people he tends to hang out with when drinking, as well as when and where it occurs. We consider these "high-risk" factors for his decision to drink.

Identify the high-risk people, places, and times associated with the common episode.

Details such as the names of the IP's friends are helpful, as they make it easy to refer to these individuals later in treatment, but they are not entirely necessary. Many CSOs do not know the names of the IP's acquaintances, since IPs often are reluctant to share the names of people involved in illegal (drug) activities.

THERAPIST: You can see that I've already got part of the first column completed—down here where it asks *when* he uses. Can we also add the time the Friday night drinking starts? (See Figure 3.1.)

CSO: Jeff's told me that they like to get the weekend started right at work. They go into the stockroom near the end of their shift, around 8:00, and have a shot of something, usually tequila, I think. When they close up shop at 9:00 P.M., they head off to one of their apartments to do the real partying.

THERAPIST: This is helpful because you're also giving me information about where the drinking takes place. I'll put this all on the form here. And if you look at the first question under "external triggers" you'll see it asks who he typically drinks with during these episodes. You said he was with his friends from work—Can you be more specific? It's fine if you don't know everyone's name.

CSO: I've met two of the coworkers he parties with: Robbie and Liz. I'm not sure about anyone else. But now that I think of it—they mostly go to Liz's place.

THERAPIST: Wonderful, Samantha. This will be plenty to work with.

External triggers	Internal triggers	Drinking/using behavior	Short-term positive consequences (rewards)	Long-term negative consequences
1. *Who* is your loved one usually with when drinking/using? Coworkers Robbie and Liz 2. *Where* does he or she usually drink/use? Starts in the stockroom at work. Continues at Liz's apartment. 3. *When* does he or she usually drink/use? Friday nights Starts 8:00 p.m. Continues until 2:00 a.m.	1. What do you think your loved one is *thinking* about right before drinking/using? This will be fun tonight. I have a few new songs to stump them on. I need an escape from my boring job. I need an escape from my mom stressing me about drinking and missing work. 2. What do you think he or she is *feeling* right before drinking/using? Happy, excited. Stressed, bored.	1. *What* does your loved one usually drink/use? Beer Tequila Cocaine? Random pills (variety) 2. *How much* (or *how many times* during the episode) does he or she usually drink/use? Tequila: 1 shot Beer: 7–8 (12-oz. size) Cocaine? Random pills? 3. Over *how long* a period of time does he or she usually drink/use? 8:00 p.m.–2:00 a.m. (6 hours)	1. What do you think your loved one likes about drinking/using with (*who*)? They admire him (feels good). They like lots of different kinds of music. Robbie will teach him guitar. 2. What do you think he or she likes about drinking/using (*where*)? Free to do drugs. Cheaper to drink than in a bar. Are in charge of the music. Sneaky/clever (not caught). 3. What do you think he or she likes about drinking/using (*when*)? Deserves to celebrate? 4. What pleasant *thoughts* do you think he or she has while drinking/using? This is a lot of fun. They think I'm cool. 5. What pleasant *feelings* do you think he or she has while drinking/using? Happy, numb (not bored or stressed).	1. What do you think are the negative results of your loved one's drinking/using in these areas [* *the ones he or she would agree with*]? a. Family Strained relationship with mom. b. Friends/partners Lost 2 good friends (Tyla and Devin). c. Physical Tired, inactive, weight gain.* d. Emotional He's grumpy. He's down (depressed?) e. Legal n/a f. Job Might lose job (calls in sick)* Only works part-time. g. Financial Can't afford own apt. h. Other

FIGURE 3.1. Completed version of Form 3.2: CRAFT Functional Analysis of a Loved One's Drinking/Using Behavior.

Point out that since the IP's substance use is preceded by reasonably predictable factors, there is hope for coming up with ways to change the CSO's behavior and thereby influence the IP's use in these situations.

THERAPIST: You've given me very helpful details about the external triggers for your son's Friday night drinking. As we continue with this exercise, we'll eventually be able to pull together a clear picture of the things that are reliably associated with his alcohol use. Then we should be able to come up with a plan for you to influence his behavior, perhaps rather subtly, so that he doesn't choose to put himself in these high-risk situations so often.

4. Outline internal triggers.

Explain that triggers also come from within the IP, in the form of thoughts and feelings, and that the CSO should give an educated guess as to what the IP's are.

Reassure the CSO that she or he is not being asked to "mind read," but instead to come up with an educated guess as to what the IP is thinking and feeling prior to deciding to use. For those CSOs who remain hesitant to guess what their IP is thinking or feeling, remind them that they know their IP better than anyone else does.

THERAPIST: Now that we've discussed the triggers in your son's surroundings, let's move on to what we call internal triggers (*points to the second column on the FA*). These triggers are Jeff's thoughts and feelings that usually lead him to use. Of course, we won't know for sure exactly what your son is thinking or feeling right before he decides to use, but you can probably make a better guess than anyone else. We're just hoping to see a pattern.

Ask the CSO to consider that the IP might be looking forward to a positive reward associated with the using behavior (e.g., socializing); discuss what the IP's anticipatory thoughts might be for that situation.

THERAPIST: It's common for individuals to look forward to drinking or using drugs because it brings them something they view as positive and rewarding. Do you think maybe Jeff says to himself something like "I can't wait to hang out with my buddies outside of work," as he anticipates the Friday night partying?

CSO: Maybe. Probably. His coworkers are a bit younger than he is, and they sort of look up to him. For one thing, he's told me they think he knows a lot about music.

THERAPIST: Interesting. How shall we describe his thoughts then?

CSO: Something like "This will be fun tonight; I have a few new songs to stump them on."

Ask the CSO to consider that the IP might be trying to escape something negative (e.g., relieving stress); discuss what the IP's anticipatory thoughts might be for that situation.

THERAPIST: It's also likely that your son looks forward to drinking because it allows him an escape of some sort, such as from the stress of work, or from boredom. Would you guess he might be thinking about getting away from something unpleasant by drinking on Friday nights?

CSO: He's definitely bored with his job, so he probably *does* see the drinking as an escape from that. And he's stressed, too—not from work so much but from me bothering him to stop drinking and to stop missing work. I don't know if he thinks about that before going out though.

THERAPIST: It's probably worth listing these thoughts here anyway, since there's a decent chance your son would say they're part of what he escapes by drinking.

Help identify the IP's feelings by discussing the IP's observable behavior prior to drinking/using.

THERAPIST: I can see why it's hard to put a label on what your son might be feeling before he parties on Friday nights, because you don't see him right before he starts to drink. But just like we did when we talked about his thoughts: Let's focus on the time when he's *anticipating* the Friday night partying and he's still home. Have you noticed any facial expressions or behaviors at those times?

CSO: It's interesting—I've noticed that he's never late when he leaves for work on Fridays, probably because he's really looking forward to the partying after work . . . and the chance to show off with his new songs.

THERAPIST: Excellent, Samantha. So how would you label that feeling?

CSO: Happy and excited.

Help identify the IP's feelings by also asking about the feelings that are probably linked with the IP's thoughts just identified.

THERAPIST: Another way we can try to guess your son's feelings is to go back to what you came up with as far as the thoughts you believed he was having as he anticipated the partying. For example, you said that he'd be looking forward to escaping—from his boring job and from the stress that he sees you playing a role in.

CSO: Yes, he's probably feeling stressed and bored then, too.

5. Clarify the IP's substance-using behavior during the episode.

Fill in the details about the substance use that were not already provided during the CSO's overview of the common episode.

The basic questions include the following: What does the IP usually drink/use during these common episodes? How much does the IP drink/use during these episodes? How long does the episode typically last? In general, if IPs are using illicit drugs, it is fairly common for CSOs to be unsure about the type of illicit drug the IP is using. Making an educated guess based on the symptoms shown is discussed in Chapter 5. Furthermore, if an illicit drug is being used and the *amount* is not known, you might instead ask, "*How many times* during the episode does the IP use the drug?" If the CSO is uncertain how to answer this question as well, simply reassure her or him that this is not a problem, and move on to the next question.

THERAPIST: Although we're focused on your son's drinking for this exercise, we should at least list the other drugs he uses on Friday nights. Now I know you said you weren't sure what kind of drugs he uses at those parties. Has he given you *any* idea? Or maybe we can tell from the symptoms he shows when he gets home?

CSO: I'm pretty sure he uses cocaine some of the times, because he's all jacked up for hours after he gets home. I hear him making all sorts of noise in his room. But he's also said something about parties where they just help themselves to random pills that people bring. Sounds scary to me. I don't know how much he uses any of these things though.

THERAPIST: And since you're not there, I'm guessing you wouldn't know how many times during the evening he uses cocaine or the other drugs—right?

CSO: I'm sorry, but I just don't know.

Stay focused on the one common episode, and cover multiple drugs only if they are regularly used together as part of the common episode.

THERAPIST: Samantha, you're doing a terrific job. Don't worry about the details for the drugs. I'm just making some general notes on the worksheet so that we have a basic record of the fact that Jeff is using other drugs on Friday nights when he's drinking. It gives us a more complete picture for those nights.

6. Outline the positive consequences of the substance use.

Explain the importance of examining the more immediate consequences of drinking/using that the IP would view as positive.

Initially, some CSOs are reluctant to acknowledge *any* positive consequences of the IP's substance use, since the CSOs can only see the pain it has caused. Once you remind them that the rewards are through the eyes of the *IP*, and that the IP would not keep using if there was no reward experienced, they are able to participate in the discussion.

THERAPIST: This fourth column (*points to the fourth column on the FA* [see Figure 3.1]) asks about the more immediate positive consequences of your son's drinking. Although *you* might not see anything positive about Jeff's drinking, we have to assume that *he* does or he wouldn't keep drinking. And if we can figure that out, we're on track to helping him find other ways to get some of those same benefits—but without drinking alcohol.

Describe the format of the short-term positive consequences column by pointing out how it incorporates the information gained in the external and internal triggers columns.

THERAPIST: You can see here that the first three questions in this column are tied back to the external triggers you came up with for your son, and the last two questions incorporate his internal triggers. As we go through it we'll fill in the blanks with your son's relevant information.

Collect specific information about the positive consequences of the substance use.

THERAPIST: So Question 1 asks, "What do you think your son likes about drinking with Robbie and Liz?" And then we'll tackle the next two questions: "What do you think your son likes about drinking in the stockroom and at Liz's apartment?" and "What does he like about drinking on Friday nights?"

CSO: I'd say he likes drinking with Robbie and Liz because they admire him, and that makes him feel good. Plus, they all seem to like a lot of different kinds of music. And Jeff mentioned that Robbie has offered to teach him to play the guitar, which I think he'd like. But I don't see why they can't enjoy music together without getting drunk or high.

THERAPIST: You're raising a great point. And maybe some of our efforts can be devoted to helping your son find ways to enjoy music—and his friends—without drinking or getting high. So I'll jot it down in the margins. But for right now, let's fill in more of this puzzle.

Note: The therapist does not follow up on the CSO's comment about finding healthy ways for her son to enjoy music with friends, other than to say it will be covered later. Instead, the therapist stays focused on the main task at hand: finishing the FA. But this *is* important information, so it would be helpful to make a note of it somewhere accessible.

CSO: Well, I think he likes drinking at Liz's apartment because then they're free to do drugs, too. And it's cheaper to drink there than in a bar. Oh, and then they're in charge of playing the music, too.

THERAPIST: Wow, Samantha, you're good at this. And what do you think your son likes about starting the evening by drinking in the stockroom at work?

CSO: I think it makes Jeff feel sneaky and clever for being able to do it without getting caught. And as far as what he likes about Friday nights . . . I don't really know. He has to work all weekend, so it's not like he's celebrating the end of a hard week. Maybe he thinks he deserves to celebrate like everyone else though.

THERAPIST: I bet you're right on target. OK. Now we'll incorporate his internal triggers. Question 4 asks about pleasant thoughts he has while drinking. Let's start by looking back at the second column in which you outlined his thoughts *before* he starts to drink. I bet some of these still hold during his drinking or right afterward.

Note: The therapist refers back to the internal triggers column, since the details from that column are incorporated into Questions 4 and 5 in the short-term positive consequences column.

CSO: He's thinking about the fun he's having; the admiration he's getting. Maybe he'd say that his coworkers think he's cool.

THERAPIST: Are you up for this last one here? What about his feelings during or right after drinking?

CSO: I'd say he's happy, because usually when he comes home late those nights he's singing or humming. And like I said before, sometimes he's jacked up and making a lot of noise in his room. But he still seems happy—sort of. Once in a while he's real quiet; seems zoned out when I check on him—like he's not feeling much of anything; maybe numb? Probably depends on what drugs he used that night.

THERAPIST: That numb feeling might be his escape that we talked about earlier.

CSO: Right—so we can say he's *not* feeling bored or stressed. Of course, I prefer the nights he's singing, because he's friendly then. On those nights I make him pancakes, even though it's 2:00 in the morning, just so I get a chance to talk with him.

THERAPIST: Well, I can certainly understand you wanting to have a pleasant time with your son whenever you can grab it. Still, we might want to take a look at that later, because we'll discuss how it would be better if you only did those extra-nice things for your son when he wasn't drunk or high. But again—that's a conversation for another time after I've had a chance to teach you some special skills.

Note: During the course of an FA it is common to hear about CSOs inadvertently reinforcing substance-using behavior. Notice the therapist does not shame the CSO for engaging in this "pancake-making" behavior, but does hint about teaching her a better time for delivering that reward to her son. This would be discussed when the CSO is taught the CRAFT procedure for delivering positive reinforcement of substance-free behavior (see Chapter 5).

Engage the CSO in a review of the connection between the IP's substance use and the factors that are maintaining it (i.e., the positive consequences).

THERAPIST: Let's look at what we have in this fourth column. I'll start it off. Based on what you've told me, Samantha, it seems like Jeff drinks on Friday nights with Robbie and Liz because their admiration makes him feel good. But he also likes their company because they have a love of music in common. What else do you see here as far as major factors that make it pleasant for your son to drink?

CSO: I think you mentioned the main reasons. But it also struck me that we figured out he's probably using the drinking as an escape from stress and boredom, too. I can't help but think there has to be a better solution!

THERAPIST: I couldn't agree with you more—and that's why you're here. Let's finish up this last column and we'll sort out some preliminary ideas for a plan going forward.

Note: Although the FA is not quite finished, the therapist takes a moment to make sure the CSO is following the critical link between the IP's substance use and the factors (rewards) that are maintaining it.

7. Outline the negative consequences of the substance use.

Explain that the final column is for outlining the areas in which the CSO believes the IP has experienced negative consequences from the substance use, <u>and</u> for identifying the ones with which the IP would agree.

It is helpful to mark with a star (*) on the FA form those negative consequences proposed by the CSO that would be acknowledged *by the IP*, as well. When an IP is aware of the connection between a particular negative consequence (e.g., the loss of something valued) and the drinking/drug use, the CSO is in a better position to negotiate some behavior change on the part of the IP. For example, if an IP agrees with the CSO that friends have been lost due to the substance use, the CSO is more likely to be successful at encouraging the IP to try some healthy social activities with non-using friends than if the IP sees no link between the substance use and the loss of friends.

THERAPIST: This last column is pretty straightforward (*points to the fifth column on the FA form*): It asks you to list the ways in which your son has suffered negative consequences from his drinking. In other words, what are some of the bad things that have happened to Jeff because of his drinking? And as much as possible we'll try to make it specific to his Friday night episodes. Some categories are listed here, but we can add our own, too. And I'll also ask you to point out which ones you think he'd agree with you on. Those will get a little star.

List the negative consequences of the substance use.

THERAPIST: We can either talk about the negative consequences more generally first and I can fill in the worksheet in the right places, or we can go down item by item. Your preference?

CSO: It's caused so many problems that I'm not sure where to start. Actually, let's start with our relationship. I think his drinking has been awful for our relationship. He knows our relationship is strained, but he'd blame it on me and not the drinking.

THERAPIST: I'll list that here under the first category, "Family." But I won't put a star next to it since you say that he wouldn't blame his drinking for the problem. Has his drinking been bad for any of his other relationships, like his friends or maybe a romantic partner?

CSO: Yes. But again, I doubt he'd agree. He's lost friends in the last year, and I think it's because they have better things to do than drink all the time. And ever since he's lost these friends, he drinks even more. The drugs are new, too.

THERAPIST: Do you want to list the names of these friends so it's easier to refer to them?

CSO: Sure: Tyla and Devin. He hasn't dated in a while, so I don't know what to say about romantic partners.

THERAPIST: No problem. What about some other negative consequences? And as I said before, we're really focusing on his Friday night drinking as much as possible. I know it might be hard to separate them out from his drinking in general, but just do the best you can.

CSO: As I look down the list here, I can honestly say he's had bad things happen in just about every category, at least from his drinking in general. For "Physical" consequences: He stays up really late every Friday night when he parties, so he's tired and grumpy the next day even when he sleeps in.

THERAPIST: I'll put "tired" under "Physical" and "grumpy" under the "Emotional" category. Would Jeff agree with you on these?

CSO: He'd agree that he was tired and grumpy the next day, but he'd say it was because he stayed up late, not because he was drinking.

THERAPIST: Fair enough. What about any other physical or emotional consequences?

CSO: He used to be more active. He'd go out and do things with his friends, like play basketball, and that kept him in better shape. He's complained to me that he's put on weight. Oh, but that's probably more related to his weekday drinking.

THERAPIST: That's OK. We should mark it down because it's really all related. If he wasn't out late drinking, he might be more inclined to get out of the house the next day and do active things with his friends like he used to.

Note: It often is difficult to make a distinction between the negative consequences for one type of substance use episode versus another. For the most part it is not essential to do so anyway, since the negative consequences tend to spill across episodes.

CSO: Makes sense. And he'd even admit that the weight gain is related to his drinking.

THERAPIST: I'll put a star next to that then. What else?

CSO: I'm still thinking about his mood. Yes, he's grumpy after he's been out late, but his mood in general is different. He seems down, maybe depressed? Again, I'm not sure if the drinking is doing this or not.

THERAPIST: It's important that you're bringing it up though, because you'll see later in therapy that this type of information is very helpful when we're looking for a variety of ways to motivate someone like your son to come into treatment. In other words, Jeff might not want to get treatment for his drinking problem, but he might agree to see someone for his depression. Besides, alcohol is a depressant, so at the very least it's making his depression worse. I'll add it to the worksheet. I'm guessing I shouldn't star it?

Note: The therapist is mentioning one of the CRAFT motivational hooks for entering treatment: the fact that the IP can work on non-substance use problems. This hook and others are discussed in detail in Chapter 11. Before the CSO presents any hooks verbally to the IP, at the very least the CSO is taught positive communication skills (see Chapter 4) so that the message can be delivered skillfully.

CSO: Right. I'm not sure he'd even admit he's depressed. As far as the "Legal" category; he hasn't had any legal problems . . . yet, so I'll skip that. At least he doesn't drive when he's been drinking. But his job is a different story. Jeff calls in sick after a really late night. I know his boss has spoken to him about this already. And he only works 20–25 hours a week. He's not motivated to look for anything full-time. He'd never be able to afford his own apartment again. I think he'd agree that the job problem is drinking related—well, at least the part about missing work.

THERAPIST: Sounds like we can fill in both the "Job" and the "Financial" categories. We're just left with "Other." Can you think of any other negative consequences from his drinking? And by the way, Samantha, you've been incredibly good at this entire exercise.

Note: The therapist keeps the conversation upbeat and positive throughout the exercise and takes advantage of opportunities to compliment the CSO (e.g., for her knowledge about the IP).

8. Get the CSO's reaction to the completed FA and assist with summarizing the main findings.

Help the CSO step back and look at the information contained in the completed FA form by asking for the CSO's overall reaction to the exercise and what it produced.

THERAPIST: Samantha, thank you for your hard work on this today. Now let's step back a minute and talk about what this process has been like for you. What's your reaction to what you see here and what we've discussed?

CSO: I'm not sure why, but seeing it all laid out like this makes me feel more hopeful that something can be done to help Jeff.

THERAPIST: I'm glad to hear that, because that's how I feel, too. This road map will help us set up a solid plan for trying to influence Jeff's behavior.

If the CSO has not already mentioned the main triggers, ask the CSO to do so and assist if necessary.

This does *not* mean you (or the CSO) should go question by question down the first two columns on the FA. Instead, simply find out what made an impression on the CSO.

THERAPIST: Based on this information, how would you sum up your son's main triggers for drinking on Friday nights?

CSO: I'm not surprised that it's related to being around a few coworkers. But I hadn't thought about him looking forward to those evenings with Robbie and Liz because he feels good when he's around them.

THERAPIST: You said earlier that you think he's depressed, and so maybe this is his attempt to feel better about himself.

CSO: Maybe so. And I also hadn't thought about it being a way for him to escape from things he doesn't want to deal with, like the stress I'm causing him.

THERAPIST: Samantha, it's important that you don't blame yourself for your son's decision to drink. Most people choose much healthier ways to deal with stress and depression. This isn't your fault! But information can be powerful, so if we work together we can create some positive changes.

Note: The therapist took the opportunity to remind the CSO that she is not responsible for her son's substance use problem. This message is repeated multiple times throughout CRAFT, when clinically indicated.

Ask the CSO to comment on the consequences, and at least cover the main positive ones.

THERAPIST: Now let's summarize the main consequences for Jeff's Friday night drinking. Can we start with the positive ones? This will be fast, because you'll see that the positive consequences usually go along with the internal triggers for wanting to drink in the first place. So, what are the positive things Jeff gets out of drinking on Friday nights?

CSO: It makes him happy. Robbie and Liz make him feel good and he enjoys listening to music with them.

THERAPIST: Excellent summary. And what do you see as the main negative consequences?

CSO: Do you mean the ones that just I see or the ones he also agrees with?

THERAPIST: Let's make it simple and just stick with the main ones that *you* see.

CSO: He's lost friends and hurt our relationship. And he might lose his job.

9. Offer ideas regarding how this FA information can be used and settle on an assignment.

Referring to the triggers or consequences, give one or two examples regarding how the information can be used in the CSO's treatment.

When illustrating the clinical utility of the information gathered, you need to decide whether to focus on the FA's triggers (external? internal?) and/or consequences (positive? negative?). Some therapists gravitate toward whatever new information seems to make the most sense to the CSO or generates the most enthusiasm. For example, if the number one priority for the CSO in our case example was to help her son get a new job, then her therapist probably would emphasize both the positive and negative consequences of the drinking (noted above). Specifically, while the CSO might focus only on the negative consequences (the son being in danger of losing his current job), the therapist would remind the CSO of the positive consequences of the IP's drinking episodes (being admired for his music knowledge) so that it could be taken into consideration when planning for a new job (such as in a music store).

In offering examples of how the FA information can be used to guide the development of a plan that will ultimately influence the IP's behavior, keep in mind that it might be premature to immediately turn these ideas into homework assignments at this early stage in CRAFT. Generally, the ideas are meant to (a) provide a bigger picture of the direction you are likely headed with the particular CSO and IP, (b) show the CSO that she or he has already provided valuable information regarding the IP, and (c) offer hope and motivation for the CSO. Still, some of the examples you supply *are* apt to be developed into assignments later in therapy once CSOs have been taught skills through additional CRAFT procedures. And other examples possibly *could* be formed into homework for the upcoming week if they include a basic first step toward a more long-term goal mentioned. Since a homework assignment *will* need to be given before the session ends, some therapists opt to highlight information that lends itself to formulating an assignment for the week.

Several examples of the therapist generating preliminary therapy directions based on information gained from the completed FA are listed below. Each description identifies the relevant column of the FA form (e.g., external triggers, positive consequences). The therapist probably would provide only one or two of these examples, but they are included here to demonstrate multiple options for making the most of the FA information.

THERAPIST (*external triggers*): It's clear that Robbie and Liz are big triggers for drinking on Friday nights. But do they *have* to be? Can we somehow break that connection? Sure, ideally, we'd like to get Jeff to choose nondrinking friends to hang out with—like maybe old friends he's lost contact with. But for starters, can we help him come up with fun things to do with his current coworkers that don't totally revolve around drinking?

THERAPIST (*internal triggers*): Since stress and boredom are two of your son's main triggers to drink on Friday nights, we should look at healthy ways for Jeff to handle those feelings. The easy part will be coming up with some other coping strategies; the trick will be to find ones that Jeff is willing to choose over drinking.

THERAPIST (*positive consequences*): You said Jeff was excited that one of his coworkers, Robbie, offered to teach him to play the guitar. One possibility is that you eventually decide to negotiate with him around the guitar. For example, maybe you'd offer to buy him a guitar if he agrees to attend treatment.

THERAPIST (*negative consequences*): You've named several problem areas, aside from substance use, that would be great things for Jeff to work on in treatment. For example, he might want help finding a job he loves, or dealing with depression or his inactivity. I'm mentioning this because sometimes we can entice a person to enter treatment to work on other areas first. The substance use issues always follow at some point.

THERAPIST (*positive and negative consequences*): I think it will be important for us to find a way for Jeff to continue his involvement in music, but in a healthier setting. And it would be ideal if his involvement allowed him to be recognized for his music knowledge. Just off the top of my head: What about a job at a music store? That would also address some of the negative consequences you mentioned if the job happened to be full-time. And he'd be more likely to show up to work if he liked the job, and of course, if he was drinking less.

In collaboration with the CSO, make a specific homework assignment.

The complexity of the assignment will vary depending on the CSO's capabilities and drive, and the IP's anticipated reaction to the change in the CSO's behavior. In this current case, the therapist and CSO likely would generate an assignment similar to Option 1 or 2 below (or an equivalent assignment; see Box 3.1). Regardless, this homework (also called an "assignment," "practice," "home exercise/task," or "experiment") is designed to be relatively easy, given that this is one of the first CRAFT sessions and the CSO has not yet learned the necessary skills for more complicated assignments.

Sample Assignment Option 1

The CSO will develop and bring to the next session a list of:

- Ten non-substance-using local activities that the IP might enjoy doing with his coworkers (Robbie and Liz).
- Five non-substance-using coping strategies that the IP has used successfully in the past to deal with his stress and boredom.

BOX 3.1

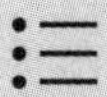

Homework Assignment Guidelines

Overview

- An assignment should be made in every session.
- The assignment (from the previous week) should be reviewed at the start of every session.

Assignment Procedure: The First Assignment

- Offer a rationale:
  - Practicing the new skills outside of therapy will ensure that the CSO improves these skills.
  - Carrying out the task in the real world is the key to influencing the desired changes at home.
- Ask the CSO which term is preferred: "homework," an "assignment," a "practice," an "experiment," a "task," and so forth.

Assignment Procedure: Every Assignment

- In collaboration with the CSO, develop an assignment and offer the clear expectation that it should be tackled in the upcoming week.
- Once the CSO has settled on an assignment, ask her or him:
  - To "walk" you through it, or to imagine carrying out each step of it.
  - To notice problems/obstacles/barriers that arise in doing so (assist if necessary).
- Resolve these potential problems/obstacles/barriers to completing the assignment (or select a different one).
- Ask the CSO to state in her or his own words exactly what the final assignment is.
- Remind the CSO how this assignment is in line with her or his therapy goals.
- At the *start* of the next session, review how the assignment went (start with the assumption that it was at least attempted).
  - If the assignment was completed or attempted, find out whether it went as planned and whether it had the desired outcome.
  - If the assignment was not attempted or only partially completed, find out why and determine whether the CSO is invested in it still.
- Troubleshoot any problems with the assignment and together with the CSO, decide whether to reassign, modify, or drop the assignment.
- Update the Goal Setting form (once it has been introduced; see Chapter 10, Form 10.3).

Assignment Format

- The assignment itself should be:
  - Concise and uncomplicated.
  - Described with positive/action-oriented wording (what the person *will* do, as opposed to what she or he won't do).
  - Based on specific (measurable) behaviors.
  - Reasonable.
  - Under the CSO's control.

Note: The first three points under the assignment format are the same ones used in positive communication training (Chapter 4) and in goal setting (Chapter 10).

Sample Assignment Option 2

The CSO will bring to the next session the following:

- Contact information for any of the IP's three closest friends from the past who are still in town.
- Job listings for any basic/starter job that involves music.

COMMON PROBLEMS TO AVOID

Although FAs appear rather straightforward to administer, there are a number of problems you may encounter in the process. Several of these are outlined below.

Problem: Clinicians sometimes refer to the entire FA exercise as a "form," "worksheet," or "chart" when introducing it, saying something like "Now we're going to do this form." While the FA form is a valuable tool for the exercise, referring to the entire FA procedure in this manner tends to minimize its importance by making it sound comparable to "paperwork."

Safeguards:

- Simply refer to all CRAFT procedures as, well, . . . procedures, or skills-training exercises/tasks.
- Exhibit enthusiasm when introducing CRAFT procedures so that CSOs get a sense of their importance from the start.

Problem: New CRAFT therapists often mistakenly go through the FA form in a highly mechanical style. In other words, they get so caught up in asking the series of questions and recording the CSO's responses that they sacrifice empathy and support in the process.

Safeguards:

- Keep good eye contact throughout the exercise, spending more time looking at the CSO than looking at the FA form.
- Encourage CSOs to take their time and provide as much detail as possible when they are describing a common substance use episode. Fill in the relevant parts of the FA form during this more conversational format, and be prepared to jump around on the form in order to do this. Recording this information in a more natural style early in the FA process will reduce the number of questions to be asked in a more formal manner as the remainder of the form is finished.
- Resist the urge to get an answer to every question if the CSO is struggling to generate responses, or if the process is simply taking an uncomfortably long period of time. There will be sufficient information to make the most of the FA even if there are blank spaces on the form.
- Feel free to conduct the interview in any order that feels comfortable; do not feel

compelled to go in the order shown on the FA form if the interview is moving along well in a conversational style.

Problem: Therapists periodically deviate significantly from the FA exercise in an attempt to follow up on potentially important pieces of information the CSO is sharing. The flow of the FA is compromised if the CSO is allowed to go off on too many tangents, since the FA is set up to clearly demonstrate the path from triggers to substance use to consequences. Nonetheless, often there *is* clinically valuable information reported in the course of doing the FA, information that could be quite helpful at a later point in treatment. For example, assume a CSO starts to describe fun, healthy activities the IP used to enjoy prior to abusing substances. Since at a later session you will be asking the CSO to recall activities such as these from the IP's past, it helps to have them already noted briefly, particularly in the event that the CSO cannot generate them again readily.

Safeguards:

- If the CSO is providing a lot of IP-related details that do not seem suitable for the FA form, gently interrupt the CSO. Explain that while the information is valuable, it is important to finish the task at hand first—that the additional information being provided will be revisited at a later session.
- Jot down the potentially useful information either in the margins of the FA form or on a separate piece of paper so that it can be followed up on sometime after the FA has been completed.

Problem: One of the most salient problems shown by CRAFT therapists entails selecting a supposedly common episode for the FA that is, in fact, a unique (*nonrepresentative*) one. As explained earlier (see the section "2. Settle on a common using episode . . . ," above), choosing an *uncommon* episode will result in spending considerable therapy time on an exercise that is bound to yield less clinically useful findings.

Safeguards:

- Before the CSO spends too much time describing a purportedly common episode, inquire about how often that particular type of episode occurs. Some CSOs automatically report on a recent episode, or one that stands out due to its intensity, regardless of whether it is a frequently occurring episode.
- If it is unclear whether the episode first being described by the CSO at the start of the FA exercise is truly a common one, go directly to the third column of the FA form ("drinking/using behavior") and ask those questions. Emphasize the word "usually" in the questions and see whether it raises issues with the CSO's choice of episode.

Problem: It is not unusual for new CRAFT clinicians to combine two common (yet different) episodes into one FA. For example, some clinicians might attempt to combine both daily *weekday* cocaine use and weekly *Saturday night* cocaine use episodes into one FA, even though the triggers (and perhaps the consequences) are very different for the episodes. An FA form that contains two completely different sets of triggers and consequences is nearly impossible to use when developing a plan, and as a result its impact is minimized.

Safeguards:

- As a general rule, simplify the FA exercise as much as possible.
- While still working with the CSO to settle on the common episode, ask yourself: Is this one or two episodes? If it is clearly two distinct episodes, help the CSO narrow it down to one.

Problem: Clinicians sometimes conduct more than one FA within one session *or* in consecutive sessions. First of all, it is unusual to ever need more than one FA to address the IP's substance use. After CSOs have gone through the FA exercise once, you can discuss triggers and consequences involved in another type of episode without going through the formal FA exercise. Also, although clinicians sometimes are most comfortable resorting to a CRAFT procedure that is very structured (like the FA), CSOs tend to find multiple FAs burdensome.

Safeguards:

- Instead of reaching for another FA form at a time when one seems required, pull the initial completed form from the CSO's file. After the CSO provides a brief overview of the new episode, refer to the initial (completed) FA form and inquire about the ways in which the new episode's triggers and consequences are the same or different from the initial episode. It is not necessary to review each question; both you and the CSO will have learned enough from the first FA exercise to move quickly to a plan.
- To fight the urge to administer a second FA (especially if one has been conducted recently), simply observe whether the CSO's eyes glaze over or the CSO emits sighs as soon as you mention the FA or present a new FA form. These are cues that rapport will be compromised if a formal FA is attempted.

SUMMARY

This chapter introduces a comprehensive method for outlining a CSO's perception of the triggers that lead up to the IP's substance use, the factors that maintain it, and the ways in which the IP's use has negatively impacted both the IP and others. This FA/road map begins the process of finding creative ways for the CSO to help the IP select new responses to problematic triggers and healthier ways to obtain some of the same rewards typically associated with the substance use. Importantly, the FA is only one of the CRAFT procedures that focuses on these objectives; an entire "toolbox" remains. Furthermore, the FA format can be used to outline the context of other problem IP behaviors (e.g., angry outbursts) *and* healthy behaviors that the CSO would like the IP to increase (see Chapter 6).

FORM 3.1

Functional Analysis of a Loved One's Drinking or Using Behavior: Checklist

1. Introduce the FA and explain its purpose.

- ☐ a. Link the FA with two CRAFT goals (to decrease the IP's use and get the IP into treatment) and with the CSO's general role.
- ☐ b. Explain how the CSO's knowledge of and contact with the IP makes her or him well suited for doing the FA.
- ☐ c. Describe some of the specific information that will be collected (external/internal triggers, positive/negative consequences) and explain how it will be used.
- ☐ d. Give the CSO a copy of the FA form and point out the column headings so that she or he can follow along.

2. Settle on a common using episode for the IP and begin to collect information.

- ☐ a. Ask the CSO to describe a common/typical substance use episode of the IP's—a pattern that happens fairly often.
- ☐ b. Before the CSO spends too much time describing an episode, check to make sure the type of episode occurs regularly.
- ☐ c. Focus on *one* common episode; do not jump around between multiple episodes describing different drugs and/or occasions.
- ☐ d. Complete the FA form as much as possible once the CSO begins to describe the episode.
- ☐ e. When next proceeding to clarify and fill in gaps in the FA form, use a conversational style whenever possible and do not feel compelled to fill in every blank.

3. Outline external triggers.

- ☐ a. Explain the concept of a high-risk situation—how it is important to look at the IP's environment (external triggers) at the time of the episode because triggers "set the stage" for the IP's substance use.
- ☐ b. Identify the high-risk people, places, and times associated with the common episode.
- ☐ c. Point out that since the IP's substance use is preceded by reasonably predictable factors, there is hope for coming up with ways to change the CSO's behavior and thereby influence the IP's use in these situations.

4. Outline internal triggers.

- ☐ a. Explain that triggers also come from within the IP, in the form of thoughts and feelings, and that the CSO should give an educated guess as to what the IP's are.
- ☐ b. Ask the CSO to consider that the IP might be looking forward to a positive reward associated with the using behavior (e.g., socializing); discuss what

(continued)

the IP's anticipatory thoughts might be for that situation.

- ☐ c. Ask the CSO to consider that the IP might be trying to escape something negative (e.g., relieving stress); discuss what the IP's anticipatory thoughts might be for that situation.
- ☐ d. Help identify the IP's feelings by discussing the IP's observable behavior prior to drinking/using.
- ☐ e. Help identify the IP's feelings by also asking about the feelings that are probably linked with the IP's thoughts just identified.

5. Clarify the IP's substance-using behavior during the episode.

- ☐ a. Fill in the details about the substance use that were not already provided during the CSO's overview of the common episode.
- ☐ b. Stay focused on the one common episode, and cover multiple drugs only if they are regularly used together as part of the common episode.

6. Outline the positive consequences of the substance use.

- ☐ a. Explain the importance of examining the more immediate consequences of drinking/using that the IP would view as positive.
- ☐ b. Describe the format of the short-term positive consequences column by pointing out how it incorporates the information gained in the external and internal triggers columns.
- ☐ c. Collect specific information about the positive consequences of the substance use.
- ☐ d. Engage the CSO in a review of the connection between the IP's substance use and the factors that are maintaining it (i.e., the positive consequences).

7. Outline the negative consequences of the substance use.

- ☐ a. Explain that the final column is for outlining the areas in which the CSO believes the IP has experienced negative consequences from the substance use, *and* for identifying the ones with which the IP would agree.
- ☐ b. List the negative consequences of the substance use.

8. Get the CSO's reaction to the completed FA and assist with summarizing the main findings.

- ☐ a. Help the CSO step back and look at the information contained in the completed FA form by asking for the CSO's overall reaction to the exercise and what it produced.
- ☐ b. If the CSO has not already mentioned the main triggers, ask the CSO to do so and assist if necessary.
- ☐ c. Ask the CSO to comment on the consequences, and at least cover the main positive ones.

9. Offer ideas regarding how this FA information can be used and settle on an assignment.

- ☐ a. Referring to the triggers or consequences, give one or two examples regarding how the information can be used in the CSO's treatment.
- ☐ b. In collaboration with the CSO, make a specific homework assignment.

FORM 3.2

CRAFT Functional Analysis of a Loved One's Drinking or Using Behavior

External triggers	Internal triggers	Drinking/using behavior	Short-term positive consequences (rewards)	Long-term negative consequences
1. *Who* is your loved one usually with when drinking/using? 2. *Where* does he or she usually drink/use? 3. *When* does he or she usually drink/use?	1. What do you think your loved one is *thinking* about right before drinking/using? 2. What do you think he or she is *feeling* right before drinking/using?	1. *What* does your loved one usually drink/use? 2. *How much* (or *how many times* during the episode) does he or she usually drink/use? 3. Over *how long* a period of time does he or she usually drink/use?	1. What do you think your loved one likes about drinking/using with (*who*)? 2. What do you think he or she likes about drinking/using (*where*)? 3. What do you think he or she likes about drinking/using (*when*)? 4. What pleasant *thoughts* do you think he or she has while drinking/using? 5. What pleasant *feelings* do you think he or she has while drinking/using?	What do you think are the negative results of your loved one's drinking/using in these areas [* the ones he or she would agree with]? a. Family b. Friends/partners c. Physical d. Emotional e. Legal f. Job g. Financial h. Other

Chapter 4

Improving Concerned Significant Others' Communication Skills

Frequently there are communication issues in relationships in which one individual has a substance use problem (Haverfield, Theiss, & Leustek, 2016; Hussaarts et al., 2011; Mancheri et al., 2019; McCrady et al., 2016). These issues can manifest as episodic angry outbursts or chronic belittling, blaming, and shaming. But communication problems also may involve periodically offering the silent treatment or avoiding the other person altogether. Both the CSOs and IPs typically play a role in maintaining the problematic communication. Not surprisingly then, communication skills training is used routinely in many cognitive-behavioral and behavioral couple therapy programs for individuals with alcohol or drug problems (Epstein et al., 2007; McCrady, Owens, & Brovko, 2013; McCrady et al., 2016), and is part of the CRA relationship protocol (see Chapter 12; see also Meyers & Smith, 1995, pp. 163–170). Teaching CSOs positive ways to communicate is an integral procedure in CRAFT, in part because it forms the foundation for several other CRAFT procedures. Some of these procedures involve CSOs explaining to their IPs why non-using behavior is now being rewarded, and CSOs inviting their IPs to treatment.

In addition to enhancing the CSO–IP relationship and providing the IP with a supportive environment, the improvement of the CSO's communication skills also offers benefits directly to the CSO. The benefits might include opening the doors to larger support systems and providing the CSO with a skill that can increase satisfaction in other (non-IP-related) life areas, such as the CSO's job.

THE BASICS

General Description

CRAFT's communication skills training focuses on the *beginning* of difficult conversations that are usually (but not exclusively) with the IP. Getting these challenging conversations started on a positive note is extremely important, because otherwise the IP might walk away, or respond negatively and then walk away. If the beginning of the conversation goes well, the remainder of the conversation should fall into place more naturally, since presumably the other person will be more open to listening.

CRAFT communication skills training is a step-by-step approach to building a positive conversation by following a set of communication guidelines. Although CSOs do not need to incorporate all of the guidelines in their practiced conversations, the objective is for CSOs to learn and use a sufficient number of the guidelines so they are heard and understood by the other person. Typically, this entails CSOs overlearning their conversations through repeated role plays and detailed feedback sessions. Carrying out the planned communication assignments in the real world is a particularly important homework assignment.

Procedure Timing

Communication skills training commonly is introduced in one of the earlier CRAFT sessions, given that it is the foundation for several other CRAFT procedures. Despite the interest in getting communication skills training covered early in CRAFT, it is still preferable to introduce the procedure when there is a clinical reason for doing so. With practice, you will get in the habit of watching for signs of the need for communication training. This need becomes apparent when the CSO reports a problem that requires having a difficult conversation in order to resolve it, or when incomplete homework assignments can be linked to communication problems. Occasionally, CSOs simply ask for help in discussing a topic with the IP.

Forms

- Improving CSOs' Communication Skills: Checklist (Form 4.1)
- Planning Positive Communication (Form 4.2)
- Making Communication Positive (Handout 4.1)

CLINICIAN GUIDANCE AND SAMPLE DIALOGUE

The specifics regarding how to conduct communication skills training with CSOs are presented below in detail. A sample case is followed throughout as a way to illustrate the training process. All of the components for conducting this exercise are outlined in Form 4.1, Improving CSOs' Communication Skills: Checklist, found at the end of this chapter.

Case Description

The CSO (Jackie) is a 23-year-old single, female friend of the IP (Rachel). These Latino women have been close friends for many years and became roommates approximately 1 year ago. During this year, Jackie has grown increasingly concerned about Rachel's cocaine use. Initially, Rachel was a weekend partier who primarily used alcohol. About 6 months ago, Rachel started to spend all of her free time with new friends: several fellow tattoo artists who were known for their drug habits. Rachel quickly cut off all contact with her other friends and began getting high daily. Jackie has tried to talk with Rachel about her concerns, but Rachel's response was that Jackie should move out if she was unhappy with the living environment.

1. Discuss why positive communication is addressed.

In order to get *buy-in* from CSOs to work on mastering a new skill, it is necessary to offer compelling reasons. The three most commonly presented reasons for teaching communication skills are illustrated separately in the dialogue below, but the entire list is outlined here. Positive communication (a) is "contagious," (b) makes it more likely CSOs will get what they want, (c) is the foundation for other CRAFT procedures, (d) opens the door to larger social support networks, (e) increases CSOs' life satisfaction in other areas aside from IP interactions, (f) can serve as a powerful reward for a loved one, and (g) is limited in most relationships when one individual has a substance use problem. Of these, only those reasons that appear most relevant to an individual case are used.

Explain that positive communication is contagious.

THERAPIST: Have you ever noticed that positive communication is "contagious"? In other words, if someone speaks to us in a pleasant way, it's natural for us to answer back in that same positive way. I'm thinking it could be helpful to prepare for upcoming challenging situations with your roommate by practicing to communicate in a positive way.

State that individuals tend to be more successful in getting what they want from another person if they communicate in a positive way.

THERAPIST: It's also helpful to be positive when we communicate because we're more likely to get what we want that way. I imagine it's partly because people tend to listen to us when spoken to in a friendly way—we don't automatically get shut out.

Discuss how good communication is the foundation for other CRAFT procedures.
From the examples that follow, briefly mention one or two that are most relevant to the CSO. Good communication is essential, particularly in the following cases:

- When CSOs are explaining to their IPs (a) why rewards are being linked with their non-using behavior (Chapter 5), (b) why rewards are being withdrawn during times of substance use (Chapter 7), (c) why the natural consequences of IP substance use are being allowed to occur (Chapter 8), and (d) why they are in treatment (Chapter 11).
- When CSOs are looking to increase their social support network (Chapter 10).
- When CSOs are inviting their IP to sample treatment (Chapter 11).

THERAPIST: Another reason why I focus on communication skills training is because good communication is critical for many of the other CRAFT procedures. For example, you'll find it helpful when you explain to Rachel why you're doing pleasant things with her only when she's not using, and you'll also need it when you get to the point of inviting her to treatment.

Select a specific situation in which to practice the communication skills.
Communication skills training typically is introduced when a clinical situation is presented that calls for improved communication. Although the exercise often involves

practicing a conversation between the CSO and the IP (and which frequently, but not always, is at least indirectly related to the IP's substance use), in reality it can be a conversation between the CSO and any other individual about any topic.

THERAPIST: I brought up the idea of practicing communication skills today because you said you weren't sure how to handle the fact that Rachel has recently started to party late every night with her new friends at the house, and you're having trouble sleeping. How about we use that situation today to practice a new way to communicate?

CSO: Sure. But it's not just that I can't sleep. I'm worried about Rachel. How long can she keep this up? It's *so* unhealthy. But then there's the problem of me needing to find another place if she kicks me out after talking to her about this.

THERAPIST: I know you're concerned about Rachel, because that's what brought you to the CRAFT program in the first place. Keep in mind that one of the goals of CRAFT is to help the people we care about to decrease their use even before they agree to treatment. So if you get Rachel to limit her partying at night so that you can get more sleep, can you see that you're still helping Rachel decrease her substance use? It's a win–win situation.

CSO: Yes, sure. Makes sense.

THERAPIST: As far as the possible negative consequences of this conversation with Rachel, I'm glad you brought it up. Yes, Rachel might ask you to move out as a result of this conversation. But I'm hoping that if we come up with a positive way to make your request, she'll be OK with it. Since you brought it up though, how *would* you handle it if she asked you to move out?

CSO: It would be a pain to find a new place, but I don't want to stay living with Rachel if she keeps living the way she has been. It's too hard to see her struggle.

Note: Often you would discuss the possible negative ramifications of a homework assignment after the conversation has been practiced in role plays and the time for it has been planned, since this tends to make the upcoming conversation seem more realistic. Nonetheless, the therapist decided to briefly discuss the potential fallout at this earlier point in the session, given that the CSO brought it up.

2. Describe the positive communication guidelines and develop examples of each.

Although it is not necessary to start by presenting Guideline 1 for positive communication (be brief) and then proceeding down the list for all seven of them in order (see Box 4.1; Forms 4.1 and 4.2), this is how the exercise is commonly done. An exception to this would be made if you did not want to overwhelm the CSO, and thus only presented a few of the seven guidelines. Another exception would occur if you believed certain guidelines were more relevant to the CSO's case than others and therefore you presented only the more pertinent ones.

Present and develop an example of Guideline 1: Be brief (uncomplicated).

THERAPIST: Here's a set of guidelines we use when teaching communication skills (*points to Form 4.2* [found at the end of this chapter]). This form can be used as a worksheet

BOX 4.1

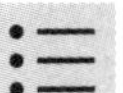

Positive Communication Guidelines

1. Be brief (uncomplicated).
2. Use positive/action-oriented wording (indicating what you would like to see happen).
3. Mention specific behaviors.
4. Label your feelings.
5. Offer an understanding statement.
6. Accept partial responsibility (for something related to the problem situation, *not* for the substance use).
7. Offer to help.

Note: The first three guidelines are the same ones used in goal/strategy setting (see Chapter 10).

at home, too, once you've learned the guidelines. OK. Let's start with 1: Be brief (uncomplicated). That means it's good to get right to the point of what you're trying to say. If you start to drag in a lot of old history and things that aren't directly relevant to what you really want to talk about, the other person is likely to get distracted and either lose interest or get annoyed. Jackie, go ahead and give it a shot. Using this first guideline, just state briefly what the problem is. We'll build on it from there.

CSO: How about something like "Rachel, don't get mad, but can you maybe ask your friends to leave a little earlier at night?"

THERAPIST: Great start. You were brief and to the point, so you followed the first guideline.

Note: The therapist and the CSO are *not* engaged in a role play . . . yet. The CSO is simply generating some conversation segments/snippets. These segments will soon be pulled together and used as part of an actual role play. Also note that since only the first (very basic) guideline had been covered at this point, the therapist did not offer the CSO specific feedback regarding how she could improve the conversation segment. This becomes more important as the conversation segments grow and develop into full role plays (see Box 4.2).

Present and develop an example of Guideline 2: Use positive/action-oriented wording (indicating what you would like to see happen).

The notion of using positive wording in a way that does not simply imply being "nice" is often confusing to CSOs, and so examples are tremendously helpful.

THERAPIST: Looks like you already did the second guideline, too, because Guideline 2 says use positive, action-oriented wording, indicating what you would like to see happen. This guideline means two things. Of course, we want you to say things in a positive and friendly way, with no blaming or name-calling, because a loved one is less likely to get defensive and stop listening if you speak this way. But Guideline 2 also means that we want you to spell out what you *do* want, not what you *don't* want anymore. In your case, this means you would tell Rachel what you *want*, not what

BOX 4.2

Is It a Role Play?

A role play involves an interaction (a "back-and-forth," a conversation "volley") between you and the CSO, during which you each act out a scene either as yourselves or a significant person in the CSO's life. These role plays/interactions are brief: typically under 2 minutes. In contrast, conversation segments/snippets (which CRAFT somewhat jokingly refers to as "one-sided role plays") merely represent the wording that is being considered for one individual as a small part of a conversation. Since they do not entail practicing the simulation of a real conversation, they do not "count" as role plays.

you *don't* want anymore. But as I said, you're already doing this, because you asked Rachel to ask her friends to leave earlier at night. What kind of questions do you have about the second guideline?

Note: The therapist asks an open-ended question that invites the CSO to inquire about the guideline (thereby normalizing questions), as opposed to asking a "yes/no" question that tends to shut down the conversation.

CSO: I wasn't sure what you meant until you gave the example. But I guess I'm still not sure why it's important.

THERAPIST: Excellent question. If we simply tell people what we don't want, then that part is clear, but how will they know what we *do* want instead? We need to help them see exactly what we're asking for. If you told Rachel that you had a problem with all the late night partying at the house, she might not know if you were asking her to stop having friends over altogether, or to limit it to weekends, or to just ask them to leave early. By telling her what you *do* want, it eliminates the confusion.

Present and develop an example of Guideline 3: Mention specific behaviors.

THERAPIST: Guideline 3 says mention specific behaviors. The more specific you are with a request, the less confusion there is in terms of what you want. It doesn't necessarily mean the other person is going to go along with your request, but at least that person will know what you're asking for. I bet we could get more specific about the behavior you're requesting. How could you make your request more specific when you ask Rachel if she can have her friends leave a little earlier? How can you make it specific enough so she knows exactly what you're asking for?

CSO: I could ask her to have her friends leave by midnight, because that's when I go to bed.

THERAPIST: Very good. Is that how you'd say it? What words would you use?

CSO: I'd say something like "Rachel, can you ask your friends to leave by midnight during the week? That's when I go to bed and it's hard to sleep with all the noise."

Note: CSOs should practice each conversation segment by using the words they think they would like to use in the real-world situation. This gives CSOs the opportunity to try out the language of the conversation, and to modify it afterward if it does not feel natural to them or if they think it will not be well received.

Present and develop an example of Guideline 4: Label your feelings.

THERAPIST: OK, good. Your request is definitely more specific. Ready for Guideline 4? It says label your feelings. It's helpful to tell the person how you're feeling about the thing you're requesting. It's like saying why it's important to you. So how might you add your feelings to your request for Rachel to ask her partying friends to leave by midnight?

CSO: I'm not sure what you mean. Do you mean I should tell her I'm tired the next day if I don't get enough sleep?

THERAPIST: Telling her how you feel physically could be part of it, but if we add something about your *emotional* feelings it will be more powerful.

CSO: Maybe I could say that I'm nasty or grumpy the next day if I'm tired.

THERAPIST: That sounds good. Hey, in case you're getting worried about remembering to add all of these statements to your conversation, you should know I'm giving you a lot of options for things you *can* add, but you're not expected to use all of them. When you're in the real situation with Rachel you'll probably be nervous, so chances are you won't remember them all anyway. Before we finish up today we'll get some good practice with the ones you feel the most comfortable with.

CSO: That's good to hear. I *was* starting to get nervous, and I know we have a few more to learn yet.

Note: Since this CSO is picking up on the guidelines quickly and is generating good conversation segments, the therapist will present all seven guidelines. Nonetheless, even skilled CSOs would feel apprehensive if they thought they had to remember and incorporate each of the seven guidelines into the conversation assigned for homework.

THERAPIST: Yes, we have three to go. Also, I'm going to send you home with both the worksheet that we've been using (*points to Form 4.2*) and a handout that gives examples of each of the communication guidelines in action (*points to Handout 4.1* [found at the end of this chapter]). Anyway, at this point you have a good basic start to a conversation.

Present and develop an example of Guideline 5: Offer an understanding statement.

THERAPIST: These last three guidelines are comments that are often very helpful in getting the other person to listen. See what you think of them. Guideline 5 is offer an understanding statement. This means you should try to understand where Rachel is coming from in the situation. Maybe you've heard of the expression to "Put yourself in another person's shoes"?

CSO: Yeah, I've heard that. What exactly am I trying to understand though? Am I trying to understand why she likes to get high?

THERAPIST: Partly, because getting high is related to your request that she ask her friends to leave by midnight. But, the best understanding statements are the ones that are directly related to the behavior you want the person to change. Can you put yourself in Rachel's shoes as far as her wanting her friends to be partying at the house late at night?

CSO: Oh definitely. Rachel used to be a lot of fun when her partying only involved drinking. I used to have a great time with her. She'd sort of get wild, but not out of control like she does now. Sometimes in the middle of the day we'd really blast the music when a heavy metal song came on, and we'd get crazy and jump all around singing and stuff. We haven't done that in a long time (*gets quiet and looks sad*).

THERAPIST: Is that something you miss about your relationship with Rachel?

CSO: Sure. She used to yell, "Jackie, come over here and dance with me!" Boy, that was fun! She doesn't do that anymore. Either she just lies around, high, with the music blasting, or she and her friends talk nonstop . . . loudly. We used to do a lot of fun things.

THERAPIST: You obviously care a lot about Rachel. And with a little more training, both in communication skills and a few other procedures, I think we can get to the point where you and Rachel have some fun together again, even if she doesn't get right into treatment.

Note: The therapist checks in with the CSO as far as how she is feeling, and uses the opportunity to highlight the CSO's compassion and to offer hope. The therapist also makes a mental note to inquire at a later time about the various enjoyable activities that the CSO and IP apparently shared previously, since these activities might be good targets for other CRAFT procedures (e.g., positive reinforcement of substance-free behavior; see Chapter 5).

THERAPIST: Using this information then, I bet you can come up with a great understanding statement.

CSO: Here goes: "Rachel, I know how much fun it is to get all crazy with your friends at night, but I wonder if you could ask them to leave by around midnight, since that's when I go to bed?" Oh—I forgot to add the part about being tired and grumpy: "Rachel, you've seen me tired and grumpy the next day if I don't get enough sleep . . . and it's not pretty."

Present and develop an example of Guideline 6: Accept partial responsibility (for something related to the problem situation under discussion, not for the substance use).

You should proceed cautiously with Guideline 6, accept partial responsibility, because CSOs have the most difficulty with it. Some CSOs have a negative emotional reaction to the thought of taking responsibility for anything related to the IP, despite understanding that the purpose of this skill is to increase the likelihood that the IP will be open to listening. If CSOs are quite resistant to practicing the incorporation of this guideline into their conversation, you can simply skip it and move on.

THERAPIST: Impressive! You definitely used all of the guidelines. Now let's talk about Guideline 6, accept partial responsibility, for something related to the problem situation under discussion, *not* for the substance use. Notice it specifically says that you're not supposed to accept responsibility for Rachel's substance use, but instead some small thing about the problem situation you brought up. What do you think?

CSO: Am I supposed to say it's my fault that she's got friends over late and she's playing the music too loud, or maybe that it's my fault that I have to get sleep?

THERAPIST: In some ways it doesn't matter so much *what* you're accepting partial responsibility for. What's most important is that you're not blaming the entire problem on Rachel; you're blaming a little bit of the problem on yourself. Why do you think this might help Rachel listen to you . . . and maybe even go along with your request? How might accepting partial responsibility help?

CSO: I guess she wouldn't feel like I was dumping everything on her. Maybe it wouldn't feel as much like an attack.

THERAPIST: Right. And as a result, we're counting on Rachel feeling more like listening to you. So, is there something you'd feel comfortable accepting partial responsibility for?

CSO: I could say that I might not be as much fun to hang out with as I used to be, ever since my shift at work changed and I have to be there by 8:00.

THERAPIST: That's really good. You're accepting responsibility for needing to go to bed earlier than in the past, and consequently needing to ask her to cut the partying short.

CSO: But you'd think she'd *know* that I need my job; how can I pay my share of the rent if I don't work? And besides, even if I didn't have to get up early, I'd still be worrying about all the drugs in the house and the neighbors calling the police.

THERAPIST: Jackie, try to keep in mind that you're only accepting partial responsibility for this one small thing because you're more likely to get what you want—namely, Rachel agreeing to end her parties early. You and I, and Rachel, too, I imagine, know that none of this is your fault. We're just trying to open up the lines of communication, and this is one pretty effective way of doing it. But we can skip this guideline if you really aren't comfortable following it. There are plenty of others!

CSO: I'll try it now, but I have the feeling it will be the first thing to "accidentally" drop off the conversation when I talk to Rachel.

Present and develop an example of Guideline 7: Offer to help.

THERAPIST: Fair enough. Here's the final one, Guideline 7: offer to help. This one can be kept real simple, because you can just say, "How can I help?" That statement is another great way to get people to listen, because it comes across as very supportive. Or you can offer to do something specific that works toward a solution to whatever the problem is that you raised. Can you think of some way you can offer to help Rachel solve this problem of there being lots of friends over partying late every night?

CSO: Hmm. That's a tough one. I guess I could offer to sleep somewhere else in the house, away from the noise, but I don't really want to do that.

THERAPIST: Good, because I wouldn't want you to do that either! That would, in some ways, make it a little easier for Rachel to keep partying, right? We're looking for things you could do to make it easier for the partying to *stop* earlier in the evening. Sometimes it's hard to make the distinction between these two different actions. Don't worry though; I know you only want the best for Rachel, and I'm here to help!

CSO: Oh, that's right. Duh! I guess I just panicked in trying to come up with something.

Note: This is a prime example of a CSO wanting to help, but instead coming up with an idea that inadvertently could make it easier for the IP to continue using. Inadvertent support of substance use is touched upon during the introductory session of CRAFT (Chapter 2) and is covered in detail when the CSOs are taught how to withdraw reinforcers during IP substance use (Chapter 7), and how to allow for the natural negative consequences of their IP's use (Chapter 8). Since the topic came up during this session, the therapist used it as an opportunity to address it briefly.

THERAPIST: Don't panic! We can figure this out. Let's see. Is there anything you could offer to do that would make it easier for Rachel to ask her friends to leave by midnight?

CSO: She might be OK with me coming out and saying that I'm headed to bed soon. That would give her a heads-up. And maybe she could blame the earlier night on me then. I'd be OK with that.

THERAPIST: You're very creative. I like it! Guess what? We've covered all seven guidelines.

3. Conduct a reverse role play and provide feedback.

Role plays in general are the most useful when they make CSOs feel, as much as possible, as if they are actually in the real-world situation—that it is happening right then. So CSOs should pretend during the role play that the therapist *is* that other person in their life (usually the IP) and that they (the CSOs) are speaking directly to that person in the moment. Importantly, it is not uncommon for both CSOs *and* therapists to be intimidated by the thought of doing role plays, and consequently to avoid them. You will feel more comfortable doing role plays once you (a) embrace the fact that role plays are an essential part of CRAFT, (b) practice them with colleagues, and (c) realize that it is not necessary for you to play the roles flawlessly. Apprehensive CSOs will be less resistant to doing role plays when *you* (a) appear comfortable doing the role plays, (b) automatically start the role play each time, and (c) use a nonthreatening word to describe the role plays (e.g., a "practice"?).

Describe the purpose and format of the reverse role play.

A *reverse* role play is one in which the CSO is played by the therapist, and the CSO plays the target of the conversation (e.g., the IP). A reverse role play often is conducted *prior* to doing a standard role play (in which the CSO plays her- or himself) because it allows you to do the following:

- Demonstrate what is expected of the CSO in a role-play exercise, thereby commonly reducing some of the CSO's anxiety.
- Provide a model of what it would look like to pull the entire conversation together.

- Gain a sense of how the person who is the target of the CSO's conversation might normally act (since the CSO is playing this person), and thus have this information available when assuming that role during an upcoming standard role play.
- Offer the CSO an opportunity to put her- or himself in the other person's shoes (normally the IP's) and to increase empathy as a result.

Note: Occasionally reverse role plays are skipped altogether, such as when the CSO's communication and empathy skills are quite advanced, or when session time constraints do not allow for it. Whenever possible though, it is advisable to conduct one.

THERAPIST: It's time for us to practice this conversation now as if you're really having it with Rachel. We can take turns playing her part, but I think it might help to have me play *you* first, and for you to play Rachel. This way I can demonstrate the type of conversation I'm talking about, using what you've come up with.

CSO: Good. I'm glad you're going to show me what you mean. Am I supposed to act like I think Rachel would in this situation? It could be harsh.

THERAPIST: Yes, definitely act the way you think Rachel would. Not only will it help me see what you're up against but it will allow me to better play Rachel's part when we get to that in a little while. I also think this reverse role play, with me playing you and you playing Rachel, might help you see things from Rachel's perspective. If you develop more empathy for her, it will give you some ideas as to what you might say in your understanding statement to her.

Engage in the reverse role play.

THERAPIST (*as CSO*): Rachel, got a minute?

CSO (*as Rachel*): What do you want?

THERAPIST (*as CSO*): I know you have a lot of fun when your friends come over at night, so this might be hard to do, but I'm wondering if you could ask them to go home earlier during the week? I have to get up pretty early, and if I don't get sleep because of the noise, I can be kind of nasty the next day—and nobody wants to see that.

Note: While playing the role of the CSO, the therapist's *initial* statement did not follow all the communication guidelines, nor did it include each conversation segment that had been prepared. If you do "too good" a job, your performance might overwhelm the CSO. As is commonly done, additional conversation segments that adhere to the seven guidelines are added as the conversation progresses.

CSO (*as Rachel*): You're asking for a lot! I don't want to give up my friends.

THERAPIST (*as CSO*): Oh, I'm not asking you to give them up. I'm just hoping you'll ask them to leave by midnight.

CSO (*as Rachel*): What's in it for me? Sounds boring.

THERAPIST (*as CSO*): I guess *I've* gotten boring, because my new shift makes me get up at an ungodly hour each morning.

CSO (*as Rachel*): I can't really hold your job against you. But I'm not sure I want to kick everyone out at midnight. And I wouldn't be able to promise I'd even remember. It's not like I have my eye on the clock when I'm partying.

THERAPIST (*as CSO*): What if I came out of my room at about 11:30 to give you a heads-up that it was getting near midnight?

CSO (*as Rachel*): That would help remind me, but I'm still not sure I'd want to do it.

THERAPIST (*as CSO*): Fair enough. But would you be willing to try it just once this week?

CSO (*as Rachel*): I guess so. Sure, why not?

Note: The therapist introduced the "sampling" technique (see Box 4.3) by asking the IP to try out the request (i.e., asking the friends to leave by midnight) just *one* night that week, as opposed to asking her to make a permanent commitment to it.

Discuss the CSO's reaction to the reverse role play.

Before focusing on which precise communication guidelines were followed, it is worthwhile to check on the CSO's reaction to being part of the reverse role play. Generally, it is helpful to inquire about (a) the CSO's overall reaction, (b) whether the CSO can picture her- or himself having such a conversation, and (c) what the CSO learned about the other person's perspective and how it might influence the CSO's actions going forward.

THERAPIST: Jackie, let's review what we just practiced here, and talk about your reaction to it. First, what do you make of the conversation?

CSO: It seemed pretty realistic to me. And it made me think that Rachel might agree to this. Of course, I don't know if she'll follow through and do it, but that's another story.

THERAPIST: Good. I'm glad it seemed realistic and that you're feeling optimistic. Did you learn anything about where Rachel is coming from by playing her part? What do you make of what she's probably thinking or feeling in this situation?

CSO: It felt like maybe she's conflicted—like she wants to give me what I want, but doesn't want to give up her fun.

THERAPIST: Interesting. Any idea how you might use that information going forward?

CSO: I could say something about that in my conversation. That might show I understand the tough spot I'm putting her in.

BOX 4.3

Sampling Technique

"Sampling" occurs when reluctant individuals try ("sample") something different, such as a new activity, just *once* on the outside chance that they might like it and thus decide to engage in it more regularly. Sampling is used for various types of CRAFT requests, including when the IP is invited to "try out" one treatment session, and when either the CSO or IP are encouraged to attend a new social activity one time.

THERAPIST: You get an A+ for that. Very good work. Now, can you picture yourself having a similar conversation with her?

CSO: I wouldn't say it exactly the way you did, but yes.

THERAPIST: Excellent. In a few minutes you'll have the chance to put the conversation in your own words when we switch rolls and I play Rachel and you play yourself.

Ask the CSO to specifically identify the communication guidelines followed and assist as needed.

THERAPIST: First we should look at the list of seven communication guidelines and see if you can tell me which ones you think you heard me use when I was playing your part (*points to Form 4.2*). I'll jump in and help if you get stuck.

CSO: You said you might get nasty if you don't get enough sleep, so that's number 4, the one about feelings. And I think you did 5, the understanding statement, because you used the line about knowing it would be hard to give up some of the fun times. You asked Rachel to have people leave by midnight, so that was 3. I'm not sure what else you did. It was a little hard to keep track.

THERAPIST: On the contrary, you did a great job keeping track. Let me help a little here. What about 1 and 2 on the list? Did I do them?

CSO: Oh sure. You were brief and positive, too, so that's 1 and 2. Wow—you did a lot of them! And later you did 7 by offering to come out and give her a heads-up.

THERAPIST: I tried to do 6, too, the partial responsibility statement, but maybe it didn't come through clearly.

CSO: I can't really remember. But that's the one I wasn't so keen on in the first place, so maybe I've conveniently forgotten it!

THERAPIST: I said something about my shift changing and being boring now since I have to get up early each day.

CSO: Smooth. I didn't even know you were accepting partial responsibility. But it sounded good.

THERAPIST: Jackie, although I didn't use them all at once, I did eventually follow all the guidelines. But as I said before, I don't want you to think that *you* have to use them all. Given your high skill level I just wanted to show how you *might* use them.

CSO: It didn't make me worry. We'd planned out everything in advance, and then you made it seem easy. I don't know. Maybe it's because the conversation was broken up into pieces—like I wouldn't have to say it all at once.

Note: This CSO was good at identifying the guidelines followed by the therapist during the reverse role play. You would assist more in pointing them out for those CSOs who have difficulty.

4. Conduct a role play and provide feedback.

Describe the purpose of the role play.

CSOs tend to be even more hesitant to engage in standard role plays (simply called "role plays") in which they play themselves (as opposed to reverse role plays in which they play someone else), because they are concerned about their ability to conduct a conversation that incorporates the communication guidelines. In addition to providing reassurance, it is helpful to offer a solid rationale for using role plays. You would commonly describe two or three of these therapeutic benefits (below) to the CSOs. A role play allows CSOs to do the following:

- Try out the planned conversation in a safe environment to see whether it feels natural, and to then make desired modifications.
- Demonstrate their skill level, allowing you to offer specific feedback for improving the wording and/or delivery style.
- Gauge the IP's reaction to the conversation by watching you play the IP's role, and use that input for modifications or processing.
- Experience some of the natural feelings (anxiety, anger) that will be present in the delivery of the conversation, thereby highlighting areas requiring attention.
- Anticipate potential barriers to delivering the planned communication, and to generate solutions.

THERAPIST: We're all set now. Let's go ahead and practice the conversation again, but this time with you playing yourself and me playing Rachel. Since you'll be acting as if you're really in the situation with Rachel, you'll have a chance to see what the planned conversation feels like and how Rachel might react, *and* whether you want to change it in any places as a result.

CSO: I already have some ideas for how I want to say things, based on playing Rachel just now.

THERAPIST: Good for you! And I should mention that if you find yourself a little nervous during this conversation in here, it will give you an idea of what you'll probably be feeling when you have the conversation at home. I think you'll see that some of this nervousness will go away as we go through the conversation several times. And if it doesn't, we should take a look at what else may be going on, since we wouldn't want it to get in the way of you doing the communication assignment.

CSO: I *do* get nervous before these things, but I know they're important, so I'll go ahead with it anyway.

THERAPIST: That's the spirit! And I can tell already that you're going to do great. OK. So one final reason for doing these practice conversations is that your skill in delivering the message should improve, in part because I'll be providing feedback. Before we jump into it: What kind of questions do you have about this?

CSO: None really. Oh, I guess I'm not sure about starting it off.

THERAPIST: No worries. I'll start it. And since I have a good idea of what this whole conversation is about, I think I can just go ahead with it. Oh—remember to pretend this situation is happening *right now*.

Note: If more details were needed about the situation being played so that the therapist could fully understand it or the CSO could more clearly picture it, this would have been the time to ask for them. In line with the Role-Play ("Practicing") Guidelines (Box 4.4), the therapist reminds the CSO to imagine that the situation is actually happening right then (i.e., as opposed to merely talking about it) and then starts the brief role play (below).

Engage in the role play.
Refer to the Role-Play ("Practicing") Guidelines in Box 4.4.

THERAPIST (*as Rachel*): What's up, Jackie?

CSO (*in role play*): Nothing much. Hey—got a minute? I wanted to ask you something.

THERAPIST (*as Rachel*): Uh-oh. What makes me think this isn't going to be good?

CSO (*in role play*): I *hope* it isn't bad. I wanted to see if you could ask your friends not to stay so late every night. My new shift is a pain, because I have to go to bed quite a bit before you do and get up early, and it's hard to sleep if there's a lot of loud noise.

THERAPIST (*as Rachel*): Wow. That's a lot to ask.

CSO (*in role play*): I know. And I feel bad asking. But you know how nasty I get if I'm tired.

THERAPIST (*as Rachel*): Right. And I know how nasty *I* get if *I'm* tired, so hmm. I don't know. Maybe we could try it for a night and see how it goes. No promises though.

CSO (*in role play*): Great! Thanks.

Note: The therapist shows minimal resistance to the CSO's request while playing the IP for the first time (see Box 4.4).

BOX 4.4

Role-Play ("Practicing") Guidelines

- Get a basic understanding of the situation being portrayed.
- Encourage the CSO to imagine the situation is actually happening.
- Start the role play yourself.
- Play your role with minimal resistance at first, but offer more resistance with repetitions of the scene.
- Keep it brief (under 2 minutes).
- Ask what the CSO liked about her or his own performance and what would be important to address yet.
- Compliment the CSO for some aspect of good communication demonstrated.
- Ask the CSO to specifically identify the communication guidelines followed and assist as needed.
- Help the CSO build in additional communication guideline components.
- Repeat the role play.
- Repeat the feedback cycle.
- Repeat again?
- Assign the conversation for homework.

Ask what the CSO liked about her or his own role-play performance and what would be important to address yet.

You will notice in the Role-Play ("Practicing") Guidelines (Box 4.4) and in the dialogue below that the feedback process for a standard role play is more comprehensive than that for a reverse role play. In part, this is because the former is a more effortful process that explicitly revolves around enhancing the CSO's performance. With that said, it is important to start on a positive note when beginning a review of a role play by asking CSOs what they *liked* about their performance. Many CSOs are critical of themselves and their skills, and so this sends the confidence-building message that there certainly were aspects of their performance that were commendable. Next, ask CSOs what they would like to change in their conversation. This gives you an idea as to how skilled the CSOs are at evaluating their own performance, including noticing the shortcomings requiring attention.

THERAPIST: Good for you, Jackie. Can you tell me what you liked about your practice conversation just now? And then maybe you can tell me what you'd like to work on yet to improve it.

CSO: I know what I *didn't* do; I forgot to see if they could leave by midnight.

THERAPIST: Good for you to notice that. But no problem. You'll have another shot at it in a minute. And what about the things you did well?

CSO: I think I asked in a nice way. I really don't want her to walk away.

THERAPIST: Yes, you were definitely nice. Can you think of anything specific you did that showed how nice you were?

CSO: I don't know. Well, I said I felt bad for asking her to get her friends to leave early. I don't think that fits in with anything we practiced, but I'm pretty sure I used some of the guidelines.

Note: As often happens, the CSO was quite vague when first asked to comment on her performance. As part of this, she did not mention that she had adhered to at least one of the seven communication guidelines: she had used an understanding statement (Guideline 5). The therapist will make a point of helping the CSO identify the communication guidelines she uses in these role plays, since this should increase the likelihood of them being incorporated into her real-life situations.

Compliment the CSO for some aspect of good communication demonstrated.

Although most CSOs are interested in receiving feedback about their communication style, nonetheless it is sometimes difficult for them to hear multiple suggestions regarding what they should consider changing. The message is easier to hear if the feedback segment begins with you offering a positive remark about their communication style that was shown in the role play. In the event that at least one of the seven communication guideline components was used by the CSO, it is appropriate to mention it (leaving the remaining ones for the *CSO* to identify). Instead (or in addition) you might opt to mention a basic aspect of positive communication skills, such as good eye contact, a friendly tone of voice, or appropriate speech volume.

THERAPIST: Jackie, I think you did better than you realize. When you agreed with me that you *were* asking for a lot, and you said you felt bad for asking, you were saying that you *understood* where I was coming from. It wasn't the line we'd practiced for our understanding statement, but it felt natural and sincere. So you're right, it *did* make the conversation sound nice, but I'm guessing it's because it was an understanding statement.

CSO: I'll take credit for it then!

THERAPIST: I also liked how you used a good tone of voice. You sounded assertive—not too soft-spoken and not too aggressive.

CSO: And I didn't even have to think about doing that one—good!

Ask the CSO to specifically identify the communication guidelines followed and assist as needed.

As noted, it is preferable to try to get the *CSOs* to identify the communication guidelines they followed rather than simply telling them. But you should supplement the CSO's reports with your own observations.

THERAPIST: You *did* follow several other of the communication guidelines we'd practiced. Which ones do you remember using?

CSO: I used the one about feelings when I said I'd be nasty if I didn't sleep. I tried to use the partial responsibility one when I said my new shift was a pain. Was that one right?

THERAPIST: Yes, that sounded like number 6, a partial responsibility statement. Good job! I think you used at least one more. Any ideas?

CSO: I guess I was brief enough, so 1, too.

Help the CSO build in additional communication guideline components.

Shaping the CSO's planned conversation typically entails building in some of the seven communication guideline components that were not used in the first role play. However, you should not feel obligated to point out every guideline that was omitted, as it may be experienced as overwhelming by the CSO. Additionally, some CSOs will benefit from practicing particular communication segments (e.g., their understanding statement) before the full role play is repeated, but others will not need to do so. You should strike a balance between making sure the communication components are overlearned and wearing out the CSO in the process.

THERAPIST: You mentioned that you forgot to be specific in terms of having the friends leave by midnight. We can add that in. Is it OK if we talk about a few other ways in which you might make this good conversation even better?

CSO: Sure. I bet you've got some ideas (*smiles*).

THERAPIST: You know me all too well! Let's start by looking at the guidelines that you didn't end up using. Maybe they're good candidates for adding. For example, how would you feel about adding in the offer to help, too?

CSO: I forgot that one too? Right. I guess I did.

THERAPIST: Jackie, keep in mind that your conversation was very good. We're just fine-tuning it now. And as I've said before, you don't have to use all seven pieces anyway. I'm only bringing them up because you're so good at this and I know you're capable of adding them if you want to. So should we go over the offer to help before we do the practice conversation again?

CSO: No, I don't think we need to. I remember what it *is*, I just didn't remember to include it.

Note: The CSO had not followed Guideline 2, as she did not state her request in positive/action-oriented words (i.e., what she wanted to see happen as opposed to what she did not want to see any longer). In other words, ideally the CSO would have requested that the IP ask her friends to leave earlier each night (by midnight) instead of asking that they not be allowed to stay so late. Given that this particular infraction of the second guideline was minor in this context, and the CSO had several other guidelines she was already using (or planned to add), the therapist decided to let it go. Furthermore, these minor infractions tend to self-correct in the course of the role-play repetitions.

5. Repeat the role play and provide feedback.

Engage in the role play.

CSOs should be encouraged to incorporate as many of the seven communication guideline components with which they feel comfortable, while also making it clear that they are not expected to use them all. Also, some therapists let CSOs know in advance that the IP will be portrayed as a bit more resistant the second time.

THERAPIST: Let's do round two for our practice conversation. Try to use as many of the positive communication components as you comfortably can, including the ones we just reviewed, but don't worry about using them all! And in my role as Rachel, I'll give you a little bit of a harder time this round, just in case Rachel does when you talk to her.

CSO: OK. I'll do my best.

THERAPIST (*as Rachel*): What's up Jackie?

CSO (*in role play*): Not much. Actually, I wanted to ask you something.

THERAPIST (*as Rachel*): Uh-oh. What's the matter?

CSO (*in role play*): I'm wondering if there's any way you could ask your friends to leave a little earlier at night, like around midnight? I know how much fun you have when your friends come over, so I'm putting you in a tough spot. Ever since my shift changed at work I've had to get to bed earlier, and sometimes the noise from the partying makes it hard to sleep. And you've seen me all nasty when I haven't gotten much sleep; it ain't pretty. I know it's a pain, and it *is* your house, but I really like living here with you.

THERAPIST (*as Rachel*): I like you living here, too. And I don't like you losing sleep. But I *really* like having people over. It's an awful lot to ask.

CSO (*in role play*): I know. And I've had a lot of fun partying with you, too. Is there anything I can do to help out though? I don't know if it will work, but maybe I can ask my boss to switch me back to the later shift.

Note: This is another example of the CSO offering to help in a way that definitely is *not* in line with the CRAFT objectives, as it could inadvertently support the IP's substance use. Since the CSO has done this twice during the session, the chances are high that she would do it in the real situation as well. Thus, it might be best for the therapist to steer the CSO away from using Guideline 7, an offer to help, for now.

THERAPIST (*as Rachel*): No, I wouldn't want you to have to do that. I know you like getting home earlier in the day. It probably wouldn't hurt for me to get to bed earlier, too. I've had some trouble getting up and into work on time the next day lately.

CSO (*in role play*): Great! Thanks for being open to the idea. If you want, I could come out and give you a heads-up at around 11:30 so that you know it's almost time to shut down the partying. What do you think?

Ask what the CSO liked about her or his own role-play performance and what would be important to address yet.

THERAPIST: Let's stop right here, Jackie. Again, let's start this review by you telling me what you liked about your conversation here, and then what you want to work on yet.

CSO: I felt more comfortable this time. I added the part about liking to live with Rachel—that just kind of came to me. And I think I used most of the pieces we practiced. I'm not sure what I need to work on yet.

Compliment the CSO for some aspect of good communication demonstrated.

THERAPIST: It *was* a really good conversation, so don't feel badly about not knowing what needs work yet. Yes, I really liked how you added that personal part about wanting to stay living with Rachel despite the problem. It was sort of a feelings statement.

Ask the CSO to specifically identify the communication guidelines followed and assist as needed.

THERAPIST: Can you tell me which of the communication guidelines you followed this time? You *did* use a lot of them again.

CSO: Didn't I use the first three: brief, positive, and specific? I remembered to ask Rachel to have them leave by midnight this time.

THERAPIST: You sure did. You did many things extremely well. What else?

CSO: I talked about feeling nasty, so that's number 4, and I offered to help when I said I could give her an 11:30 heads-up.

THERAPIST: Yes, those were very good. Do you remember offering to help in another way, too? It was earlier in the conversation. It was about getting your shift changed.

CSO: Right, but I was really hoping she wouldn't agree to that. I like getting home from work earlier in the day.

THERAPIST: Can you think of any other reason why it might not be a good idea to offer to get your shift changed as a way to solve the problem of the late-night partying? How might that not actually be helpful?

CSO: If I ended up working a later shift, I guess Rachel wouldn't have to get people to leave by midnight because I wouldn't have to get up early for work. Oh. That's not good. I did it again! What's wrong with me?

THERAPIST: There's nothing wrong with you—you just like to help, and you got caught up in the moment. We have to be careful in this type of situation though, because what if Rachel actually agreed to something like this? I wonder if it would be safer to stay away from 7, the offer to help, for now?

CSO: Good idea. I don't want to blow it.

THERAPIST: There's nothing you could say that would blow it. But it would be easier to get what you want—namely, to have everyone leave by midnight—if you don't make Rachel any tempting offers that result in her *not* having to change her own behavior. OK, so I definitely heard at least one other guideline being followed.

CSO: Didn't I use an understanding statement? I remembered to use the line I'd come up with earlier about putting her in a tough spot.

THERAPIST: I noticed! That was the one you came up with after you played Rachel's part during our reverse role play. Nice. You actually used two other understanding statements.

CSO: Really? I can't remember them.

THERAPIST: You acknowledged that it was a pain to ask her to change *and* you understood it was her house. Can you see why these would be considered understanding statements?

CSO: Yes, because I'm trying to see things from her point of view.

Note: Although the therapist might have felt awkward pointing out for a second time that the CSO had improperly used Guideline 7, offer to help, it was important to do so. The therapist did not dwell on the issue, but quickly resolved it and made a point of highlighting the excellent job the CSO had done in using Guideline 5, offer an understanding statement. Guideline 7 would be revisited in a later session.

Help the CSO build in additional communication guideline components and/or repeat the role play once more.

Normally you would have CSOs prepare for and then do at least one more repetition of the role play. Even if their conversation was very good in terms of their use of the communication guidelines, additional practice allows the conversation to flow more automatically, which is helpful when CSOs are anxious in real-life situations.

6. Decide on the day and time for the assigned conversation.

It is imperative that session time be devoted to deciding when the planned conversation will occur. This is done because the CSO (a) can be coached to avoid times when the other person (e.g., the IP) is likely to be less receptive due to mood or substance use; (b) can more clearly visualize the conversation taking place, and thus can anticipate potential problems worth addressing; and (c) hears the explicit expectation that the conversation *should occur* in the upcoming week (i.e., that it *is* an assignment).

Select a time when the other person is likely to be receptive.

THERAPIST: Let's figure out a good time for you to have this conversation this week. When do you think Rachel will be in a mood where she's likely to listen? As you might imagine, it's best to avoid times when people are already drinking or high, or when they are coming down off the high.

Make the assignment explicit.

Be sure to make the assignment explicit. The CSO may not make the connection between the practiced conversation in the session and the fact that the homework assignment for the week is to have that conversation in the real world. Leave nothing to chance! And as with all assignments, inquire about and resolve potential barriers to completing the assignment. See Homework Assignment Guidelines (Chapter 3, Box 3.1).

THERAPIST: You seem ready to take this on! As we always do with assignments before you head out the door here, can you tell me exactly what you're going to do? Now you can include when it will take place, too. Oh, and of course we'll need to talk about barriers that might get in the way of you having the conversation this week.

7. Consider the consequences of the conversation.

In all probability, the most worrisome potential negative repercussion for a CSO engaging in newly learned positive communication that week is domestic violence. Therefore, the final step in communication skills training involves the same type of safety questioning of any homework assignment. Essentially you need to be sure that CSOs are not putting themselves in harm's way by carrying out the assignment. This point is emphasized in the CRAFT introductory session (Chapter 2) when domestic violence precautions are discussed, when CSOs are taught how to withdraw rewards/reinforcers during IP substance use (Chapter 7), and when CSOs are taught to allow for the natural negative consequences of their IP's use (Chapter 8).

Explore potential problems that might occur upon having the planned conversation.

In addition to addressing issues of violence, other potential negative consequences of the homework assignment should be explored as well.

THERAPIST: Jackie, I know you've said that Rachel never gets violent, but is there a chance that she might when you have this conversation with her? As we've discussed before, this treatment sometimes asks you to do things that Rachel doesn't like, and this conversation may represent one of those things.

CSO: No, I'm 100% sure that Rachel won't get violent.

THERAPIST: That's good to hear. But we still need to talk about other possible negative consequences that might result from this conversation. I know you've already considered that she might ask you to move out, and you have a plan in place in case she does. But are there other problems to sort through?

CSO: If Rachel starts telling her friends that they need to leave earlier than usual so that I can sleep, these friends might be upset with me.

Develop a plan to address the concerns.

THERAPIST: How *would* you handle it if Rachel's friends got upset with you?

CSO: I'm not worried. They're pretty tame people. If they're really upset with me they'll just ignore me, and I'm OK with that.

COMMON PROBLEMS TO AVOID

Although communication skills training is a structured procedure, it requires considerable clinical skill for its proper implementation. You need to know when to introduce it, how much to expect of the various CSOs as they learn the skill, how to give worthwhile feedback, and how to both motivate and support the CSOs throughout the entire process. Similar to CSOs learning communication skills, you will improve your own communication *training* skills with practice. Tips for avoiding several common difficulties are outlined below.

Problem: The most salient problem exhibited by CRAFT therapists when doing communication skills training is offering vague feedback after a role play. While it is important for you to be friendly and supportive, CSOs need to hear the specifics in terms of what they should retain and change in their conversations. Giving feedback such as "That was really good," and "Great job," is not helpful if it is not followed up with specifics regarding *what* was done well and what needs work.

Safeguards:

- When offering feedback to the CSO, ask yourself, "Can I be more specific?"
- Also ask yourself, "Is the CSO going to know what I mean in terms of what was done well *and* what should be changed in the conversation?"

Problem: Another common feedback-related problem entails the therapist jumping in and telling the CSOs what they did well (and less well) in the role play instead of asking *them* first. By first asking *CSOs* it allows you to see whether they truly understand what they are attempting to accomplish. It is not that unusual for CSOs to respond with "I was just trying to sound positive," which then raises questions as to whether they actually learned the communication skills. If not, it is unlikely that they will be able to replicate the positive conversation in the real world, and eventually generalize it to other (unpracticed) conversations.

Safeguards:

- Keep the Role-Play ("Practicing") Guidelines (Box 4.4) close at hand during a role play and go down the bulleted list point by point. Note that at the end of a role play, the instructions say to start the feedback phase by asking CSOs what *they* liked about their conversation and how *they* would like to improve. The guidelines also state that you should *assist* CSOs in identifying the specific positive communication components they used. In other words, you should not automatically spell them out without allowing CSOs the opportunity to speak first.

Problem: Therapists who are unaccustomed to doing role plays often allow CSOs to *talk about* what they would say to the other person (e.g., the IP) as opposed to pretending they are *in* the situation with that person—that the situation is really happening at that moment. As noted, these so-called one-sided role plays are not technically role plays at all, as they lack any interaction with the therapist playing a role. As a result, these CSOs do not experience a conversation that feels similar to what their real-world conversation will present.

Safeguards:

- Assume that if the procedure calls for a role play, both you and the CSO will be playing roles.
- Before starting a role play, remind the CSO (and yourself!) that it should feel as if the conversation is actually happening out in the real world.

Problem: Another problem therapists have when doing role plays is letting them run too long. Role plays typically should last less than 2 minutes. It is difficult to provide specific feedback on longer role plays, in part because it is hard to remember exactly what was said. Longer role plays also tend to deviate from the main task at hand, such as the CSO making a specific request of the IP. Finally, long role plays do not allow time for repetition of them, which is an important part of learning the communication skill.

Safeguards:

- You should head into role plays with the idea that there only need to be a few conversational "volleys" between you and the CSO.
- If it starts to feel like it will be hard to provide specific feedback on the role play, it is time to stop the role play.

Problem: Therapists sometimes opt to practice a role play only once, primarily due to time constraints or the belief that the CSO has mastered the skill. This is problematic, as role-play repetitions allow you to provide feedback multiple times, which in turn affords opportunities for CSOs to watch their skills improve and to feel their anxiety decrease. Repetitions also help make the CSOs' responses more automatic, which is useful when they are in the real-world situations.

Safeguards:

- Always assume that a role play will need to be repeated at least once, and so keep an eye on the session time when starting the exercise.
- If time constraints prohibit the repetition of a role play during the session, part of the homework assignment can be for the CSO to do several repetitions of it at home with someone other than the target of the conversation (typically this would mean with someone other than the IP). You might consider asking the CSO to record the practice role play and to bring it to the next session so that feedback can be provided.

Problem: Therapists frequently assume CSOs will realize that the well-rehearsed conversation that was the focus of the communication skills training is, in fact, the homework assignment for the upcoming week. CSOs certainly know that eventually they are expected to engage in that conversation out in the world, but for various reasons, such as avoidance, they do not always treat it as their immediate assignment for that week.

Safeguards:

- This problem can be prevented by taking care to check off both items under Step 6 on the Improving CSOs' Communication Skills: Checklist (Form 4.1)—"Decide on the day and time for the assigned conversation." Specifically note that the second item clearly says, "Make the assignment explicit."
- All CRAFT sessions should have a homework assignment. Consequently, it would be good to get in the habit of always asking yourself, "Was homework assigned?" and to ask the CSO to repeat back the assignment at the end of the session.

Problem: Therapists may find themselves automatically using therapy terms that elicit reactions of apprehension or annoyance in some CSOs. Likely candidates for such words are "role play" and "homework." For some CSOs, a "role play" suggests that one needs to be an actor, and being an actor involves performing. Self-conscious, anxious CSOs will react strongly to the term, and as a result they may have great difficulty focusing on the spirit of the exercise. The term "homework" conjures up unpleasant memories for certain CSOs, and thus might make them more inclined to avoid it altogether.

Safeguards:

- Feel free to steer clear of these potentially problematic words by substituting words like "practice" or "exercise" for role play, and "assignment," "weekly task," or "experiment" for homework.
- Ask CSOs which words they would like to adopt for the tasks of "role plays" and "homework."
- Start out using the words "role play" and "homework" if you prefer them, but ask the CSOs whether they are comfortable with them and note both their verbal and nonverbal reactions.

SUMMARY

This chapter provides the rationale for teaching communication skills to CSOs and offers a detailed structure for doing so. Explicit guidelines for conducting those all-important role plays are included. Given that many of CRAFT's procedures rely on positive communication skills, including the procedure in the next chapter (Rewarding Non-Using Behavior), the need to devote sufficient attention to practicing these skills with CSOs cannot be stressed enough.

FORM 4.1

Improving CSOs' Communication Skills: Checklist

1. Discuss why positive communication is addressed.

- ☐ a. Explain that positive communication is contagious.
- ☐ b. State that individuals tend to be more successful in getting what they want from another person if they communicate in a positive way.
- ☐ c. Discuss how good communication is the foundation for other CRAFT procedures.
- ☐ d. Select a specific situation in which to practice the communication skills.

2. Describe the positive communication guidelines and develop examples of each.

- ☐ a. Present and develop an example of Guideline 1: Be brief (uncomplicated).
- ☐ b. Present and develop an example of Guideline 2: Use positive/action-oriented wording (indicating what you would like to see happen).
- ☐ c. Present and develop an example of Guideline 3: Mention specific behaviors.
- ☐ d. Present and develop an example of Guideline 4: Label your feelings.
- ☐ e. Present and develop an example of Guideline 5: Offer an understanding statement.
- ☐ f. Present and develop an example of Guideline 6: Accept partial responsibility (for something related to the problem situation under discussion, *not* for the substance use).
- ☐ g. Present and develop an example of Guideline 7: Offer to help.

3. Conduct a reverse role play and provide feedback.

- ☐ a. Describe the purpose and format of the reverse role play.
- ☐ b. Engage in the reverse role play.
- ☐ c. Discuss the CSO's reaction to the reverse role play.
- ☐ d. Ask the CSO to specifically identify the communication guidelines followed and assist as needed.

4. Conduct a role play and provide feedback.

- ☐ a. Describe the purpose of the role play.
- ☐ b. Engage in the role play.
- ☐ c. Ask what the CSO liked about her or his own role-play performance and what would be important to address yet.

(continued)

- ☐ d. Compliment the CSO for some aspect of good communication demonstrated.
- ☐ e. Ask the CSO to specifically identify the communication guidelines followed and assist as needed.
- ☐ f. Help the CSO build in additional communication guideline components.

5. Repeat the role play and provide feedback.

- ☐ a. Engage in the role play.
- ☐ b. Ask what the CSO liked about her or his own role-play performance and what would be important to address yet.
- ☐ c. Compliment the CSO for some aspect of good communication demonstrated.
- ☐ d. Ask the CSO to specifically identify the communication guidelines followed and assist as needed.
- ☐ e. Help the CSO build in additional communication guideline components and/or repeat the role play once more.

6. Decide on the day and time for the assigned conversation.

- ☐ a. Select a time when the other person is likely to be receptive.
- ☐ b. Make the assignment explicit.

7. Consider the consequences of the conversation.

- ☐ a. Explore potential problems that might occur upon having the planned conversation.
- ☐ b. Develop a plan to address the concerns.

FORM 4.2

Planning Positive Communication

Describe a specific situation that requires positive communication planning:

For each of the positive communication guidelines (below), keep in mind the situation you just described and write a conversation segment (usually a sentence) that satisfies the guideline. Be sure to use wording that you can picture yourself saying.

1. Be brief (uncomplicated).

2. Use positive/action-oriented wording (indicating what you would like to see happen).

3. Mention specific behaviors.

4. Label your feelings.

5. Offer an understanding statement.

6. Accept partial responsibility (for something related to the problem situation, *not* for the substance use).

7. Offer to help.

Drawing from the conversation segments you listed above, now write your planned conversation in the lines below (*put the number of the guideline used in parentheses next to it*). Sample: "*I know you need to unwind after a stressful day at work (5), but would you be willing to come right home tomorrow and take a half hour walk with me and Otter (1, 2, 3) instead of stopping at the pub first? I'll have an icy glass of lemonade waiting for you (7).*"

HANDOUT 4.1

Making Communication Positive

For each of the seven guidelines for positive communication listed below, there is first an example of a conversation that does *not* follow the guideline, and then one in which the conversation has been improved by following the guideline. Feel free to refer to these examples for ideas when developing your own positive communication.

1. **Be brief (uncomplicated).**

   Problematic wording: "It seems like I'm always having to remind you to help your mom with simple things around the house and with the grocery shopping. Let's see, yesterday it was to take the garbage out. And the day before it was to clean out the shed. You're 17 years old—can't you do these things without being asked?"

   Improved wording: "I'd really appreciate it if you'd pick up the few items on your mom's grocery list today."

2. **Use positive/action-oriented wording (indicating what you would like to see happen).**

   Problematic wording: "If you're planning to show up high to dinner at your friend's tonight, I'm just going to stay home. It's too embarrassing."

   Improved wording: "You're so much fun to be with when you're not high. I'd really appreciate it if you'd come to the dinner tonight without smoking first."

3. **Mention specific behaviors.**

   Problematic wording: "You never help out with the kids. I feel like I'm a single mom most of the time."

   Improved wording: "It would really help me out if you'd get the kids a snack and read to them for a half hour tonight."

4. **Label your feelings.**

   Problematic wording: "Why would you talk to me that way? Can't you see what it does to me?"

   Improved wording: "I feel put down and hurt when you're short with me."

(continued)

5. Offer an understanding statement.

Problematic wording: "It seems like you never get out of that chair to do anything with me on the weekends. I'm surprised the TV hasn't worn out."

Improved wording: "I can tell you really need your 'downtime' on the weekends. Maybe we can do something relaxing together?"

6. Accept partial responsibility (for something related to the problem situation, *not* for the substance use).

Problematic wording: "You missed your therapy appointment again? What's wrong with you?"

Improved wording: "Ya know, I could easily have texted you to remind you about your appointment today. I don't know why I didn't."

7. Offer to help.

Problematic wording: "Wait, didn't you just see your mom? Remember how much we ended up having to pay the babysitter because you stayed so late last time?"

Improved wording: "Can you wait until Thursday night to go to your mom's? I can get home from work a little early that night so we wouldn't need to hire a sitter."

Chapter 5

Rewarding Non-Using Behavior

One primary behavioral principle upon which CRAFT is built is that a behavior that is positively reinforced (rewarded) will be repeated. A salient example of this learned behavior is substance use. As outlined already in Chapter 3, Functional Analysis of a Loved One's Drinking or Using Behavior, individuals repeatedly engage in excessive drinking and/or illicit drug use *despite* experiencing problems, largely because of the short-term positive consequences (rewards) they receive for the substance use. CRAFT relies on the application of these same principles to non-using behavior or activities. This chapter focuses on teaching CSOs how to reward their IP's *non-substance-using* behavior. The objective is to increase these healthy behaviors such that they eventually can compete with the drinking or drug use.

THE BASICS

General Description

CRAFT's procedure for Rewarding Non-Using Behavior begins with an explanation of positive reinforcement, which includes a clarification of the distinction between "enabling" and the rewarding of non-using behavior. Guidelines for generating a list of suitable rewards for the IP's non-using behavior are introduced, an explicit plan for delivering a reward is developed, and potential complications are addressed. Positive communication skills are reviewed and practiced so that CSOs will be prepared to explain to the IP, if the need arises, the new practice of rewarding certain behaviors.

Procedure Timing

Clinicians commonly introduce the procedure for Rewarding Non-Using Behavior in about the third CRAFT session. One reason for this early introduction is that CSOs initially are more amenable to doing something pleasant for their IPs, as opposed to doing something that withdraws rewards and risks elevated turmoil at home. It is also important to introduce this positive reinforcement procedure because this basic principle is the foundation for other CRAFT procedures, such as when CSOs are taught to allow for natural, negative consequences (Chapter 8), and to reward themselves (Chapter 10).

Forms

- Rewarding Non-Using Behavior: Checklist (Form 5.1)
- Common Free Rewards for a Loved One (Form 5.2)
- Common Signs of Alcohol and Illicit Drug Use (Handout 5.1)

CLINICIAN GUIDANCE AND SAMPLE DIALOGUE

The components for the CRAFT procedure for Rewarding Non-Using Behavior are presented below. A sample case complete with clinician–CSO dialogue is used throughout the chapter to demonstrate the clinician's role and typical CSO responses. The components for conducting this exercise are outlined in Form 5.1, Rewarding Non-Using Behavior: Checklist, found at the end of this chapter.

Case Description

The CSO (Jasmin) is a 28-year-old woman who is the partner of the 34-year-old IP (Darnell). The couple, who identify as Black, has been cohabitating for 3 years, but they have been dating for almost 6 years. In the early stages of their relationship, both Jasmin and Darnell routinely enjoyed getting high on the weekends. Jasmin gave up marijuana use when she started a professional job, but Darnell's marijuana use continued to increase over the years. At the time of the CSO's assessment, the IP was smoking marijuana at least three times a day, and it appeared to be interfering with both his professional advancement and his relationship with Jasmin.

1. Define a positive reinforcer/reward and when to use it.

Describe a positive reinforcer as a reward or as something that is experienced as pleasurable by a person.

THERAPIST: I'd like to start off today by explaining what the term "positive reinforcer" means. It's sort of an odd-sounding term, but it really just stands for something that an individual finds enjoyable or rewarding.

Explain that a positive reinforcer makes the person want to repeat the behavior that got the person the reward in the first place.

THERAPIST: Probably the best way to decide whether something is a reward is to see if the person willingly repeats the behavior that got her or him the so-called reward in the first place. For example, you mentioned that you pay the teenage neighbor to do yard work on the weekends. One way to tell whether the money you give the neighbor is a good reward is whether he routinely shows up looking for work each weekend.

Explain that the CSO will be asked to reward the IP at times when the IP is not using substances.

THERAPIST: The reason we're spending time talking about positive reinforcers and rewards is that one of the basic CRAFT procedures involves finding ways to reward Darnell *when he is not smoking or high*. And in order to do this, we need to have a good understanding of what constitutes a reward.

Ask the CSO about any questions or concerns she or he has about using positive reinforcers, and address them.

CSOs sometimes state that they are opposed in principle to rewarding someone for doing the "right thing," or they believe they have already given their IP many rewards, but these rewards have not helped decrease the substance use. You should remind these CSOs that in the CRAFT program CSOs are taught the following:

- To deliver rewards *consistently* and *only* when the IP is substance-free.
- How to enhance the association between the rewards and the substance-free behavior by using positive communication skills to explain the behavior (if desired).
- To work toward the goal of getting the IP ultimately to value the *natural* rewards that go along with decreased substance use.
- To keep their "eye on the prize"—getting the IP to enter treatment—while they learn new skills and introduce and refine behavior changes at home.

THERAPIST: What kinds of questions or concerns do you have as you hear me talking about finding ways for you to reward Darnell for *not* getting high?

CSO: I just don't like the idea of giving him a reward for not smoking. It sounds like bribing a little kid for being good; Darnell is a grown man!

THERAPIST: I agree that it might seem odd to reward Darnell for doing something he should be doing anyway. But Darnell is stuck right now, which is why you're here. We're assuming that down the road Darnell will experience some of the natural rewards for avoiding marijuana, such as having a better relationship with you. In the meantime, I'm hoping you'll be willing to hang in there a bit longer and work with me so that we can achieve the ultimate prize: Darnell getting the help he needs.

2. Make the distinction between enabling and positive reinforcement.

CRAFT avoids the term "enabling" because of the pejorative, judgmental way it is often used. In the addiction field more generally, "enabling" is used to characterize CSO behavior that results in supporting drinking/drug use (albeit, often unintentionally), primarily by giving the IP money for alcohol/drugs or shielding the IP from the negative consequences of the substance-using behavior. In contrast, CRAFT's "positive reinforcement" represents CSO behavior that increases the IP's *non-drinking-* or *non-drug-using* (prosocial) behavior.

Appropriately distinguish between enabling and CRAFT's positive reinforcement.

THERAPIST: Occasionally people get upset when they hear me talking about rewarding their loved one, because the word "enabling" comes to mind. I think it's important to make the distinction between enabling and the type of rewards I'm talking about. Enabling means doing things that would make it easier for Darnell to smoke, whereas *we'd* be using positive reinforcement to support his *nonsmoking* behavior. Rewarding Darnell's nonsmoking behaviors should increase those healthy behaviors.

CSO: I'm not really sure *what* I've been doing, but it hasn't been working so I guess I've been enabling.

Stress that enabling is typically accidental—that it is <u>not</u> done with the intention of increasing the IP's substance use.

THERAPIST: Jasmin, even if you *have* engaged in some behaviors that periodically have made it a little easier for Darnell to keep smoking, it's certainly been accidental. You weren't *intentionally* trying to support his marijuana habit. In fact, from what you've told me, you've been doing everything you possibly could to get Darnell to cut back on his smoking. And now you're here—so that's another huge, positive step.

Explain that CRAFT's positive reinforcement will be planned out carefully in terms of when it will be used.

THERAPIST: Going forward now, we'll carefully plan out both the rewards you give Darnell and *when* you deliver them. In this way, there will be no question about whether they are serving the right purpose—namely, to reward his nonsmoking behavior.

3. Discuss whether the CSO would recognize signs of substance use and why it is important.

Explain why it is important to be able to recognize signs of the IP's use.

THERAPIST: We should spend a little time now talking about how confident you are in knowing when Darnell is using or high. Because as we've been discussing, it will be important for you to only give him the rewards we come up with when he's not using. We want to be sure you're supporting his *nonsmoking* behaviors and activities.

Ask the CSO to identify the signs that her or his IP is using or high, and provide examples, if necessary, for each of the <u>four main areas</u>: speech, mood, behavior, and appearance.

There are several options for assisting CSOs to become more aware of when their IP is under the influence. The main ones include (a) giving CSOs a copy of Common Signs of Alcohol and Illicit Drug Use (Handout 5.1, found at the end of this chapter); (b) having CSOs carefully observe the IP's speech, mood, behavior, and appearance the next time the CSO is certain the IP has used; and (c) having CSOs review their IP's triggers for substance use on the CRAFT Functional Analysis of a Loved One's Drinking or Using

Behavior (Chapter 3, Form 3.2) so that the IP's behavior can be monitored the next time the triggers are present (a high-risk time).

THERAPIST: Can you tell me how you know that Darnell has been using? What stands out? For example, what's different about how he looks and acts?

CSO: His eyes look bloodshot for sure. Sometimes I notice that his pupils look huge. And I can really smell the smoke on his clothes.

THERAPIST: Very good. You're aware of many of the things we often notice about people who've been smoking marijuana. What about the way he acts?

CSO: That's hard to say, because sometimes he gets real talkative when he's high, and other times he sort of withdraws and doesn't seem to have the energy, or motivation, to do much of anything. Does that make sense?

THERAPIST: Absolutely. All of the things you mentioned are common signs of someone being high on marijuana. You've actually covered all four of the main categories: his appearance, his speech, his behavior, and his mood. As far as this last one, his mood, does he ever get giddy or silly when he smokes? Laughing at the slightest thing might be the behavior you'd see if he's in a silly mood.

CSO: Yes! I find it so annoying. But then I feel bad because he seems so happy.

THERAPIST: You certainly have the right to feel annoyed, considering how much anguish his smoking has caused you. OK. Even though you seem to have a very good understanding of the ways in which Darnell looks and acts differently when he's high, I'm going to give you a comprehensive list of the common signs of marijuana and other drug use, including alcohol (*hands the CSO Handout 5.1*). You'll have this handy then in case you need a reminder.

4. Generate a list of potential rewards and plan the delivery of one.

Help the CSO generate a list of potential rewards for the IP.

In the process of helping CSOs think about potential rewards, it is useful to provide them with examples of some common *free* IP rewards in three general categories: verbal (e.g., complimenting the IP), physical (e.g., squeezing the IP's hand), and behavioral (e.g., joining the IP to watch one of the IP's favorite TV shows). You should offer CSOs a form that lists examples of free rewards, and the space to write in additional rewards that are specific to the particular case (see Form 5.2, found at the end of this chapter).

THERAPIST: Before I ask you to start developing a list of possible rewards for Darnell, I want to mention that these rewards don't have to cost a lot of money. Some of them won't cost anything at all. Is it OK if I show you a list of commonly used free rewards? It could give you some ideas for things that might work with Darnell.

CSO: Sure. I'd love to see what other people have come up with (*looks at Form 5.2*). I think I understand. But how will Darnell know *why* I'm doing these nice things for him?

THERAPIST: Excellent question. Once we settle on which reward you'd like to use, we can discuss whether you want to come right out and tell him why he's getting the reward. And we'll practice the conversation using your positive communication skills. So, shall we work on that list? Let's just generate a bunch of ideas before narrowing it down and selecting one. We can add them to the form [Form 5.2] if you'd like.

Note: The therapist remains focused on the task at hand while reassuring the CSO that the issue of whether she will explain to the IP *why* the reward is being given will soon be addressed (see the section "5. Discuss how to explain to the IP . . . ," later in this chapter).

CSO: I could picture using just about every item on that list of common rewards. I'd probably just leave off the last one—we're not into walking unless there's a specific purpose.

THERAPIST: Great! And how about adding a few rewards that might be specific to Darnell? Let's stick with the free ones for now.

CSO: Oh, OK. I was going to say that he always wants me to go out on the weekends—to dinner or a movie. Or to listen to music. But I'm usually too tired from work. I was thinking I could agree to do one of those things.

THERAPIST: Those activities will end up being great things to do with Darnell, as long as he doesn't get high first. Since they will require more planning *and* money, it's good to proceed cautiously with them. For now, let's stick with the easier and cheaper ones. But I'm making a note of your other ideas so we can get back to them later.

CSO: Makes sense. Let's keep this simple. I'll add two things to the free list then. First, I could help him relax by rubbing his shoulders. He likes that, and I don't do it much anymore. Second, I could invite him to help me make dinner. We used to do that a lot and really enjoyed it. But I got sick of him being high all the time; I couldn't stand to have him around me. So I pretty much banned him from the kitchen before dinner.

THERAPIST: Those seem like good additions. And I can tell that you're really "getting it" because you mentioned that Darnell enjoyed the activities—you're not just picking any old thing to do.

Help the CSO select one reward from the list to use in the upcoming week.

THERAPIST: Alright, Jasmin, you've got a very good list here. Which one do you want to start with? Keep in mind that the plan will be for you to deliver the reward *this week*, but only if Darnell hasn't been using at that time. Once you pick one, we'll talk it over to make sure it seems like it will work.

CSO: I'd like to pick the one where I ask him to help me make dinner, but I'm worried he'll come into the kitchen smelling like pot. *Then* what?

THERAPIST: You're smart to be concerned if you think there's a decent chance that will happen. What do you think your options are?

Note: The therapist compliments the CSO and asks how *she* envisions handling the potential problem situation rather than telling her what to do. The therapist would assist if necessary.

CSO: I could tell him at the time I invite him that he's only welcome if he doesn't smoke. Or maybe I could just catch him as he walks through the front door and steer him toward the kitchen.

THERAPIST: Those sound like some good ideas. In a few minutes we'll explore them further. If you decide to talk to him in advance, we can polish up your delivery of that message by using the positive communication elements we've worked on. But before we decide on that, let's talk about whether this type of activity seems like it will act like a reward for Darnell.

Check to make sure the selected reward is something that would be pleasurable for the IP.

It is helpful to remind CSOs that the selected reward should act like a positive reinforcer for the *IP* (see Box 5.1). In other words, the reward for a non-using behavior *should increase the non-using behavior.* Occasionally CSOs select rewards that are more suited for themselves instead of the IP.

THERAPIST: Are you pretty sure that Darnell would still find it fun to help you make dinner? Because if we're planning this as a reward for him on days when he's not using, we need to be convinced that he'll experience it as a reward.

CSO: Yes, I think so. We always used to have fun; we'd listen to the news or to music while cooking. And he really likes to cook. We don't drink alcohol like some couples do when they're cooking, so he wouldn't be trading one problem for another.

THERAPIST: I'm glad you brought this up; it shows you really understand what we're trying to do. I'm going to circle back to this in a little bit to discuss what to do if Darnell *does* start to drink while doing the dinner prep.

Check to make sure the selected reward is inexpensive or free, and relatively easy to deliver.

Rewards that are expensive in terms of money or time commitments are particularly problematic for CSOs to manage emotionally when they suddenly cannot be delivered as intended (due to the IP having used) or they do not seem to be having the desired effect (reduced IP use). An example of a costly reward that could prove problematic is a large extended family dinner planned by the CSO to celebrate the IP's first week of abstinence. If the IP were to use drugs earlier in the day, it would be difficult for the CSO to cancel the dinner at the last minute, and it would take an emotional toll on the CSO.

As far as obstacles to delivering the reward: If there are obvious barriers, such as cost or inconvenience, the CSO is less likely to follow through and deliver the reward as planned. Sometimes these barriers become clear only when CSOs are asked to describe

BOX 5.1

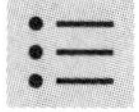

Reward/Reinforcer Selection Guidelines

The rewards should be comments/behaviors/activities that are:

- Pleasurable for the IP
- Inexpensive or free
- Relatively easy to deliver
- Comfortable for the CSO to deliver

(as they are with any homework) how they will execute the assignment for the week (see Homework Assignment Guidelines in Chapter 3, Box 3.1).

THERAPIST: It's always good to think about whether it will be too much of a hassle, or too expensive, to deliver a particular reward. Maybe we'll notice some problems as we talk through your exact plans for inviting Darnell to join you in the kitchen to cook dinner.

CSO: It shouldn't cost any more than a regular dinner, so that's good. And I'll probably just grab him as he walks in the door from work and invite him into the kitchen before he has a chance to smoke. If he ends up helping to get the dinner ready, it will be easier on me.

THERAPIST: Sounds like a win–win situation.

Ask the CSO if she or he feels comfortable delivering the reward.

THERAPIST: Can you tell me how you feel about doing this? What's it going to feel like to reward Darnell for not using? I'm mostly asking if you'll be comfortable doing this.

CSO: It'll feel good if it works. As I said, he likes to cook, and I've resented doing it on my own. But that seemed better than having to deal with him high.

5. Discuss how to explain to the IP why the reward is being given.

Determine what the CSO will tell the IP about why a reward is being offered.

Some CSOs prefer to tell their IP prior to delivering a reward that the reward is being given to support the IP's non-using behavior. These CSOs either have already told their IP that they are in treatment (and why), or they use this as an opportunity to tell their IP about being in treatment. Other CSOs elect to deliver rewards, for a period of time, without providing the IP with the reason. Many of these CSOs are curious as to whether the reward will be effective without the IP even being informed about its purpose. Other CSOs are reluctant to tell their IP that they are in treatment, and thus do not want to raise any questions about their new behavior. CSOs therefore have a number of options as far as what they might tell their IP about why a reward is being delivered. They include:

- Saying nothing, and watching to see whether the IP's non-using behavior increases in response to the reward anyway.
- Simply emphasizing the importance of the IP not drinking or using before or during the reward—leaving it up to the IP to make the connection.
- Explaining that the reward is the CSO's effort to support the IP's non-using behavior.
- Revealing that the CSO learned about Rewarding Non-Using Behavior in therapy.
- Responding to inquiries about the CSO's therapy by inviting the IP to sample treatment.

THERAPIST: You said you're going to catch Darnell as soon as he comes home so that he hasn't had a chance to smoke yet. We should talk about whether you're going to tell him *why* he's suddenly being invited to help with dinner again, and what the conditions are—namely, that he shouldn't smoke. Or you might opt to say nothing and see what happens. We just have to figure out what works best for you.

CSO: I think I'd have to tell him that he can't smoke before or during the dinner prep, otherwise I'm sure he will. Is that what you mean?

THERAPIST: Yes. In a minute, we'll practice how you're going to say that to him. Do you want to also say something about the fact that you're trying to support him for not smoking by inviting him back into the kitchen at dinner prep time?

CSO: I could do that. It would help me be more positive when I say that he can't smoke while we're cooking.

THERAPIST: Wonderful! Now what do you think about telling him where you got this idea from, to reward him when he's not smoking? You absolutely do *not* have to do this, but sometimes people use this as an opportunity to tell their loved one that they are in therapy.

CSO: I wasn't planning on telling him quite yet, but I will in another week or so.

THERAPIST: No problem. It's important for us to move at a pace that's comfortable for you. And this will give you time to learn more communication skills.

Note: The therapist used this opportunity to gently suggest that the CSO might bring up the topic of her own therapy to the IP while in the process of telling him why she was rewarding him. "Windows of opportunity," such as these, are addressed in Chapter 11, Inviting the Identified Patient to Enter Treatment. Notice that the therapist dropped the subject when the CSO did not appear to be ready to have that conversation with her IP.

Engage in a role play that explains to the IP why a reward is being given.

Even if a CSO does not plan to tell the IP why a reward is being given, it is helpful to do a role play of such a conversation so that the CSO is prepared in case the IP comes right out and asks. For those CSOs who *do* plan to tell their IP the reason for the reward, the best time to have this conversation should be discussed with their therapist.

THERAPIST: Since you *are* going to ask Darnell not to smoke before joining you in the kitchen, and you're OK with the idea of telling him that you're trying to support him when he's not using, let's practice how you'll say all that. And you might try to use some of your positive communication skills that we've practiced.

CSO: Yes, I know I need the practice in saying it in a positive way. OK. I'm ready.

THERAPIST (*as Darnell*): Hey Jasmin, how ya doing?

CSO (*in role play*): Pretty good. I wanted to see if you'd like to help me make the fajitas tonight. I know you're probably tired after a long day at work, but I'd like the help.

THERAPIST (*as Darnell*): Wow, you haven't asked me to help with the dinner in a long time. What's up?

CSO (*in role play*): I was thinking it would be nice to try doing it together again. But there's one condition: You can't smoke first. You're a lot more fun to be around when you're not high, so I'm trying to do what I can to make that happen more.

THERAPIST (*as Darnell*): Well, I like the invitation to help, but I don't particularly like being told what I can and can't do. It's my house, too!

CSO (*in role play*): I can see why you don't like being told what to do. But I'm really *asking* you, not telling you. It would mean a lot to me. Here, why don't you come on over and sit down. I've made some of that iced tea you like. And the veggies look great for the fajitas. How about giving it a shot?

THERAPIST: Let's stop the role play and talk about it. What did you like about how you handled the conversation?

CSO: I caught myself getting negative and tried to turn it around. I know I used some of the communication skills, like an understanding statement and an offer to help.

THERAPIST: Yes, I thought you did a great job using positive communication skills. I heard several understanding statements: You recognized that he was probably tired after work, and that he didn't like being told what to do. And your offer to help; giving him the iced tea he likes, was good, too. You sort of shared a feelings statement. Do you remember what you said?

CSO: I told him it would mean a lot to me. But I'm stuck on the fact that I said, "There's one condition." I think you played Darnell perfectly when you acted upset in response to being told he couldn't smoke.

THERAPIST: Yes, but as you said yourself, you turned it around when you said you were actually *asking* him. And then not only did you coax him with the feelings statement and the iced tea and fresh veggies, you also asked him to give it a try, to "sample" it. Oh, and you complimented him for being fun when he's not high, and said you wanted to support that. Masterful! Let's talk about what you want to do differently, and we'll try it again.

Note: Refer to Chapter 4 for (a) Role-Play ("Practicing") Guidelines (Box 4.4), and (b) Positive Communication Guidelines (Box 4.1).

6. Address potential complications when delivering the reward.

Discuss the CSO's options if it is clear that the IP has been using when it is time to deliver the reward, or if the IP starts using during the reward delivery.

The conversation should cover the following CSO options:

- Withhold the reward (a) if the IP is unaware of an impending reward anyway, or (b) if the IP is aware of the reward in advance, but the CSO is not concerned about any extremely negative IP behavior in response.
- Give the reward (a) if an extremely negative IP reaction might result from withholding the expected reward (e.g., aggressive behavior toward the CSO), or (b) if a significant financial loss for the CSO would result from withholding the reward (e.g., expensive tickets for a social event).

If the reward is given despite the substance use, in most cases the CSO would discuss the situation with the IP once the IP is no longer under the influence of alcohol or other drugs (see Chapter 7 for a sample role play of such a conversation).

THERAPIST: Jasmin, you've got a great plan here. It sounds like you and Darnell used to have a lot of fun preparing dinner together while listening to music. Let's think about what you'll do if Darnell agrees to help with dinner without smoking, but halfway through the prep he leaves for a few minutes and comes back high. What's a good way to handle that?

CSO: I could see that happening—probably not the first time, but after we got comfortable doing this together again. I guess I'd tell him to leave the kitchen.

THERAPIST: You'd feel comfortable and safe addressing the issue directly?

CSO: Definitely. He might get upset, but he'd leave.

Engage in a role play that addresses the IP being under the influence when it is time to deliver the reward.

THERAPIST: As you know, I always like us to practice what you're going to say to Darnell. So let's pretend that the event I mentioned just happened. I'll play Darnell. And it's usually helpful to use positive communication skills when dealing with difficult situations like this.

CSO: I'll do my best.

THERAPIST (*as Darnell*): OK. I'm back. What else do you need help with?

CSO (*in role play*): Darnell, it sure looks like you've been smoking. I know you're used to smoking when you get home, but I thought we had an agreement? That's the end of you helping me tonight.

THERAPIST (*as Darnell*): I'm fine though. Come on, let's keep working. This is fun.

CSO (*in role play*): It was fun for me, too, but it's not anymore. Now I'm upset because you gave me your word that you weren't going to smoke tonight. Whatever. Maybe we can try again tomorrow.

Note: The "debriefing" of this role play would cover these points:

- The CSO made the appropriate decision to withdraw the reward, given that she felt comfortable and safe doing so, and there was no large negative financial consequence.
- Two positive communication skills elements were used: (a) understanding statement ("I know you're used to smoking when you get home"), and (b) label your feelings ("Now I'm upset because you gave me your word. . . . ").
- The CSO did not allow herself to get drawn into an argument with the IP. She simply suggested that they try preparing dinner together again the next day.
- The therapist might suggest that the CSO enhance her response by adding, for example: (a) a partial responsibility statement ("Maybe it wasn't fair of me to expect

you to change all at once and without more notice"), and (b) an offer to help ("Is there something I can do to make it easier for you to help me with dinner tomorrow night without you smoking?").

Discuss the CSO's options if the IP becomes suspicious or upset about the CSO's motives for offering a reward.

THERAPIST: Based on what I've seen with other clients, it wouldn't be unusual if Darnell started asking questions about why you're acting differently, or why you're being so nice, when you start to link rewards with his nonsmoking behavior. I know you plan to tell him you're trying to support him when he doesn't smoke. Do you think he'll be satisfied with that?

CSO: I don't know. He might just think I'm trying something totally different, because so far I've mostly just gotten on his case for smoking so much, and that obviously hasn't worked.

THERAPIST: Fair enough. Occasionally clients tell me that when they start rewarding their loved one they get accused of trying to make up for something "bad" they did, like spend too much money. Or they get accused of being extra nice so they can get something they want, like some new electronic gadget. I don't get the impression that this will play out this way for you and Darnell though.

CSO: No, I don't think so. What do *you* think? *Should* I tell him more about what I'm up to?

THERAPIST: That's really up to you. In another couple of weeks we're going to talk specifically about how you can invite Darnell to attend treatment, and we'll be practicing different conversations you can have with him. One option would be to refer back to these times when you've been rewarding his non-using behavior, and to tell him how that got started.

Note: Refer to Chapter 11 for (a) windows of opportunity and (b) motivational hooks.

COMMON PROBLEMS TO AVOID

Here we highlight frequent difficulties encountered by new CRAFT therapists when administering the procedure for Rewarding Non-Using Behavior, and we outline tips for avoiding these problems.

Problem: CSOs can be reluctant to *withdraw* carefully planned-out rewards if their IP starts to use or shows up high, and clinicians sometimes "let it slide" because they feel sorry for the CSOs. Nonetheless, you should follow up by talking (empathically) with the CSOs again about the importance of withdrawing rewards when indicated, given the critical association being nurtured between positive reinforcement and *non-using* IP behavior.

Safeguards:

- When reviewing homework on positive reinforcement, make a point of automatically asking CSOs whether their IP was under the influence when it was time to deliver the reward, and if so, how the CSOs handled it.
- Practice role plays with another CRAFT clinician on this topic of addressing CSOs' reluctance to withdraw rewards during times of IP use.

Problem: Clinicians occasionally get caught up in the excitement of helping CSOs plan rewards for substance-free IP behavior such that the rewards end up being too costly in terms of money, time, or energy.

Safeguards:

- Make a point of always asking CSOs to start with free or inexpensive rewards (refer to Form 5.2, Common Free Rewards for a Loved One).

Problem: Clinicians miss opportunities to remind CSOs to use their positive communication skills (and to practice role plays that highlight them) when they are considering telling their IPs *why* they are rewarding non-using IP behavior.

Safeguards:

- Regardless of the CRAFT procedure, try to get into the habit of checking to see whether the homework assignment likely entails any type of conversation with the IP. If it does, remind the CSO about the benefits of incorporating positive communication into the conversation; review the skills if necessary, and do a role play if time permits.

Problem: Clinicians periodically forget to remind CSOs that meaningful change in the IP's behavior takes time. Successfully rewarding substance-free behavior just once does not guarantee that the substance-free behavior will continue.

Safeguards:

- It can be helpful to remind CSOs at every session that CRAFT usually works by building upon small changes over time.

SUMMARY

This chapter presents the CRAFT procedure for rewarding positive (non-substance-using) IP behaviors. The objective is to significantly increase these behaviors such that the IP has enticing alternatives to substance use. Furthermore, many of these new IP behaviors should directly compete with the substance-using behavior in terms of their similar positive consequences and their occurrence during the day and time when the use generally takes place. The next chapter introduces the complementary procedure for *withdrawing* rewards when the IP is using.

FORM 5.1

Rewarding Non-Using Behavior: Checklist

1. Define a positive reinforcer/reward and when to use it.

- ☐ a. Describe a positive reinforcer as a reward or as something that is experienced as pleasurable by a person.
- ☐ b. Explain that a positive reinforcer makes the person want to repeat the behavior that got the person the reward in the first place.
- ☐ c. Explain that the CSO will be asked to reward the IP at times when the IP is not using substances.
- ☐ d. Ask the CSO about any questions or concerns she or he has about using positive reinforcers, and address them.

2. Make the distinction between enabling and positive reinforcement.

- ☐ a. Appropriately distinguish between enabling and CRAFT's positive reinforcement.
- ☐ b. Stress that enabling is typically accidental—that it is *not* done with the intention of increasing the IP's substance use.
- ☐ c. Explain that CRAFT's positive reinforcement will be planned out carefully in terms of when it will be used.

3. Discuss whether the CSO would recognize signs of substance use and why it is important.

- ☐ a. Explain why it is important to be able to recognize signs of the IP's use.
- ☐ b. Ask the CSO to identify the signs that her or his IP is using or high, and provide examples, if necessary, for each of the *four main areas*: speech, mood, behavior, and appearance.

4. Generate a list of potential rewards and plan the delivery of one.

- ☐ a. Help the CSO generate a list of potential rewards for the IP.
- ☐ b. Help the CSO select one reward from the list to use in the upcoming week.
- ☐ c. Check to make sure the selected reward is something that would be pleasurable for the IP.
- ☐ d. Check to make sure the selected reward is inexpensive or free, and relatively easy to deliver.
- ☐ e. Ask the CSO if she or he feels comfortable delivering the reward.

(continued)

5. Discuss how to explain to the IP why the reward is being given.

- ☐ a. Determine what the CSO will tell the IP about *why* a reward is being offered.
- ☐ b. Engage in a role play that explains to the IP why a reward is being given.

6. Address potential complications when delivering the reward.

- ☐ a. Discuss the CSO's options if it is clear that the IP has been using when it is time to deliver the reward, or if the IP starts using during the reward delivery.
- ☐ b. Engage in a role play that addresses the IP being under the influence when it is time to deliver the reward.
- ☐ c. Discuss the CSO's options if the IP becomes suspicious or upset about the CSO's motives for offering a reward.

FORM 5.2

Common Free Rewards for a Loved One

Read the sample rewards for each category below and decide which rewards may be suitable for your loved one. Cross out any that are not relevant. For each category, see whether you can add several rewards that are *specific to your situation*.

Verbal Rewards

- Complimenting your loved one.
- Expressing warm feelings toward your loved one.
- Conversing about topics your loved one enjoys discussing.
- ______________________________
- ______________________________
- ______________________________
- ______________________________

Physical Rewards

- Squeezing your loved one's hand.
- Hugging or kissing your loved one.
- ______________________________
- ______________________________
- ______________________________
- ______________________________

Behavioral Rewards

- Doing one of your loved one's chores.
- Sitting down with your loved one to listen to music.
- Joining your loved one to watch one of his or her favorite TV shows.
- Playing an online game with your loved one.
- Inviting your loved one to go along on a walk.
- ______________________________
- ______________________________
- ______________________________
- ______________________________

Common Signs of Alcohol and Illicit Drug Use

	Depressants (e.g., alcohol, barbiturates, benzodiaz-epines)	**Marijuana**	**Hallucinogens** (e.g., LSD and PCP)	**Stimulants** (e.g., cocaine, crack, meth-amphetamine, Ecstasy)	**Opiates** (e.g., heroin, morphine, OxyContin, Percocet)
Speech	• Slurred • Odor on breath	• Talkative • Loud • Outbursts • Smoky breath	• Slowed • Loud • Outbursts • Garbled	• Accelerated • Lacks conti-nuity • Frequent change of subject	• Slurred • Slow
Mood	• Agitated • Labile • Depressed • Irritable • Elated • Passive	• Silly • Passive • Withdrawn • Labile • Euphoric • Anxious	• Labile • Anxious • Depressed	• Violent • Erratic • Anxious • Elevated • Euphoric	• Sullen • Flat affect • Withdrawn • Euphoric
Behavior	• Unsteady gait • Impaired judgment • Impaired motor skills • Drowsiness • Slowed breathing • Confusion • Memory lapses • Nausea • Blackouts • Tremors	• Relaxed state • Enhanced sensations • Impaired coor-dination • Slowed reflexes • Increased appetite • Inappropriate laughter • Impaired atten-tion • Impaired memory • Lack of energy • Low motivation • Flashbacks • Increased heart rate • Coordination problems	• Distorted reality • Confusion • Impaired coordination • Flashbacks • Hallucina-tions • Agitation • Disorienta-tion • Delusions • Increased heart rate • Dizziness • Loss of appetite	• Restlessness • Increased breathing • Increased alertness • Confusion • Paranoia • Insomnia • Loss of appetite • High energy • Elevated blood pres-sure • Increased heart rate • Distorted perceptions • Teeth grinding	• Nodding off • Drowsiness • Lethargy • Slowed breathing • Chronic constipa-tion • Nausea • Vomiting • Decreased blood pres-sure

(continued)

	Depressants	Marijuana	Hallucinogens	Stimulants	Opiates
Appearance	• Bloodshot eyes • Poor hygiene • Flushed skin	• Dilated pupils • Bloodshot eyes • Dry mouth • Smoky-smelling clothes	• Dilated pupils • Bloodshot eyes • Dry mouth • Poor grooming	• Dilated pupils • Dry mouth • Runny nose • Extreme weight loss	• Constricted pupils • Needle tracks • Scars • Droopy eyelids • Dry mouth

Main Resources

Falkowski, C. L. (2003). *Dangerous drugs: An easy-to-use reference for parents and professionals* (2nd ed.). Center City, MN: Hazelden.

National Institute on Drug Abuse. (2018, June). Commonly abused drugs. Retrieved from *www.drugabuse.gov/drugs-abuse/commonly-abused-drugs-charts*

Additional Resources

Sanchez-Samper, X., & Knight, J. R. (2009). Drug abuse by adolescents. *Pediatrics in Review, 30*, 83–93.

Substance Abuse and Mental Health Services Administration. (2006). *Detoxification and substance abuse treatment: A treatment improvement protocol TIP 45*. Rockville, MD: Author.

Chapter 6

Functional Analysis of a Loved One's Fun, Healthy Behavior

This chapter expands on Chapter 5, which outlined CRAFT's procedure for Rewarding Non-Using Behavior. In Chapter 6, we present the CRAFT Functional Analysis of a Loved One's Fun, Healthy Behavior—a unique approach for examining and increasing the frequency of a non-using IP behavior or activity. As discussed in Chapter 3, there are two types of FAs: one that targets an unhealthy behavior in order to decrease it (e.g., substance use), and one that targets a healthy behavior in an attempt to increase it. The objective of this latter FA is to understand the context in which the IP selects and enjoys the fun, healthy behavior, and to determine what the CSO can do to enhance the odds of the IP selecting this healthy behavior more often.

THE BASICS

General Description

The FA for increasing a fun, healthy IP behavior is used with CSOs who have a specific IP behavior in mind that they hope to increase *and* for which they are uncertain about the factors that influence their IP's decision to select this behavior. Similar to the FA for a problem behavior, the FA for a healthy behavior is a semistructured interview (see Form 6.1, Functional Analysis of a Loved One's Fun, Healthy Behavior: Checklist, found at the end of this chapter) that utilizes an FA form (Form 6.2), referred to here as "the FA form for healthy behavior." The FA form for healthy behavior flips the last two columns such that you ask about the *problems* associated with the largely pleasant behavior prior to asking about (and thereby finishing with) the many *enjoyable* aspects of it. In line with the procedure for the FA for a problem behavior, the information gathered for this FA should be recorded on the form (a paper version or perhaps a whiteboard representation of it). A copy of the completed form should be sent home with the CSO for future reference.

Procedure Timing

The Functional Analysis of a Loved One's Fun, Healthy Behavior is an optional CRAFT procedure that is often introduced in conjunction with the more general procedure for Rewarding Non-Using Behavior. It is common for this FA to be completed at some point *after* the CRAFT Functional Analysis of a Loved One's Drinking or Using Behavior has been done. Under what circumstances might the Functional Analysis of a Loved One's Fun, Healthy Behavior be the *first* FA administered? If the CSO is extremely eager to start rewarding the IP's non-using behavior *and* is reluctant to examine the substance use more directly, then this FA might be introduced early in CRAFT. Interestingly, in the process of focusing on increasing a positive behavior or activity, worthwhile information about the IP's substance use pattern also tends to surface. As a rule, the two different FAs are *not* conducted back-to-back within a session or in consecutive sessions.

For which CSOs might this optional FA not be used at all? Certain CSOs have little difficulty generating solid ideas of fun, healthy IP behaviors *and* methods for supporting them, and thus for them this FA is not needed. With some other CSOs (including those who find doing an FA a daunting task), it simply is more efficient to rely on other CRAFT techniques (e.g., Problem Solving) when identifying an IP behavior to reward.

Forms

- Functional Analysis of a Loved One's Fun, Healthy Behavior: Checklist (Form 6.1)
- CRAFT Functional Analysis of a Loved One's Fun, Healthy Behavior (Form 6.2)

CLINICIAN GUIDANCE AND SAMPLE DIALOGUE

The components for the FA for a fun, healthy behavior are presented below. Given that this procedure often supplements the procedure for Rewarding Non-Using Behavior, the same case from Chapter 5 is continued here. Once again, clinician–CSO dialogue is used to demonstrate your role and typical CSO responses. The components for conducting this exercise are outlined in Form 6.1, Functional Analysis of a Loved One's Fun, Healthy Behavior: Checklist.

Case Description

As a reminder, the CSO (Jasmin) has been living with the IP (Darnell) for 3 years. When she began CRAFT, Darnell was smoking marijuana at least three times a day. An initial plan was developed for rewarding his non-using behavior (Chapter 5): Jasmin was going to invite Darnell to help her prepare dinner while listening to music or the news without being high. At the start of the next session, Jasmin happily reports that she carried out the assignment as planned. Darnell had eagerly joined her to help with the dinner preparation without smoking first, and they had enjoyed listening to and discussing the news while cutting vegetables several times that week. When the therapist inquires whether Darnell had shown up high for *any* of the dinner prep times, Jasmin states that this had occurred once, and she had delivered the rehearsed conversation about him needing to leave the kitchen. Darnell had complied and had shown up substance-free to help with dinner on the remaining nights that week. Jasmin and the therapist conclude that the activity appears to be sufficiently rewarding to compete with Darnell's marijuana smoking before dinner, and consequently should be continued indefinitely.

Jasmin next states that although she is pleased with the time she is spending with Darnell during the week, she cannot understand why he does not seem particularly interested in pursuing some of the weekend drug-free activities they had always enjoyed. She is frustrated because she has no idea what is driving his decision to select smoking marijuana over spending time with her. In response, the therapist suggests (see case below) that the CRAFT Functional Analysis of a Loved One's Fun, Healthy Behavior (Form 6.2) would be an ideal exercise for reintroducing another healthy, pleasant activity from Jasmin and Darnell's recent past. The case example assumes an FA (for Darnell's using behavior) was already conducted in an earlier session. If one had *not* been conducted yet, the therapist would have spent additional time orienting Jasmin to the FA process and objectives.

1. Introduce the FA and explain its purpose (rationale).

Provide a general overview of how the FA information will be used.

Part of introducing this FA exercise for identifying a fun and healthy IP activity entails letting the CSO know that it will result in a homework assignment for the week.

THERAPIST: Jasmin, sounds like you're saying that you can't figure out why Darnell chooses to stay home and smoke marijuana instead of engaging in some of the fun weekend activities with you more often. I think it might be helpful to do another one of those "road map" exercises that maps out his behavior, like we did for his smoking. By mapping out a healthy and fun behavior we'll be able to see what influences it, and what role you might play in helping to make it happen more often. From that, we'll turn it into an assignment for you for the upcoming week.

Describe some of the specific information that will be collected (external/internal triggers, positive/negative consequences) and explain how it will be used.

THERAPIST: We'll be talking about triggers for this healthy behavior. In other words, what seems to set the stage for Darnell to choose the healthy behavior over an unhealthy one, like smoking? And how can we use this information to encourage him to make the healthier choice? We also will be looking at consequences of the healthy behavior. For negative consequences, we'll want to see the types of things that get in the way of him choosing that behavior more often, and what we might do to address them. As far as positive consequences, maybe there's something you can do to make the activity feel even better.

Give the CSO a copy of the FA form for healthy behavior and point out how it differs from the FA form for substance use behavior.

THERAPIST: This worksheet for a healthy behavior (*refers to Form 6.2*) is set up the same way as the one for Darnell's substance use behavior. The main difference is that the last two columns are reversed—it asks about short-term *negative* consequences in the fourth column and long-term *positive* consequences in the last column. This minor change simply lets us end on an upbeat note for the behavior that we're hoping to increase. This change also suggests that the negative consequences for this healthy behavior are short term, whereas the positive consequences are longer lasting.

2. Settle on an occasionally occurring fun, healthy behavior/activity for the IP.

Ask the CSO to describe one occasionally occurring fun, healthy IP behavior/activity—preferably one that can be increased during "high-risk" times.

A fun and healthy behavior or activity that is available during a high-risk time is best poised to directly compete with the substance-using behavior. However, this timing is not a strict requirement, since *any* increase in fun, healthy behavior is likely to combat the desire to use substances. As far as identifying the IP's high-risk times, they can be found in the triggers' columns of the CRAFT Functional Analysis of a Loved One's Drinking or Using Behavior (see Chapter 3, Form 3.2).

THERAPIST: As far as doing something fun with Darnell on the weekend, which pleasant weekend activity that Darnell only periodically engages in now would be a good one for us to focus on? Keep in mind that the goal is to get him to do it more often in general, and ideally at a time that would compete with his smoking. It would be great if we could get Darnell to choose the fun, healthy activity over smoking at a high-risk time.

CSO: The first thing that comes to mind is how Darnell really likes to relax and listen to old record albums. He has a big collection. We used to go poking around in old dusty stores on weekends to find "treasures," as he called them. We haven't done that in a long time, even though I've suggested it more than once.

THERAPIST: This has good potential because you're actually talking about two separate but related pleasant activities.

Make sure the behavior/activity has occurred at least once in the last 6 months, but it is <u>not</u> occurring so frequently that it cannot reasonably be increased.

THERAPIST: Before we select one of these activities, I'd like to get a sense of how often they've been happening lately. As far as you know, when's the last time Darnell listened to his old albums or shopped for them?

CSO: I doubt he's shopped for them lately. We mostly went together, and we haven't shopped for albums for a few months. But we used to do it about every other weekend.

THERAPIST: So it's been a few months? That could work. For this exercise, I like to start with an activity that's occurred within the last 6 months, because we'll be able to get more valuable, detailed information about a more recent activity. Also, it's sometimes easier to get loved ones to try out a pleasant activity again when it hasn't been such a long time since they last did it. Of course, if we pick an activity that *you'd* be involved in, you'd have more control over seeing that it happens anyway.

CSO: I'd be happy to go with him. I usually shopped for other things while he sifted through the dusty albums. But we always had fun.

THERAPIST: Excellent. Let's keep the shopping for albums as a strong possibility then. What about the other pleasant activity you mentioned: Darnell relaxing while listening to his old albums?

CSO: That one he does more often—about twice a week.

THERAPIST: That could work, too. If he already was doing this activity a lot, like every other day, there wouldn't be much room to increase it.

Ask whether the behavior/activity is one in which alcohol or drugs are typically involved—if so, reevaluate for appropriateness.

Since ideally the proposed IP activity is one that *could* occur during a high-risk time such that it would compete (timewise) with the substance use behavior, it is not surprising that many of these activities *have* involved substance use in the past. This association with substance use should not automatically rule out the activity going forward. In general, you and the CSO together would try to determine the likelihood that the IP would be able to engage in the activity without resorting to substance use in the presence of external triggers. If the IP *always* associated the activity with being high, or the IP found the substance use to be the most enjoyable aspect of the activity, then it might be more difficult to get the IP to try the activity without using alcohol or drugs.

THERAPIST: Now I have to ask the all-important question about whether Darnell is typically smoking or already high while he's shopping for old record albums or listening to them at home. This can be a little tricky, because as I said earlier, ideally we want the activity to be one that *could* occur during a high-risk time, like when he might normally choose to get high. But if he *always* associates the activity with being high, then it's probably going to be harder to get him to try the activity without smoking. Have I confused you with all of this?

CSO: No, I think I see what you mean. He never used to be high when we went shopping, but now he seems to be satisfied skipping the shopping altogether and staying home so he can smoke. Lately he's *always* high when he listens to his old albums at home. In the past he'd only occasionally smoke before pulling out his albums, so I guess I was hoping we could get back to those times.

THERAPIST: And you might be able to. We just need to decide on the best place to start. It seems to me that we could possibly incorporate the activity of him listening to his old albums, without being high, into your ongoing plan to have him help you make dinner. If I'm remembering correctly, originally you said you were going to listen to music or the news then. The news seems to be working well, but I wonder if you might encourage him to put on some of his old albums during the dinner prep? That might pave the way for him to get used to the idea of listening to the albums without being high. What do you think?

CSO: I think that could work. His old record player cranks up pretty loud, so we'd be able to hear it from the other room.

THERAPIST: Then let's make that a variation on the dinner prep assignment you're carrying over from last week. If one of you isn't in the mood for that type of music, simply go with one of your original options for music, or listen to the news again. With that settled, let's do this new road map exercise on the album shopping activity. It sounds ideal, because lately he's mostly been choosing to stay home on weekend afternoons instead of going shopping for old albums, and he *used* to shop without being high.

Stay focused on just one fun, healthy activity.

CSO: He used to go to flea markets to look for albums sometimes. Should we talk about that, too?

THERAPIST: It's best to narrow it down to one specific activity for this exercise, since there might be different things that influence his decision to do one of these over the other. Let's discuss whether one of the shopping activities would be better at competing with his smoking by being at a high-risk time, and whether he simply likes one more than the other.

CSO: I think he likes shopping in the stores more. He found flea markets boring sometimes. He's not the most patient man.

THERAPIST: OK. So, he liked shopping in the stores more. And as far as these two activities conceivably occurring during a high-risk time: You said the album shopping in actual stores happened during a high-risk time—Saturday afternoons. Did the flea market shopping happen Saturday afternoons, too?

CSO: No, we'd go to flea markets in the morning. Oh, right. We should stick with shopping in the stores because that was an afternoon event, and so is his Saturday smoking now.

THERAPIST: Looks like we're settled on the album shopping in the stores then.

3. Clarify the IP's fun, healthy behavior/activity.

Once you have collected sufficient information to be satisfied that the CSO's proposed IP behavior or activity is suitable for the FA exercise, you would gather a few more details about the behavior or activity itself (middle column on Form 6.2) in order to have a broader context for exploring the healthy behavior.

Fill in the details about the fun, healthy activity that were not already obtained during the CSO's initial discussion of it.

THERAPIST: Can you say a bit more about the record album shopping that Darnell used to enjoy so much? I'll be jotting down your remarks on this form [see the completed FA sample, Figure 6.1].

CSO: We'd head out after lunch, usually on a Saturday. We'd be gone about 2 hours, I guess. If we grabbed coffee afterward, it would be closer to 3 hours.

4. Outline the external triggers.

Explain how examining the external triggers that "set the stage" for the IP's selection of the fun, healthy activity might allow the CSO to increase the IP's contact with these triggers or make them more effective.

External triggers	Internal triggers	Fun, healthy behavior	Short-term negative consequences (barriers)	Long-term positive consequences
1. *Who* is your loved one usually with when (*behavior*)? Me (Jasmin) 2. *Where* does he or she usually (*behavior*)? Downtown 3. *When* does he or she usually (*behavior*)? After eating lunch downtown when he hasn't had to wait a long time in line to be seated.	1. What do you think your loved one is *thinking* about right before (*behavior*)? Jasmin and I deserve a fun afternoon. Maybe I'll find a treasure. I wish dad could see my collection. 2. What do you think he or she is *feeling* right before (*behavior*)? Happy (to be spending time with me). Stress-free. Bored.	1. *What* is your loved one's fun, healthy behavior? Shopping in stores for old record albums. 2. *How often* does he or she engage in it? Only once in the last few months. 3. *How long* a period of time does it last? About 2 hours, but 3 hours if coffee, too.	1. What do you think your loved one dislikes about (*behavior*) with (*who*)? Kept waiting sometimes. 2. What do you think he or she dislikes about (*behavior*) (*where*)? Store too crowded sometimes. Seller won't negotiate price. 3. What do you think he or she dislikes about (*behavior*) (*when*)? Too sleepy if he's had a beer. 4. What unpleasant *thoughts* do you think he or she has while (*behavior*)? This is nuts; I've gotta get out of here. 5. What unpleasant *feelings* do you think he or she has while (*behavior*)? Annoyed, anxious.	1. What do you think are the positive results of your loved one's (*behavior*) in these areas: a. Family Memories of dad. Gifts for mom that lead to spending time with her. b. Friends/partners Spend time with me. Discuss music with Tyrone. c. Physical Walking feels good; relaxing & exercise. d. Emotional Loves old music & finding "treasures." e. Legal n/a f. Job n/a g. Financial n/a h. Other:

FIGURE 6.1. Completed version of Form 6.2, CRAFT Functional Analysis of a Loved One's Fun, Healthy Behavior.

THERAPIST: As I mentioned briefly a few minutes ago, it's helpful to look at the things that might influence Darnell's decision to choose a healthy activity, like old record shopping, over substance use. One way to do this is to first look at the things in Darnell's environment that have been associated with, or paved the way to, the album shopping. Then we'll see if we can find a way for you to help increase his contact with these external triggers. Or maybe there's a way you can help make these external triggers more effective so that he's swayed by them and makes a healthier choice as a result.

Identify the people, places, and times associated with the fun, healthy activity.

THERAPIST: Think about the more recent times that you and Darnell have decided to go album shopping on a Saturday afternoon. You said you went after lunch. Can you tell me the circumstances as far as what was going on around you guys at the time the decision was made to go shopping? Even when you were going more regularly, you didn't go every weekend. What can you think of that was more often associated with him deciding to go? And for now I'm talking about the *external* triggers: the things going on around him. We'll talk about the things going on inside of him in a minute.

CSO: That's an interesting question. Hmm. I'm not really sure. *I* was always there making the suggestion, so I guess I'm not the deciding factor.

THERAPIST: Maybe your presence alone didn't influence his decision, but it could still be related to your behavior in some way. And as you know, we're hoping your behavior *can* influence his decision going forward! We'll look at that shortly. It's certainly possible that his decision was influenced by something totally separate.

CSO: Now that I think about it, I remember he was more likely to go album shopping if we were already downtown having lunch.

THERAPIST: This sounds important; like something we can really work with. You'll see that I'm jotting all your comments down in the first column of this form (*refers to the first column of Form 6.2*).

Probe to make sure all of the external triggers are listed.

THERAPIST: Just take another moment and picture you and Darnell deciding to go album shopping. Does anything else come to mind that we can associate with him agreeing to go? For instance, did he pretty much always agree to go if you were already downtown having lunch, or did that depend on other factors?

Note: The clinician does not rush the process but asks the pertinent questions in several different ways. The clinician even suggests that the CSO use imagery so she can get a true sense of the IP's thoughts and feelings at the time he made the pivotal decision regarding whether to engage in the fun and healthy activity in the past.

CSO: If we had to wait a long time to be seated for lunch he'd be grumpy, and then he seemed to be in a rush to get home afterward.

THERAPIST: I'll make a quick note about his mood in the internal triggers column. Was a long wait associated with a particular restaurant or the time you went?

CSO: Probably both. If we went before 1:00, it was crowded at most restaurants. I like a particular restaurant that tends to be really crowded on weekends.

THERAPIST: One of the things we'll talk about in a little bit is whether it might be reasonable to plan on going at 1:00 or later, or maybe avoiding that restaurant. But let's wait on that for now.

5. Outline the internal triggers.

Explain how examining the IP's thoughts and feelings associated with the selection of the fun, healthy activity might allow the CSO to help increase the occurrence of these triggers.

THERAPIST: You mentioned that if Darnell's in a grumpy mood, he's less likely to agree to shop after lunch. This is a good example of an internal trigger—in this case, a *feeling*—that affects Darnell's decision to go shopping. Similar to the external triggers, we like to examine a person's *internal* triggers so we can see if there's any opportunity to influence them in a way that supports the selection of the fun and healthy behavior over the substance use. We'll take a look at his thoughts, too, for the same reason.

Identify the IP's thoughts and feelings that precede the fun, healthy activity.

THERAPIST: So far, I know that if Darnell is in a grumpy mood at lunchtime, he's less likely to want to go shopping afterward. How would you label his feeling when he's *more* inclined to agree to shop? I think that will be more helpful than just saying "not grumpy" (*smiles*).

CSO: Sometimes he's happy and wants to spend time with me, and other times he's just bored. But if he's stressed, he usually isn't interested in shopping. I'm not sure how to describe that, other than to say stress-free?

THERAPIST: That will work. I'm adding these feelings to the second column on the form (*refers to Form 6.2*). What do you think Darnell is *thinking* at these times when he's likely to agree to go shopping for old albums?

CSO: Something like "Jasmin and I deserve a fun afternoon," or "Maybe I'll find a treasure." He might even be thinking about his dad, because Darnell has told me his dad loved all kinds of music.

THERAPIST: And if we could hear his thoughts about his dad, what do you think they might be?

CSO: Maybe "I wish dad could see my collection." His dad passed away a few years ago.

THERAPIST: That's interesting, because he's clearly not just thinking of himself and his own happiness in this scenario. OK. Good. It's on the form now (*refers to the second column of Form 6.2*).

Probe to make sure all of the internal triggers are listed.

THERAPIST: Let's take one last moment with the internal triggers. Remember, we're trying to see if there might be certain thoughts or feelings that influence Darnell's decision to go album shopping on a Saturday afternoon versus going home to get high.

CSO: I've racked my brain over this question. I'm just not sure I've got anything else.

THERAPIST: No problem! Let's move on then.

6. Outline the negative consequences (barriers) associated with engaging in the behavior/activity.

Explain that there are barriers associated with fun, healthy activities, and the CSO might be able to help address some of them.

THERAPIST: Fun, healthy activities typically have something negative associated with them, or people would do them all the time. One way to increase the chance that an individual will choose the healthy activity over the substance use activity is to eliminate or reduce some of the problems associated with the healthy activity. And CRAFT knows that people like you can play an important part in this.

List the barriers associated with the fun, healthy activity.

THERAPIST: You'll see in the fourth column here (*refers to Form 6.2*) that there are multiple ways in which we try to get at the question about barriers that might be interfering with Darnell selecting album shopping more often than he currently is. We'll be thinking the words "album shopping" where it says "behavior" throughout this column. But before we move down the column, I'd rather just get your reaction to the question first. You've already mentioned a few things you've noticed while he's eating lunch that interfere with his decision to go shopping, like being in a bad mood, or being stressed. But what would you say are the main problems or hassles he associates with the album shopping itself based on past experience? These can also interfere with him selecting the shopping again.

Note: As was the case with the CRAFT Functional Analysis of a Loved One's Drinking or Using Behavior, it is best to make this FA into a natural conversation as much as possible. If this therapist had opted exclusively to go down the list of questions in each column of the FA (Form 6.2) in a highly structured manner, this *semi*structured interview would have appeared too mechanical and could have interfered with the rapport with the CSO.

CSO: Hmm. If he's had a beer with lunch, he sometimes complains that he's sleepy while we're shopping. He doesn't seem to enjoy it that much then. If we go to a popular shop, he gets annoyed because we have to fight to get through the crowd. He also gets annoyed if he thinks the albums are priced too high and the seller won't come down at all.

THERAPIST: Very informative. You can see I've jotted down your remarks on the form (*refers to the fourth column of Form 6.2 [see also Figure 6.1]*). Let's take a look at the remaining questions here. The first question asks what you think he dislikes about shopping with you. What do you think?

CSO: If the store doesn't have many albums or other old music stuff, he's ready to leave the store before I am. If I keep him waiting a while, he gets impatient.

THERAPIST: All right. It's on the form now. The last two questions in Column 4 ask about his unpleasant thoughts and feelings while shopping for albums. I know you mentioned he gets annoyed if the store is too crowded or the seller won't negotiate prices. Any other negative feelings?

CSO: I can see him getting anxious if he's waiting for me to finish my own shopping.

THERAPIST: What about negative thoughts?

CSO: If the store is crowded, he's probably thinking, "This is nuts. I've gotta get out of here."

7. Outline the positive consequences of engaging in the behavior/activity.

Explain that positive consequences of the behavior/activity will be examined, since the CSO might be able to enhance these effects.

THERAPIST: We'll finish this exercise by making sure we're aware of all the positive things Darnell experiences when he goes album shopping. And if some of them are similar to the reasons why he smokes on many Saturday afternoons, then it's even more likely he'll be OK with trying the shopping instead. Regardless, it's possible that there may be small things you can do to make this fun, healthy activity even *more* enjoyable for him, which will further increase the chance of him agreeing to try it instead of getting high.

List the positive consequences associated with the fun, healthy activity.

THERAPIST: Before we look at the categories in this fifth column (*refers to the fifth column of Form 6.2*), just tell me what stands out to you. Why specifically do you think Darnell enjoys the album shopping?

CSO: Like I said before, his dad liked all kinds of music. So maybe it brings back happy memories of his dad?

THERAPIST: That's certainly possible. I'll add this to the form while we're talking. What else?

CSO: Just like his dad, Darnell really loves all types of music, and these old albums honestly feel like treasures to him. And both of us enjoy antiquing, so we don't mind searching through the dusty shops. Sometimes he buys old sheet music. I know he likes spending time with me, especially since there are a lot of things I won't do with him anymore.

THERAPIST: This is good information. Maybe some additional positive consequences will come to mind as we go down this list. For the first category, "Family," I've already put the memories of his dad. Can you think of any other positive family things that come out of his album shopping?

CSO: Once in awhile he finds something for his mom, because she likes antiques, too. I know it makes him feel good when he gives her a small gift.

THERAPIST: That's wonderful, because I bet that's helpful for their relationship in general.

CSO: Definitely, because he doesn't spend that much time with her lately. I've even suggested we invite her to come with us some Saturday afternoon, but he hasn't been thrilled with the idea.

THERAPIST: If he hasn't been enthusiastic about his mom coming along, we'd better hold off on that for now. We have to stay focused on the idea that this activity should be as enjoyable as we can possibly make it, because otherwise he's likely to select staying home and getting high instead. OK. The next category is "Friends/Partner."

Note: The therapist reminds the CSO that the objective is to find pleasant activities that have a good chance of competing with her IP's substance use, and part of this task entails reducing any potential barriers to the IP selecting the healthy activity over the substance use.

CSO: He has a friend who appreciates the old music, too. I've heard the two of them talking about some of the albums Darnell has found. But I don't think that would help him choose to go album shopping again.

THERAPIST: Maybe not, but it's worth noting here. Does this friend smoke, too?

CSO: I don't think so. Tyrone is pretty conservative.

THERAPIST: Then that's all the more reason to include this on our form. Possibly we can influence Darnell in some way to spend more time with Tyrone down the road. What about the "Physical" category?

CSO: More than once while shopping, Darnell has said that it feels good to get out and walk around. He's put on some weight lately, and it bothers him. He said the walking relaxes him, too, as long as there aren't big crowds of people around.

THERAPIST: Excellent. It's on the form now. And I'm reminded that you said one of Darnell's positive consequences for getting high was to relax. So it's interesting that the smoking and the shopping have that in common. That's a good sign as far as increasing the chance that Darnell is willing to try the shopping. We should think more about how to make sure he gets to relax at least somewhat while shopping.

Note: The clinician notices the overlap in one of the functions of the Saturday afternoon substance use behavior and the planned fun, healthy activity. An effort will be made to capitalize on this overlap when helping with the details of the homework assignment.

CSO: I might be able to come up with something else if I think about it a while.

THERAPIST: Don't worry about that for now. We can revisit it when we come up with the actual assignment. What about these other categories: "Legal," "Job," "Financial"?

CSO: No, I can't think of anything for them.

8. Get the CSO's reaction to the completed FA and assist with summarizing the main findings.

Summarizing the main findings does *not* mean you (or the CSO) should go down the completed Form 6.2 item by item. The objective is to see what information made an impression on the CSO, and to help "connect the dots" so an assignment can be made.

Help the CSO step back and look at the information contained in the completed exercise by asking for the CSO's overall reaction to the exercise and what it produced.

THERAPIST: Let's sit back a minute and see what you make of this picture. What's your reaction to doing this exercise and seeing what it produced?

CSO: It was fun, because I already have some ideas of things I can do differently that should help.

THERAPIST: Excellent. Like what?

CSO: It reminded me how much Darnell hates being in crowds, whether it's at a restaurant or a shop. I should be able to plan the afternoon with those things in mind. And like you just said, if he can find the shopping to be relaxing, he'll be more likely to agree to do it again.

If the CSO has not already mentioned the main triggers, ask the CSO to do so and assist if necessary.

THERAPIST: Yes, steering away from crowded restaurants and shops sounds important. I'm just going to stick to the restaurant topic for another minute as I look at the trigger columns. You made another good observation about the restaurant you choose for lunch: that it should be downtown, since it's close to the shops then.

If the CSO has not already mentioned the main consequences, ask the CSO to do so and assist if necessary.

THERAPIST: You hit upon the main negative consequence associated with Darnell's record shopping: disliking crowded shops. As you look at these other potential barriers in the fourth column, would you say that any of them are serious enough that we should consider addressing them in order for your planned excursion to be successful?

CSO: I think he's kind of selfish when he gets impatient waiting for me to finish my own shopping, but I noticed that if I keep it to a minimum and let him know I'm aware of the time, he's usually much better about it. The beer at lunch can possibly be fixed by me suggesting we get a beer *after* we finish the shopping, or by stopping for a coffee in between shops.

THERAPIST: Wonderful. Now let's move on to the main things you said Darnell *likes* about the album shopping: the *positive* consequences.

CSO: I think I can play up the physical activity he gets from it—the walking.

THERAPIST: And we don't want to forget the enjoyment he gets from spending time with *you* on those afternoons, right? Later we can come up with a few novel ideas for Darnell spending time with you *and* listening to those old albums. We already talked about possibly doing this while he's helping you prepare dinner.

9. Offer ideas regarding how this FA information can be used.

By referring to the triggers or consequences, give several examples of how the information can be used in developing the homework assignment.

As was done for the Functional Analysis of a Loved One's Drinking or Using Behavior (Chapter 3), several examples of the therapist highlighting notable information gleaned from the completed FA form for healthy behavior (Figure 6.1) are listed below. However, for this type of FA, the ideas regarding how to use the information are directly related to the pending homework assignment, since the purpose of the Functional Analysis of a Loved One's Fun, Healthy Behavior is to get the IP to increase the pleasant activity that was just outlined. Once again, each example shows (in parentheses) the column of the FA being relied upon (e.g., external triggers, negative consequences) in generating the idea. The therapist would provide several examples to consider. Note that the examples are not yet in the format of a finalized homework assignment, as the therapist is simply presenting possibilities to the CSO.

Some of these situations might seem to be unfair to the CSO, since they are asking her to give in to the IP's seemingly unreasonable demand (e.g., to minimize her own shopping so as not to keep him waiting). However, since the immediate objective is to increase the likelihood that the IP will begin choosing a healthy behavior (e.g., album shopping) with his partner over sitting home and getting high, potential barriers should be reduced. Issues such as an IP's impatience can be addressed later in treatment if it persists once other changes have been made.

THERAPIST (*external triggers*): Going out to lunch in a downtown restaurant is important, since it places you closer to the shops. And going at a time when the restaurant won't be too crowded is key. You said something about going after the lunch rush, like around 1:00. Or maybe you could go to a place that requires a reservation.

THERAPIST (*internal triggers and positive consequences*): I wonder if it would help to talk during lunch, or even at breakfast that same day, about some of the treasures Darnell's dad collected over the years, and some of the music he liked? That might get Darnell fired up to shop.

THERAPIST (*negative consequences*): In terms of Darnell being impatient, you said earlier that you could minimize the time you keep him waiting while you're finishing up your shopping, and you could comment on being aware of the time, too. Are you OK with doing that at this point?

THERAPIST (*negative consequences*): Since crowded stores bother him, too, I wonder if you could do a little searching prior to the Saturday outing to see if maybe there are some shops that are more off the beaten path?

THERAPIST (*negative consequences*): I like your idea of suggesting that Darnell hold off on his beer until *after* you're done shopping, or that you stop mid-shopping for a coffee if he gets too sleepy.

THERAPIST (*positive consequences*): Do you think Darnell's love of old music might be enhanced if he read some books about the bands or singers, or even the composers? If so, you guys could spend time together tracking down some of those books, either old or new ones.

THERAPIST (*positive consequences*): And you mentioned that you could play up Darnell's interest in getting some physical activity. There's probably a lot of ways to do that. One idea would be to use a step counter, either a separate device or one that's on his phone or watch, so you could track the number of steps you both get while shopping. You could even set a record for the day. That could carry over to other days, too. Oh—and the walking helps him relax, too, which is one of the same reasons why he says he smokes . . . so that's a bonus.

10. Decide on a specific assignment based on the information gathered.

Ask the CSO to share ideas for a specific assignment that is based on the FA just conducted, and assist with finalizing it.

THERAPIST: As I said before, the goal of this exercise was to come up with an assignment for you for this next week based on the material you just generated. So the plan will be for you to invite Darnell to go album shopping, presumably this Saturday. Can you add the specifics like we always do for assignments? In other words, walk me through it from the start.

CSO: I am going to let him know Friday evening that I really want to go snooping around the antique stores Saturday afternoon. And I'll tell him that I want to eat lunch downtown since it's closer to the shops, and that we should go closer to 1:00 so it's not crowded. Oh, and I'll let him know I won't get too distracted in the shops and make him wait . . . at least not for too long (*smiles*).

THERAPIST: Impressive! Is there any way you might check out in advance which stores are less crowded? That might be a tough one.

CSO: I read about a section of town that has opened up some new shops but is struggling a bit. Sounds like our kind of place both in terms of the smaller crowds and better deals! And hopefully he'll then find the walking to be relaxing, too.

THERAPIST: Very good. And you also have some ideas for handling his interest in a beer at lunchtime.

Note: Depending on the CSO's communication skills, this therapist might suggest practicing a role play of the planned conversation with the IP. Regardless, the therapist would remind the CSO to use the positive communication skills she had learned already. Importantly, the remaining guidelines for homework assignments would be followed (see Chapter 3, Box 3.1).

COMMON PROBLEMS TO AVOID

The common problems to avoid that were outlined for the CRAFT Functional Analysis of a Loved One's Drinking or Using Behavior (see Chapter 3) largely apply to the current chapter's Functional Analysis of a Loved One's Fun, Healthy Behavior, as well. The one exception is the point that cautioned therapists not to use an uncommon episode as the focus of the FA. Given that the purpose of the current FA is to increase a (healthy) behavior, you *should* select a relatively uncommon activity. Additional pitfalls to avoid when administering the Functional Analysis of a Loved One's Fun, Healthy Behavior include:

Problem: Clinicians sometimes complete a beautiful FA, but then do not make the assignment explicit that CSOs should follow up with their specific role in getting the activity to happen in the upcoming week. More often than you might expect, CSOs do not assume that an assignment resulted from the exercise.

Safeguards:

- Assume every CRAFT session will result in a homework assignment, and preferably it will grow out of the main CRAFT procedure being covered that day.
- Before the end of each session, routinely check to make sure the *CSO* knows what the assignment is.

Problem: Clinicians sometimes get swept up in CSOs' enthusiasm about scheduling a healthy IP activity that, upon consideration, is probably not particularly *fun* for the typical IP (e.g., cleaning out the garage, straightening the pantry). Consequently, there would be little chance for the activity to compete with substance use.

Safeguards:

- Get into the habit of simply asking the CSO whether the IP would experience the proposed activity as fun. If the answer is "no," then it will be important to pick another activity.

Problem: Although it is not absolutely necessary for the proposed fun and healthy IP activity to be scheduled during a high-risk time for the IP (even if that is the ideal scenario), some clinicians do not make a concerted effort for this to happen.

Safeguards:

- When the CSO proposes a possible activity for this FA exercise, you immediately should ask whether the activity conceivably could take place during a high-risk period.

SUMMARY

This chapter presents the CRAFT Functional Analysis of a Loved One's Fun, Healthy Behavior. This procedure helps CSOs characterize a seemingly pleasant (and healthy) activity or behavior that the IP, for somewhat uncertain reasons, only elects to engage in infrequently. Once an understanding is reached as to when and why the IP periodically *does* select this particular activity (e.g., instead of substance use), specific plans are made for assisting the CSO in influencing the IP to select this behavior more often. The next two chapters are focused on procedures that directly target the reduction of problematic behavior.

FORM 6.1

Functional Analysis of a Loved One's Fun, Healthy Behavior: Checklist

1. Introduce the FA and explain its purpose (rationale).

☐ a. Provide a general overview of how the FA information will be used.

☐ b. Describe some of the specific information that will be collected (external/internal triggers, positive/negative consequences) and explain how it will be used.

☐ c. Give the CSO a copy of the FA form for healthy behavior and point out how it differs from the FA form for substance use behavior.

2. Settle on an occasionally occurring fun, healthy behavior/activity for the IP.

☐ a. Ask the CSO to describe one occasionally occurring fun, healthy IP behavior/activity—preferably one that can be increased during "high-risk" times.

☐ b. Make sure the behavior/activity has occurred at least once in the last 6 months, but it is *not* occurring so frequently that it cannot reasonably be increased.

☐ c. Ask whether the behavior/activity is one in which alcohol or drugs are typically involved—if so, reevaluate for appropriateness.

☐ d. Stay focused on just one fun, healthy activity.

3. Clarify the IP's fun, healthy behavior/activity.

☐ a. Fill in the details about the fun, healthy activity that were not already obtained during the CSO's initial discussion of it.

4. Outline the external triggers.

☐ a. Explain how examining the external triggers that "set the stage" for the IP's selection of the fun, healthy activity might allow the CSO to increase the IP's contact with these triggers or make them more effective.

☐ b. Identify the people, places, and times associated with the fun, healthy activity.

☐ c. Probe to make sure all of the external triggers are listed.

(continued)

5. Outline the internal triggers.

☐ a. Explain how examining the IP's thoughts and feelings associated with the selection of the fun, healthy activity might allow the CSO to help increase the occurrence of these triggers.

☐ b. Identify the IP's thoughts and feelings that precede the fun, healthy activity.

☐ c. Probe to make sure all of the internal triggers are listed.

6. Outline the negative consequences (barriers) associated with engaging in the behavior/activity.

☐ a. Explain that there are barriers associated with fun, healthy activities, and the CSO might be able to help address some of them.

☐ b. List the barriers associated with the fun, healthy activity.

7. Outline the positive consequences of engaging in the behavior/activity.

☐ a. Explain that positive consequences of the behavior/activity will be examined, since the CSO might be able to enhance these effects.

☐ b. List the positive consequences associated with the fun, healthy activity.

8. Get the CSO's reaction to the completed FA and assist with summarizing the main findings.

☐ a. Help the CSO step back and look at the information contained in the completed exercise by asking for the CSO's overall reaction to the exercise and what it produced.

☐ b. If the CSO has not already mentioned the main triggers, ask the CSO to do so and assist if necessary.

☐ c. If the CSO has not already mentioned the main consequences, ask the CSO to do so and assist if necessary.

9. Offer ideas regarding how this FA information can be used.

☐ a. By referring to the triggers or consequences, give several examples of how the information can be used in developing the homework assignment.

10. Decide on a specific assignment based on the information gathered.

☐ a. Ask the CSO to share ideas for a specific assignment that is based on the FA just conducted, and assist with finalizing it.

FORM 6.2

CRAFT Functional Analysis of a Loved One's Fun, Healthy Behavior

External triggers	Internal triggers	Fun, healthy behavior	Short-term negative consequences (barriers)	Long-term positive consequences
1. *Who* is your loved one usually with when (*behavior*)? 2. *Where* does he or she usually (*behavior*)? 3. *When* does he or she usually (*behavior*)?	1. What do you think your loved one is *thinking* about right before (*behavior*)? 2. What do you think he or she is *feeling* right before (*behavior*)?	1. *What* is your loved one's fun, healthy behavior? 2. *How often* does he or she engage in it? 3. *How long* a period of time does it last?	1. What do you think your loved one dislikes about (*behavior*) with (*who*)? 2. What do you think he or she dislikes about (*behavior*) (*where*)? 3. What do you think he or she dislikes about (*behavior*) (*when*)? 4. What unpleasant *thoughts* do you think he or she has while (*behavior*)? 5. What unpleasant *feelings* do you think he or she has while (*behavior*)?	1. What do you think are the positive results of your loved one's (*behavior*) in these areas: a. Family b. Friends/partners c. Physical d. Emotional e. Legal f. Job g. Financial h. Other

Chapter 7

Withdrawing Rewards for Using Behavior

Part of the protocol for Rewarding Non-Using Behavior (see Chapter 5) involves teaching CSOs the importance of *removing* these newly planned/offered rewards if the IP begins to use. This chapter expands the focus on the strategic removal of rewards by training CSOs to stop routinely "rewarding" their IPs in ongoing day-to-day situations in which the IPs are under the influence of alcohol or drugs. Often this problematic CSO behavior involves engaging in a pleasant activity with an IP who is inebriated or high, but it can also take the form of a material reward automatically given to an IP who continues to use. Importantly, CSOs typically are unaware of the fact that their behavior would even be considered a reward for their IP, and that this reward is playing a role in maintaining their IP's substance use.

Withdrawing Rewards for Using Behavior, or taking a "time-out from positive reinforcement," is categorized as one of CRAFT's "negative consequences" procedures. Most CSOs (and therapists) would prefer to implement a procedure that involves *giving* rewards (for substance-free behavior), but such a procedure needs to be supplemented at times with the active withdrawal of rewards. This activity does *not* entail the introduction of harsh new punishments. Instead, the procedure involves looking at current CSO responses to IP substance use and evaluating whether the responses might be experienced as rewarding by the IP and therefore should be stopped. Not surprisingly, it is a harder "sell" to get CSOs to engage in a "negative consequences" assignment, in part because CSOs are concerned (and rightfully so) that they might upset their IP in the process. Furthermore, CSOs struggle with the message that they may have been inadvertently supporting their IP's use.

THE BASICS

General Description

The Withdrawing Rewards for Using Behavior procedure opens with a discussion of some of the prominent situations in which the IP is still using or under the influence while in the CSO's company. The CSO's response to the IP in these situations is reviewed with an eye toward whether this behavior might be experienced as rewarding by the IP. The fact that the CSO may have been *unintentionally* rewarding the IP's using behavior must be discussed with great care, and with reassurance that the CSO will be taught new skills to halt this practice and support only non-using behavior going forward.

At this point in CRAFT, most CSOs have already learned the Rewarding Non-Using Behavior procedure, and so the training continues with a reminder about how that procedure includes instructions to remove the reward if the IP starts to use. CSOs are then assisted in the selection of the specific ongoing situation to target, and the details of withdrawing the reward and dealing with the consequences are covered. Finally, CSOs are taught to apply their positive communication skills to this situation so that, if they choose to, they can explain to their IP why they are removing rewards. As always, safety issues are addressed.

Procedure Timing

The Withdrawing Rewards for Using Behavior procedure is commonly introduced after CSOs have learned about reinforcement principles within the Rewarding Non-Using Behavior procedure. It is also helpful for CSOs to have been taught the CRAFT communication skills so that they are prepared to explain their change in behavior to their IPs in a positive manner. Although CSOs were introduced to the idea that they might be unintentionally rewarding some IP using behaviors during the initial CRAFT session, the Withdrawing Rewards for Using Behavior procedure is the first time this CSO behavior is explored in detail and targeted for change. Thus, it is helpful for you to have had some time to establish a good rapport with the CSO so that the message is received as intended.

Forms

- Withdrawing Rewards for Using Behavior: Checklist (Form 7.1)
- Using Positive Communication to Explain the Withdrawal of Rewards (Examples) (Handout 7.1)

CLINICIAN GUIDANCE AND SAMPLE DIALOGUE

The components for the CRAFT procedure for Withdrawing Rewards for Using Behavior are presented below, and are outlined in Form 7.1, Withdrawing Rewards for Using Behavior: Checklist, found at the end of this chapter. A sample case that illustrates clinician–CSO dialogue throughout the chapter is included.

Case Description

The CSO (Carlos) is a 45-year-old Latino male who works for a small business. He has been in a relationship with the IP (Alex), who identifies as American Indian and Latino, for 3 years. They have lived together for 6 months. The IP lost his job about 4 months ago, which is when Carlos noticed that Alex appeared high much of the time. In talking to him, Carlos learned that Alex was getting pills from various acquaintances, and Alex said he "needed" the pills so that he did not have to think about the problems he was having getting another job. Carlos asked Alex to seek help for his polydrug use, but he flatly refused.

1. Discuss the CSO's current response to the IP's substance use and the outcome.

Ask the CSO how she or he currently responds to the IP's substance use in an ongoing situation.

THERAPIST: Carlos, as we've discussed, your assignment to reward Alex's non-using behavior went well this week. And this included *not* rewarding him when he *was* using, or taking the reward away if he started to use. Now I'd like to take a look at some of the common times he's still using or high. Can you give me an example of a time this week when you were with Alex when he was using or had just used? And what did *you* do in that situation?

Note: The therapist took the opportunity to praise the CSO for a successfully completed homework assignment and to mention that it involved the withdrawal of rewards during times of IP use. This provides a segue into the topic for the current session.

CSO: I was really pissed when Alex showed up at the gym the other day while I was working out, because I could tell he was high. He wouldn't stop bothering me. He shows up like this every now and then, but this time it was really bad. He wouldn't leave. He just kept standing by me and talking in a loud voice. It was embarrassing.

THERAPIST: What did you do?

CSO: I got him to sit on a bench nearby and watch the TV monitor. And I went over about every 10 minutes to talk with him so he'd stay quiet. I still had to cut my workout short.

Ask what the CSO thought the impact of her or his response was on the IP's substance use behavior, and whether it seemed problematic.

THERAPIST: As you think about it now, what do you make of how you handled the problem?

CSO: At least I got him to sit quietly for a while. I talked to him the next day about it. I doubt he'll be trying that again anytime soon, but I guess he *could* if he's high.

THERAPIST: It's good that you're able to talk to Alex about things that are bothering you, and I like that you're talking to him when he's not under the influence. We'll talk about this more later. What about your behavior toward him while you were at the gym?

Note: The therapist uses the opportunity to compliment the CSO's open communication with his partner and the timing of the conversation, as the latter is an important consideration when explaining the withdrawal of rewards. However, the therapist immediately returns to the issue of the CSO's behavior at the time of the IP's use and its effect.

CSO: That's a good question, because if anything, he *liked* how I acted toward him then. I was going out of my way to keep him happy so he wouldn't embarrass me.

THERAPIST: That's what I'm curious about. So it got him to be quiet at the gym for a while, but do you think it will have any effect on him getting high in the future?

CSO: It definitely won't help. I paid *more* attention to him while he was high.

Explain that sometimes CSOs accidentally reward their IP's substance use behavior. Although not essential, at this point you could refer back to earlier sessions in which "enabling" was discussed (Chapter 5) or in which unintentional support of IP substance use was raised in other contexts, such as during the introductory session (Chapter 2). If the Allowing for Natural, Negative Consequences of Use procedure (Chapter 8) has been taught already, the topic would have been covered there as well.

THERAPIST: It's so interesting, because your reaction to him at the gym was probably what most people would have done. But as you've just said, you actually ended up paying *more* attention to him while he was high. What do you think all the extra attention might have said to him about getting high?

CSO: That it was OK, because I'd spend even more time than usual talking with him at the gym if he was high. Well, that's *not* the message I want him to get, that's for sure.

THERAPIST: It's clear that you *don't* want to be supporting his drug use, but you can see how tricky this gets. Also, it's important to know you're not alone. In fact, it's pretty common for people in similar situations to you to find themselves accidentally rewarding substance use. And hey—I don't know whether Alex is likely to show up high at the gym again as a result of the extra attention he got from you, but I'm thinking it might be worthwhile to look at how you respond to Alex at other times when he's high. If you're reacting in a way that makes a connection between his substance use and something enjoyable, then you're actually rewarding his behavior of getting high. Of course, you're not doing it on purpose!

Note: The therapist normalizes the CSO's response to the IP (by pointing out that it was a common CSO reaction), and at the same time suggests that it was not supporting the goal of reduced IP use.

Explore the CSO's feelings about the idea of accidentally rewarding the IP's substance use behavior.

THERAPIST: Can you tell me what you're feeling now as I'm telling you that you might have unintentionally made it a little easier for Alex to keep getting high at times?

CSO: I knew I wasn't *helping*, but I hate to think I was making things worse.

THERAPIST: But you *were* doing the best you could. And you're here in treatment for him now, right? That shows how much you care about him.

2. Stress the importance of withdrawing a planned reward if the IP uses.

The sample case dialogue assumes the CSO has already been taught the procedure for Rewarding Non-Using Behavior (Chapter 5), since in most cases it *will* have been taught prior to this Withdrawing Rewards for Using Behavior procedure. If that procedure has *not* been taught yet, you would need to spend more time explaining the importance of linking rewards with non-using behavior in order to increase them, and withdrawing rewards when associated with substance-using behavior in order to decrease them.

Give a rationale for withdrawing the reward if the IP uses.

THERAPIST: Recently we worked on a procedure for *giving* a reward to Alex when he's not high, and part of it naturally involved taking the reward away if Alex uses. You had good success with this procedure this past week. But it doesn't hurt to explore this topic a bit more, since you'd be accidentally *rewarding* his substance-using behavior if you didn't *take away* a reward when he was using or high. Are you up for taking a look at other times when you might be accidentally supporting his use, with the goal of making that stop?

CSO: Yes. I'm curious to see how much I'm doing this.

Explain that it works best to withdraw rewards right while the IP is using or is under the influence, as opposed to waiting until later.

A CSO's success in carrying out this task is attributable, in part, to her or his ability to recognize when the IP is under the influence. If this topic has not been discussed yet, it would be necessary to do that now (see Chapter 5). Depending on the CSO's skills, you might deem it worthwhile to discuss this issue even if it was addressed already. Note that the guidelines for selecting a reward to withdraw (see Box 7.1) are incorporated into the dialogue for this sample case.

THERAPIST: Great! We'll focus on times when you can take away a reward right while Alex is still using or is high, because the procedure works best when there's no question as to why you're taking away a reward. And we've already established that you're good at detecting when he's using, so we won't review that.

Emphasize the importance of being consistent about withdrawing the reward when the IP uses <u>and</u> reintroducing it when the IP is not using.

THERAPIST: Another thing to keep in mind as we move ahead is that it will be important to be *consistent* in withdrawing the reward if Alex uses. This might end up being hard to

BOX 7.1

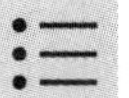

Selection of a Reward to Withdraw Guidelines

The reward being taken away should be one that the CSO:

- Can withdraw close in time to when the IP is using.
- Is willing to consistently withdraw when the IP is using and reintroduce when the IP stops using again.
- Finds relatively easy and safe to withdraw.
- Believes the IP values and will miss.

do at times, like if you and Alex are having fun and you don't want to spoil the mood. Also, the reward should be something that you'll be ready to reintroduce when he's not using. I'll help you with all of these things to remember though, so don't worry about that. I'll revisit these points once we figure out what the reward will be.

Note: The therapist mentions one of the most common reasons given by CSOs for not following the homework plan for the Withdrawing Rewards for Using Behavior procedure—namely, they did not want to spoil the good mood at the time. This issue should be raised as a potential obstacle later in the session when the assignment is being finalized for the week.

3. Plan for withdrawing an additional reward at times of IP use.

Identify a few common ongoing occasions in which the IP is using or under the influence in the CSO's presence.

Once you have a basic idea as to how the CSO unintentionally supports the IP's use at times, the next step is to investigate whether there are other occasions that might be more suitable to target for the Withdrawing Rewards for Using Behavior procedure, due to factors such as their high frequency of occurrence or the level of distress experienced by the CSO.

THERAPIST: We've been talking about the incident in the gym when Alex visited you while he was high, and where the extra attention he got from you might have felt rewarding to him. How often would you say that Alex visits you in the gym when he's high?

CSO: He probably visits every other week. Well, maybe a little more often. But those visits are nowhere near as bad as the one the other day that I just described.

THERAPIST: OK. Let's keep the gym situation in mind but consider another one, too. Is there another time when you and Alex are often together and he's high?

CSO: The one that happens the most, about three times a week, is when he joins me and my buddies during my lunch break. He's already high then, but I'm not sure the other workers can tell.

Explore whether the CSO's typical response to the IP's use on these occasions might be experienced by the IP as rewarding.

THERAPIST: Carlos, these are both good situations to explore further. As far as Alex's routine visits to the gym when he's high, what would you say is your normal reaction to him?

CSO: Good question (*pauses*). I guess I'm friendly, but mostly because I don't want to create a scene. I stop my workout for about 5 minutes and visit with him. Then he leaves.

THERAPIST: Do you think Alex finds that 5-minute conversation rewarding?

CSO: I don't know. Well, probably, because he keeps coming back for more.

THERAPIST: Exactly. It sounds like you're rewarding him in these other gym situations, too, but with smaller rewards than for the big incident the other day, because that's all the attention he's needed. And what about when he joins you for lunch when he's high?

CSO: I don't think I'm doing anything unusual. If he's high but is still functioning all right, he comes and sits with me and everyone at the large table. It's a pretty lively group. Seems pretty normal I guess. But sometimes I can tell from the way he's coming toward me when he arrives that I'd better move to a table for just the two of us because he's really "out of it."

THERAPIST: I absolutely agree that you aren't doing anything unusual here. But the important question is whether you're behaving in a way toward Alex when he's high at lunch that feels like a *reward* to him?

CSO: Maybe. It's hard to tell because he's always high when he joins me, so I don't know what to compare it to. But I *have* noticed that he seems to like eating with the larger group instead of just with me. I don't blame him—my coworkers can be really entertaining.

THERAPIST: That's interesting . . . and quite helpful. So you're already taking away the preferred reward of him eating lunch with all of your friends when he's really out of it, but it hasn't been enough to get him to reduce his substance use, right? Eating with you alone is still enough of a reward to him. We'll probably have to look at that, too, if we choose this lunch situation.

Note: The therapist helps the CSO see that his behavior toward the IP in these situations is experienced by the IP as rewarding, with some of the behaviors even more so than others.

Help the CSO select one of her or his common "rewarding behaviors" to withdraw in the upcoming week when the IP uses.

In order for you to assist CSOs in selecting rewards to withdraw, it might be helpful to view a number of examples (see Box 7.2). Therapists tend to find it useful to see the varying magnitudes of these rewards and the types of contexts in which they may occur.

THERAPIST: The lunch scene happens more often, so that might be good to focus on this week in terms of practicing how to withdraw a reward. Yet, either of these situations could work. What do you think?

CSO: The one that's been bothering me the most is Alex coming to lunch high. I've asked him again and again not to do it, but he keeps doing it anyway. I'm not sure what I'm supposed to do though if he comes to lunch high again. I mean, I know I shouldn't let him sit down and have lunch with us, but I'm not sure what that will look like.

THERAPIST: Don't worry; we'll sort that out in a minute. And this situation is in line with what I mentioned earlier about being able to take the reward away right at the time Alex is using, and then reintroducing it when he's not using. So that's good.

Have the CSO describe exactly what the new behavior of withdrawing the reward will look like.

It might be worthwhile to have CSOs stop for a moment and imagine themselves in the exact situation under scrutiny (perhaps even to close their eyes while imagining it). See what ideas pop into their head as they try to picture themselves behaving in a way that is different from their typical response to their IP. If this does not help generate useful ideas regarding a new way to behave in that situation, you could introduce (or reintroduce) the Problem Solving procedure (see Chapter 9).

BOX 7.2

Examples of Common Rewards to Withdraw

- A 35-year-old mother (CSO) of two small children lives next door to her father (IP). The CSO regularly welcomes the IP into her house after dinner to watch TV with the children or to read them a story. The CSO has noticed that the IP is acting like he is taking too much pain medication, and yet he denies it. The CSO tells the IP that he is welcome to join her family after dinner only if he has not taken more than the recommended dose of his pain medication.

- A 60-year-old man (CSO) golfs with a group of friends weekly. He routinely invites his brother (IP) to join them, but lately the IP has had a few drinks prior to the CSO picking him up, and he has several more drinks while on the course. The CSO informs the IP that he is welcome to join future golf outings only if he does not drink that day.

- A mother (CSO) recently bought her 12-year-old son (IP) a new laptop that he loves to use for playing computer games. The CSO has spoken to the IP a number of times about coming home from school smelling like marijuana. She tells him that he will no longer be allowed to use the laptop on the days that he arrives home smelling like marijuana.

- A husband (CSO) and his wife (IP) have always enjoyed Sunday brunch at his parents' house. The CSO has discussed with the IP his concern over her attending brunch when she has been using. The CSO tells the IP that she will be welcome to join him for Sunday brunch only if she is not under the influence of any drugs.

THERAPIST: Let's work out the details now. Try to picture yourself carrying this out: *not* letting Alex join you for lunch if he shows up high. What can you picture yourself doing? Feel free to close your eyes if it helps to see this clearly.

CSO: It seems obvious that I should tell him in the morning that he can't join me for lunch that day if he's high. But I've done that before and it doesn't work.

THERAPIST: Telling him in advance is a good start, so we'll practice using your new positive communication skills as you prepare to go home and tell him. But since this hasn't been enough to get him to change *his* behavior, what else can you do to change *your* behavior? Specifically, what can you do differently the next time he shows up high for lunch? And let's assume it would be good for you to try something other than simply eating with him alone when he's high, as that hasn't really been a deterrent either.

Note: The therapist stresses the importance of coming up with a *new* CSO response while also supporting the notion of the CSO telling the IP about the plan in advance (using positive communication skills).

CSO: I can't just insist that he leave. That would be embarrassing for both of us.

THERAPIST: Can you say more about that? Why would that be embarrassing?

CSO: Because then all of my coworkers would know about Alex's drug problem, if they don't already, *and* they'd know we're having problems because of it. It's nobody's business.

THERAPIST: Fair enough. So what are your options for dealing with this? For instance, is there a way to respond that doesn't let your coworkers know your business?

CSO: I guess when I see Alex coming toward me I could walk over and meet him. I'd be able to tell if he was high or not. If he *is*, maybe I could ask him to walk with me back to the street? As we're walking, I'd remind him about what I'd told him that morning. He'd be mad and just leave.

THERAPIST: It sounds like a decent plan to me so far. We have a few things to sort out yet.

Make sure the reward will be relatively easy to withdraw and address anticipated barriers.

THERAPIST: We'll still need to work through some of the barriers to pulling this off, just like with any assignment. If it turns out to be too complicated, we should try something else. So as you think about how you'll carry this out, what might get in the way?

CSO: As long as I warn him in advance, maybe both the night before *and* that morning, I can picture myself doing this—I think.

THERAPIST: What's your biggest concern?

CSO: That I'll feel bad turning him away.

THERAPIST: And how will you deal with that?

CSO: I'll remind myself as I'm walking toward him that I'm doing this because I love him, and that it might be hard at first, but that it should make things better in the long run.

THERAPIST: Impressive! And right on target. What else might prevent you from following through with this?

CSO: Nothing really. It's all up to me.

Note: As with any assignment, the therapist checks for barriers and is ready to help with developing solutions (see Homework Assignment Guidelines in Chapter 3, Box 3.1).

Check that the selected reward is something the IP will miss once withdrawn.

THERAPIST: Based on what you've said already, I think I know the answer to this important question: Does Alex value this reward of joining you for lunch enough that it will matter to him when it's taken away? Will he really miss it? Will it make an impression on him?

CSO: No question. He won't believe I'm serious about it at first. Then he'll be pissed.

Ask how the CSO feels about withdrawing the reward on a consistent basis.

THERAPIST: And what do you think it will be like to keep this up? It will be very important to be consistent in your message: If he gets high, he can't join you and your coworkers for lunch. Period. You know the old saying: If you give him an inch. . . .

CSO: I don't know. If it doesn't start working right away, I might wonder if it's worth bothering with it. But I need to do something different.

THERAPIST: And as always, we'll talk about how things went with the assignment as we start each session. I can help you troubleshoot if necessary.

4. Address potential problems created by withdrawing the reward.

Explore and address potential problems that might arise upon withdrawing the reward.

THERAPIST: Carlos, let's assume you followed through with your plan. You walked over to Alex as he was approaching you at lunchtime, and when you saw that he was high, you walked him back to the street. I know we haven't worked out the wording yet, but let's assume you told him why you were doing this. What kind of new problems might this create for you, either right then or later? For example, you said a few minutes ago that he'll be pissed?

CSO: Definitely. But he won't make a scene. He'll just leave. And then I'll get the silent treatment for a while. I can deal with that though.

THERAPIST: Are there any *other* ways in which your life could be harder for a while, once you follow through with this plan?

CSO: If Alex isn't speaking to me for a few days, it will make meals awkward.

THERAPIST: True. But since meals will be awkward for him, too, can you see why it would be important *not* to give up on your plan?

CSO. Yes. I can deal with it. I'm not worried.

Note: The therapist reminds the CSO of the importance of consistently adhering to the plan to withdraw rewards despite any problems created by the plan itself.

Specifically discuss possible safety/violence concerns and develop a plan if necessary.

THERAPIST: It might sound like I'm harping on this, but I just want to check again about any safety concerns as a result of this change in your behavior. You said Alex will be pissed when you escort him away, but that he'll just leave. Any chance at all that he might get violent at any point?

CSO: Nope. We're good.

Remind the CSO to use CRAFT problem-solving skills when needed.

THERAPIST: And don't forget that you can resort to your problem-solving exercise if you get stumped and need ideas.

Note: The therapist refers to the Problem Solving procedure (Chapter 9). In this case, the assumption was that it had already been taught to the CSO.

5. Discuss how to explain to the IP the reason for withdrawing the reward.

Many CSOs feel uncomfortable "surprising" their IP by suddenly withdrawing a reward without any warning, and thus it is common for them to tell their IPs *in advance* about the plan to withdraw a reward if the IP engages in substance use. However, some CSOs prefer to wait until after they have withdrawn a reward (in response to the IP's substance use) before they explain the reason for its withdrawal. The timing of this message is key; it should be delivered when the IP is no longer under the influence of any substances (e.g., the next day). And some CSOs choose to *never* explain why they withdrew a reward. Importantly, if there is any doubt as to whether a certain conversation with the IP (such as one regarding withdrawing rewards) might take place in the upcoming week: Conduct role plays to prepare nonetheless! Even if the conversation does not occur over the next few days, in all probability it will occur eventually.

Determine what the CSO will tell the IP about why a reward is being (or was) withdrawn.

Similar to the situation faced by CSOs when they need to determine what (if anything) they will tell their IP about why a reward is being *given* (see Chapter 5), planning for the withdrawal of a reward prompts the same discussion. In fact, most of the common conversation options are available in both situations (and also are referred to in Chapter 8, Allowing for Natural, Negative Consequences). Withdrawing a reward can entail:

- Saying nothing, and watching to see whether the IP's substance-using behavior eventually decreases in response to the CSO withdrawing a reward when the IP is using.
- Explaining that withdrawing a reward is the CSO's effort to no longer support the IP's using behavior.
- Revealing that the CSO learned about withdrawing rewards in therapy.
- Responding to inquiries about the CSO's therapy by inviting the IP to sample treatment.

THERAPIST: From what you've said before, it sounds like you're going to tell Alex ahead of time about your plan to not let him join you and your coworkers for lunch if he's high.

CSO: Right. I don't want to surprise him with the whole lunch thing.

THERAPIST: Sounds good. So now the question is whether you're going to tell him *why* you're suddenly changing your behavior? Did you have something in mind?

CSO: Not really. I guess I'll just say that I have to try something different because he won't listen to me.

THERAPIST: All right. In a minute we'll practice that conversation using your newly learned positive communication skills. Let me ask you though: Do you think this might be a good time to tell Alex that you're in therapy, and why? Or if the timing seems right, which we can talk about, you could even go one step further and invite him to attend treatment. We'd definitely work on the wording for either of these options though.

CSO: I wasn't planning on telling him that I'm in therapy yet, but it might come up anyway.

THERAPIST: If there's a chance it might come up, it would be a good idea for us to practice what you'll say.

CSO: OK. But I'm not making any promises that I'll bring it up this week.

Engage in a role play that incorporates positive communication skills when explaining to the IP why a reward is being (or was) withdrawn.

In all likelihood, the CSO already will have learned positive communication skills. Depending on the CSO's skill level, you would decide whether to proceed with the role play by simply reminding the CSO to incorporate the skills, or by reviewing the skills more extensively before starting the practice. As always, refer to the Positive Communication Guidelines and Role-Play ("Practicing") Guidelines (Chapter 4, Boxes 4.1 and 4.4).

THERAPIST: For this practice conversation that we'll do in a minute, see if you can use a few of the parts of positive communication that you learned last week. I know you really seemed to like the "understanding statement" and the "offer to help." Do you have some idea as to how you could use these in your conversation with Alex?

CSO: I think I'll start with the "understanding statement." I'm not sure about the rest. I'll confuse myself if I try to plan too much of it out.

THERAPIST: Fair enough. I'll start off our practice conversation. I'm playing Alex.

CSO: OK. Ready or not, I guess!

Note: In line with the Role-Play ("Practicing") Guidelines (Chapter 4, Box 4.4), the therapist initiates the role play. This effectively circumvents a potential conversation with an anxious CSO as to whether a role play is needed in the first place.

THERAPIST (*as Alex*): Uh-oh. You've got that serious look of yours. What did I do wrong this time?

CSO (*in role play*): I guess it *is* my serious expression. I want to talk about you coming to see me at lunchtime when you're high.

THERAPIST (*as Alex*): *That* again? I don't do it that much.

CSO (*in role play*): You don't come every day anymore, but you *do* still come a couple of times each week. And you're high each time.

THERAPIST (*as Alex*): There's *no* way your friends at work can tell, so what do you care?

CSO (*in role play*): I can understand why it might not seem like it's important, but it matters to *me*. And I've asked you again and again not to show up high. So from now on I'm going to take you aside and ask you to leave if you show up high. That's it. I'm serious. But if there's some way I can help so that you can join me for lunch without being high, you should tell me.

THERAPIST (*as Alex*): Where the heck is all of this coming from?

CSO (*in role play*): I've been talking to someone about you being high all the time. It's really been bothering me. This person has given me some ideas about what to do.

THERAPIST (*as Alex*): Who? And why are you talking to somebody about our business? *You're* always the private one!

CSO (*in role play*): This is different because this person is a therapist.

THERAPIST: Bravo! Let's stop the role play here, and start the discussion by you telling me what you liked about how you did. And in case you haven't mentioned them, we'll then see which of the positive communication components you used, and which ones you might want to add when we repeat the practice.

Note: Since CSOs tend to talk in general terms about "how they did" when they review their own conversations, the therapist deliberately mentions the components of positive communication. This reinforces the idea that the CSO should be using these components *and* be able to identify them. It also paves the way for the therapist to suggest specific ideas for improving the conversation when the role play is repeated.

CSO: I tried to use a couple of them, but I'm not sure how they came across.

THERAPIST: I thought you did very well, especially since this was your first attempt. And speaking of which: Your first attempt at revealing to Alex that you're in therapy was very good. I can offer some pointers on how to make that part of the conversation smoother and hopefully more effective, but we'll get to that later.

Note: The therapist would then offer specific suggestions for the remainder of the debriefing for this particular role play. It would entail discussing whether the CSO:

- Would consider moving his understanding statement (number 5 on the Positive Communication Guidelines list; Chapter 4, Box 4.1) to the start of the conversation in an effort to reduce the IP's defensiveness.
- Could incorporate additional positive communication elements:
  - Accept partial responsibility (Positive Communication Guideline 6) for not taking a clear stance sooner about the IP needing to leave if he showed up at lunch high.
  - Add a feelings statement (Positive Communication Guideline 4) to clarify what "it matters to me" means.
  - Use positive wording (Positive Communication Guideline 2) by saying what he loves about the IP on those visits when he is clearly substance-free.
- Would be willing to revise his wording when revealing that he is in therapy, such as by saying the therapy is for *their relationship* instead of explicitly stating it is for the IP's substance use problem (see Chapter 11).
- Would like to revisit the idea of inviting the IP to enter treatment, and if so, whether this would be a good time to do so (see Chapter 11).
- Could envision having a rather similar conversation if he had already withdrawn the reward (due to the IP's substance use) *and* the IP was no longer under the influence of alcohol or drugs.

The role play would be repeated at least two more times, with the therapist playing an increasingly more defensive IP as a way to simulate a real-life conversation and to challenge the CSO to put his new skills into practice. For additional sample conversations that might be helpful for either you *or* CSOs, see Handout 7.1, Using Positive Communication to Explain the Withdrawal of Rewards (Examples), found at the end of this chapter. For suggestions regarding the permanent removal of large rewards, see Box 7.3.

Discuss the time or occasion for having the conversation.

It is important to remind CSOs to follow through with the planned conversation with their IPs at the predetermined "ideal" time. Primarily this means avoiding times when IPs are under the influence of substances. Not only will IPs have difficulty processing CSOs' conversations at such times, but CSOs frequently go "off script" and react angrily

BOX 7.3

Permanent Removal of Large Rewards

This chapter focuses on the withdrawal of rewards that will be reintroduced at times when the IP is not using. However, in some cases, CSOs are advised to consider withdrawing "larger" rewards permanently, or at least until a period of non-use has been demonstrated for a considerable period of time. These recommendations might be introduced if an IP has not responded favorably to several other CRAFT-guided CSO attempts to get the IP to reduce or stop the using behavior, or if the IP's continued use has significant negative ramifications for the CSO's own well-being (e.g., job, health). Since more serious negative consequences are associated with the removal of larger rewards, CSOs understandably will have concerns that must be addressed. For example, note that in each sample case (below), the CSO gave the IP a reasonable amount of "notice" before the planned permanent removal of the large reward (job, housing)—time that theoretically would allow the IP to "turn around" his or her behavior and be successful.

- A dad (CSO) hired his 22-year-old son (IP) to work as an assistant in his auto body shop. The IP's marijuana use has been affecting his work performance. Since the CSO's feedback has not improved the situation, he feels the need to fire his son. The CSO gives his son 4 weeks' notice so that he has the opportunity to pass a drug test when he interviews for another job. The CSO is hopeful that his son will be motivated to reduce his smoking, given that a nonrelative employer will not tolerate his drug-related poor performance for as long a period of time as the dad did.
- An older sister (CSO) has been allowing her 30-year-old younger sister (IP) to stay in the guest room for several months while the IP earns enough money to afford her own apartment. The IP has been assuring the CSO that her "partying" is under control, and yet the IP appears to be high multiple times a week. The IP's substance use has been interfering with her plan to pick up extra shifts at work. The CSO informs the IP that she must move out in 2 weeks. The CSO is counting on this deadline to serve as an impetus for the IP to reduce her partying and to work more shifts. The CSO knows that if the IP does not have enough money for a new place in 2 weeks, she will be forced to crash on a friend's couch until she does.

as opposed to following the carefully rehearsed positive conversation. As a result, the goal of the communication is not achieved typically.

THERAPIST: Thanks for hanging in there and going over your planned conversation a few times. It's sounding really good. Now we have to nail down when and where you'll have this discussion.

CSO: He's probably going to stop by work tomorrow, so I'd better talk to him tonight.

THERAPIST: Will you be able to catch him before he's high tonight? As we've discussed before, it's always best to have these conversations when your loved one isn't high or somehow under the influence.

CSO: I think he'll be OK if I talk to him as soon as I get home from work.

THERAPIST: Good. One final thing: Let's talk about things that might get in the way of you actually having that conversation before dinner tonight, and what a good backup plan might be.

COMMON PROBLEMS TO AVOID

Withdrawing Rewards for Using Behavior is one of CRAFT's main "negative consequence" procedures, and by its very nature it is somewhat uncomfortable for therapists to introduce and for CSOs to implement. A few suggestions for therapists are covered below.

Problem: Although it is true that therapists should select the most appropriate CRAFT procedures to introduce on the basis of their clients' needs, some therapists rarely use the Withdrawing Rewards for Using Behavior procedure. These therapists essentially report that CSOs prefer to reward IP behavior as opposed to removing rewards, and therefore they are reluctant to promote it.

Safeguards:

- You routinely should ask yourself whether you are avoiding using certain procedures, and if so, why? Giving rewards (for non-using behavior) and withdrawing rewards (for substance use) are *both* essential components of the CRAFT program.
- If you only rarely use the Withdrawing Rewards for Using Behavior procedure, you will likely introduce it somewhat reluctantly and without confidence when you *do* use it. Then you will be more apt to face CSOs who resist the procedure as a result. Therefore, it is important to review the rationale for the procedure for your own edification, and to carefully rehearse its delivery.

Problem: Some clinicians immediately drop their request for CSOs to do a role play of a conversation about the plan to withdraw a reward if the CSOs state that they have no intention of telling their IP about the plan in advance (or at all). This decision on the part of clinicians is problematic, given that many CSOs *do* end up telling their IP regardless. Without role-playing the conversation in advance during a session, the real-life conversation tends to proceed in a less than ideal fashion.

Safeguards:

- Simply present the role play as the next step in the Withdrawing Rewards for Using Behavior procedure that you are teaching. Assure CSOs that the topic is bound to come up sooner or later with their IP, and so it is best to have practiced what they will say.
- Ask yourself whether *you* are actively avoiding role plays, or if you routinely seem to run short on time in sessions to do them. It is worth examining any reluctance on your own part to do role plays, and to practice them with a trusted colleague.

Problem: Clinicians sometimes do not ask follow-up questions when CSOs report that they had the conversation with their IP about *why* they were withdrawing a reward, but their conversation *and* the actual implementation of the withdrawing rewards task did not go particularly well. Determining exactly what happened and where the assignment went wrong is crucial for future planning.

Safeguards:

- Always assume that homework assignments, particularly "unsuccessful" ones, require follow-up. Simply plan on beginning this discussion by asking CSOs whether they had the conversation *at the designated time*. Often CSOs state that they did *not*—instead, they delivered a variation of the rehearsed conversation at a time when the IP did something that upset them. As one can imagine, the resulting conversation was not a good example of positive communication.
- Another type of automatic follow-up for an assignment that involved a conversation is to ask CSOs to demonstrate the wording they used. The problem in the delivery of the communication often becomes readily apparent. For instance, you might witness CSOs only half-heartedly conveying the message about withdrawing rewards. Upon further inquiry, the CSOs conceivably could confess that they were reluctant to spoil the day because their IP was in a good mood, or the CSOs were unsure as to whether they wanted to follow through with the reward withdrawal anyway. Not surprisingly, CSOs who have conversations such as these with their IPs about the Withdrawing Rewards for Using Behavior procedure often experience difficulty in their implementation.

SUMMARY

The Withdrawing Rewards for Using Behavior strategy in this chapter goes hand-in-hand with the CRAFT procedure for Rewarding Non-Using Behavior (Chapter 5). Withdrawing Rewards for Using Behavior is the first of two CRAFT procedures that teaches CSOs how to skillfully pair negative consequences with their IP's substance use. Although CSOs tend to agree in theory with the idea of helping their IPs experience negative consequences when using substances, nonetheless many CSOs still have trouble carrying out these plans for a variety of reasons. Thus, additional therapist support and guidance are required. The next chapter presents the second of these CRAFT procedures that links negative consequences with the IP's substance-using behavior.

FORM 7.1

Withdrawing Rewards for Using Behavior: Checklist

1. Discuss the CSO's current response to the IP's substance use and the outcome.

- ☐ a. Ask the CSO how she or he currently responds to the IP's substance use in an ongoing situation.
- ☐ b. Ask what the CSO thought the impact of her or his response was on the IP's substance use behavior, and whether it seemed problematic.
- ☐ c. Explain that sometimes CSOs accidentally reward their IP's substance use behavior.
- ☐ d. Explore the CSO's feelings about the idea of accidentally rewarding the IP's substance use behavior.

2. Stress the importance of withdrawing a planned reward if the IP uses.

- ☐ a. Give a rationale for withdrawing the reward if the IP uses.
- ☐ b. Explain that it works best to withdraw rewards right while the IP is using or is under the influence, as opposed to waiting until later.
- ☐ c. Emphasize the importance of being consistent about withdrawing the reward when the IP uses *and* reintroducing it when the IP is not using.

3. Plan for withdrawing an additional reward at times of IP use.

- ☐ a. Identify a few common ongoing occasions in which the IP is using or under the influence in the CSO's presence.
- ☐ b. Explore whether the CSO's typical response to the IP's use on these occasions might be experienced by the IP as rewarding.
- ☐ c. Help the CSO select one of her or his common "rewarding behaviors" to withdraw in the upcoming week when the IP uses.
- ☐ d. Have the CSO describe exactly what the new behavior of withdrawing the reward will look like.
- ☐ e. Make sure the reward will be relatively easy to withdraw and address anticipated barriers.
- ☐ f. Check that the selected reward is something the IP will miss once withdrawn.
- ☐ g. Ask how the CSO feels about withdrawing the reward on a consistent basis.

(continued)

4. Address potential problems created by withdrawing the reward.

- ☐ a. Explore and address potential problems that might arise upon withdrawing the reward.
- ☐ b. Specifically discuss possible safety/violence concerns and develop a plan if necessary.
- ☐ c. Remind the CSO to use CRAFT problem-solving skills when needed.

5. Discuss how to explain to the IP the reason for withdrawing the reward.

- ☐ a. Determine what the CSO will tell the IP about *why* a reward is being (or was) withdrawn.
- ☐ b. Engage in a role play that incorporates positive communication skills when explaining to the IP why a reward is being (or was) withdrawn.
- ☐ c. Discuss the time or occasion for having the conversation.

HANDOUT 7.1

Using Positive Communication to Explain the Withdrawal of Rewards (Examples)

1. Be brief (uncomplicated).
2. Use positive/action-oriented wording (indicating what you would like to see happen).
3. Mention specific behaviors.
4. Label your feelings.
5. Offer an understanding statement.
6. Accept partial responsibility (for something related to the problem situation, *not* for the substance use).
7. Offer to help.

Note: The number of the positive communication guideline used in the examples below is in brackets.

Example 1: The Concerned Significant Other (CSO) is the partner of an Identified Patient (IP; treatment refuser) who misuses a variety of drugs. The IP has lost his job recently, and so regularly visits the CSO at his workplace at lunchtime:

CSO: "I know you like joining me for lunch [5], and I love it when you do, too [4], but only when you haven't been using [3]. I know it's partly my fault because I've been giving you mixed signals about whether it's OK to visit when you're high [6]. From now on I'll ask you to leave if you arrive high. In the meantime, I'm wondering if there's something specific I can do to make it easier for you to still visit often, but only when you're not under the influence [1, 7]."

Example 2: The CSO is the sister of a 55-year-old woman who misuses marijuana (IP). The IP enjoys assisting the CSO in the running of a small shop on weekends:

CSO: "I love it when you work with me on weekends, because it gives us time to catch up [1, 3, 4]. And I'm sure you're probably right that it makes it less stressful for you if you're high when the shop gets busy some afternoons [5]. But I'm really uncomfortable having you in the shop with me after you've been smoking [3, 4], so I'm now asking you to stay home if you *have* been [1]. I probably should have mentioned how I felt sooner [6]. I'd *really* love to have you keep coming in though [4]. What if we look for some other ways to help you stay relaxed when the store gets busy [2, 7]?"

(continued)

Example 3: The CSO is the father of a 21-year-old young man who misuses alcohol (IP). The IP has always enjoyed going with his dad up into the mountains to fish or hunt, but for the last few fishing trips the son has insisted on bringing alcohol and drinking throughout the day.

CSO: "I think you know how much I've always enjoyed your company when I go fishing or hunting [4]. But I'm not happy with you bringing beer now, because like I've said before, it has gotten out of hand [1, 4]. Maybe it was wrong for me to bring beer for myself all those times when you were little [6]. Anyway, I know you're 21 now and it's fun to drink. I remember turning 21 [5]. But since I'm worried about your drinking in general, I think it's important for us to go out on the streams and have a good time without beer [2]. I'm serious about this, so I'm asking you to sit it out next time if you show up with alcohol or you've been drinking already [1, 3]. Maybe it will help if I bring a bunch of other kinds of things to drink [7]?"

Chapter 8

Allowing for Natural, Negative Consequences of Use

In Chapter 7, on withdrawing rewards, we pointed out that the positive reinforcement of the IP's substance-free behavior often needs to be supplemented with the appropriate use of negative consequences for IP substance use. This chapter focuses on a CRAFT procedure called Allowing for Natural, Negative Consequences of Use. It entails having CSOs examine their current immediate responses to their IP's using behavior, and deciding whether that particular CSO behavior might, in fact, be making it a little easier for the IP to continue using. If so, interested CSOs are assisted in developing a plan in which they refrain from engaging in a behavior that appears to be "taking care of" their IP in the short term (e.g., helping an inebriated IP up the stairs and into bed), but inadvertently is facilitating substance use overall. As noted in Chapter 5, the popular term for this type of CSO behavior is "enabling," but CRAFT traditionally steers clear of this word because it can be pejorative, and because it often is used incorrectly to more broadly describe CSOs' use of rewards for *non-using* IP behavior as well (which CRAFT explicitly encourages).

When clinicians introduce this particular procedure, it frequently evokes strong reactions from CSOs. Despite CRAFT therapists' reliance on a nonjudgmental and supportive style, CSOs sometimes think the therapist is blaming them for the IP's use, whereas other CSOs automatically blame themselves when enabling behaviors are discussed. Many CSOs feel helpless because they do not readily see any alternatives to how they have been responding to the IP in these situations. Other CSOs express doubt that changing their behavior (such as by *not* stepping in to take care of a problem created by the substance use) will serve as a deterrent to the IP's drinking or drug use. Finally, some CSOs simply express concern over behaving in a way that might upset their IP. Regardless, if you have good clinical skills, you should be able to address these concerns and move forward with this important procedure.

THE BASICS

General Description

CRAFT's procedure for Allowing for Natural, Negative Consequences of Use begins with a gentle explanation of how CSOs in general may unintentionally support their IP's substance-using behavior at times. The procedure moves to an exploration of the CSO's *own* such behavior. CSOs' strong reactions to this notion are processed while blame is minimized. Possible CSO behaviors to target (i.e., CSO behaviors to *stop* doing) are discussed, and ultimately one is tentatively selected for this exercise.

A significant amount of time is spent exploring whether CSOs can picture themselves following through with this change in their behavior, and whether the behavior change will be experienced as negative by their IP *and* linked to the substance use. New problems that might be created for CSOs as a result of these behavior changes are considered very carefully, and if these hardships are significant such that they outweigh the potential gain if the procedure succeeds, then a different behavior that allows for the natural consequences of the IP's use is selected and scrutinized. Importantly, communication skills are reviewed and practiced so that CSOs are prepared to explain to their IPs *why* they suddenly have changed their immediate responses to the substance-using behavior. Finally, CSOs are reassured that although this one intervention certainly will not solve the drinking or drug problem, in all probability it *will* be noticed by the IP and the effect *can* be quite profound (especially with repetitions over time).

Procedure Timing

Allowing for Natural, Negative Consequences of Use commonly is introduced somewhat later in the series of CRAFT procedures, as it is helpful for you to already have discussed reinforcement principles, such as within the Rewarding Non-Using Behavior procedure. Also, it is preferable for CSOs to have learned communication skills so that they can offer the rationale for their new behavior in a positive manner. As explained earlier, CSOs often have rather strong negative reactions upon first hearing about this procedure, so it is worthwhile for you to have had ample time to establish good rapport before suggesting that it be tackled.

Form

- Allowing for Natural, Negative Consequences of Use: Checklist (Form 8.1)

CLINICIAN GUIDANCE AND SAMPLE DIALOGUE

The components for the CRAFT procedure that allows for IPs to experience natural, negative consequences of their use are presented below. A sample case is again included. The components for conducting this exercise are outlined in Form 8.1, Allowing for Natural, Negative Consequences of Use: Checklist.

Case Description

The CSO (Charlie) is the 66-year-old husband of the 62-year-old IP (Kate). Each individual identifies as non-Hispanic white. This is the second marriage for both Charlie and Kate; they have been married for 12 years. Kate has a grown daughter by her first husband, and two grandchildren, ages 6 and 3. Alcohol routinely played a small role in both

Charlie's and Kate's lives during the first 11 years of their marriage. Upon retiring from an administrative assistant job she had held for 34 years, Kate increased her alcohol consumption considerably. Her occasional nights out with a few female friends grew into late evenings 3 nights a week, and marijuana smoking became part of those evenings as well. Kate's inability to get up some mornings to babysit her youngest grandchild prompted the CSO to seek CRAFT treatment.

1. Offer common examples of CSOs' unintentional support of substance use and the resulting consequences.

Explain how it is common for CSOs to support their IP's substance use unintentionally.

THERAPIST: Individuals like yourself who are extremely worried about their loved one's drinking or drug use often go out of their way to protect their loved one from any negative consequences of the substance use. It's totally understandable because it sidesteps immediate problems, but in the long run it *unintentionally* makes it a little easier for the person to keep using substances.

Describe one or two examples of unintentional support of an IP's substance use that result from blocking the negative consequences of the use.

It is useful to give CSOs a few concrete examples of how CSOs "block" the negative consequences of their IP's substance use and the way this behavior inadvertently supports the drinking or drug use.

THERAPIST: Let me give you a few examples of what I mean by "unintentional support" of a loved one's substance use. Let's say a mother calls her teenage son's wrestling coach to say he's sick when, in fact, he's sleeping off a night of partying. The mom has unintentionally made it a little easier for her son to keep up the partying, since she's stepped in and reduced the likelihood that he'll get cut from the wrestling team as a result of his substance use. Or consider a wife who cleans up her husband's mess after he gets home late from a night of drinking and vomits in the bathroom. The bathroom is more tolerable the next morning, but the "price" is that the husband doesn't have to deal with the cleaning, and the embarrassment, himself. It makes it more likely that he'll drink heavily again.

2. Explore the CSO's unintentional support of the IP's substance-using behavior.

Ask whether the CSO may sometimes be supporting the IP's substance use unintentionally.

THERAPIST: Charlie, what do you think? Is it possible that you're doing something similar with your wife periodically? Do you think you might be stepping in and doing things to prevent problems from happening when she's been out drinking?

CSO: You've got me wondering if that's what I'm doing when I take charge of the babysitting of our granddaughter on the mornings when Kate can't get out of bed. I'm not sure I have a choice though. My granddaughter is only 3.

Ask the CSO to describe in some detail an example of her or his own behavior that might result in unintentional support of the IP's substance use.

THERAPIST: You might *not* have a choice in that situation, or in others for that matter, but it's worth taking a look. Can you give me a few details about what happens on those mornings?

CSO: Kate won't get out of bed on time even though she knows it's our day to babysit. I guess she knows I'll handle things. Anyway, her daughter drops little Tillie off at 8:00. I get her some breakfast and then try to keep her entertained until my wife joins us at about 9:30.

THERAPIST: Do you say anything to Kate's daughter about where her mom is when she drops off Tillie?

CSO: I usually just say she didn't sleep well, or that she's still getting dressed. I don't know if she's suspicious or not. But I guess I can see your point—I *am* making it easier for Kate to sleep it off. I'm just not sure what my options are.

THERAPIST: We'll talk about this situation more in a few minutes. Maybe it will turn out that it's *not* a good one to focus on in terms of you changing your behavior.

Reassure the CSO that she or he is not at fault for engaging in this type of behavior.

THERAPIST: I know I've said this before, but it's worth repeating: It's not your fault that your wife is drinking. Notice that I've been talking about ways in which people *unintentionally* support their loved one's substance use. If we find some things you're doing that might be making it a little easier for Kate to keep drinking, we'll come up with a plan for addressing them. Just by being here in therapy I know you're going out of your way to take care of your wife—you can't be blamed if some of the things you've tried at home haven't worked.

3. Discuss how to change a particular CSO behavior in order to allow for the natural, negative consequences of substance use.

Help select a CSO behavior to change in order to allow for the natural consequences.

There are several ways you can help identify a suitable CSO behavior to target. For example, you can (a) refer back to comments made by the CSO earlier in the session (or on other occasions) when unintentional support of the IP's use was discussed, (b) ask specifically about the CSO's immediate and delayed responses to the IP's substance use and watch for behaviors that are blocking negative consequences, (c) refer to the already-completed FA (see Chapter 3, Form 3.2) and review the Negative Consequences column. Ask whether the CSO is doing anything to block or minimize the impact of these negative consequences, and (d) refer to the Positive Consequences column of the FA and ask whether the CSO is doing anything that might be allowing these "rewards" to be enhanced.

THERAPIST: I'd like to find a situation for which you'd be comfortable stepping back and allowing your wife to experience the natural consequences of her drinking. When we did your "road map" a few sessions ago, we outlined your wife's evenings out with her friends. And now you've mentioned again the mornings when you take charge of the babysitting while she sleeps in after these nights out, and you make excuses for Kate to her daughter. What are your thoughts as we consider possibly using this situation in which you've been taking over the babysitting?

CSO: I don't know about that one. If I'm *not* going to watch Tillie until my wife eventually gets up, I'd either have to drag Kate out of bed or tell her daughter not to bring over Tillie that morning. Her daughter would want to know why. Plus, she'd have to find another sitter at the last minute. It sounds really complicated. Or I guess I could keep babysitting but stop making excuses to Kate's daughter. Not sure I like that option either.

THERAPIST: Yes, it does sound like a complicated thing to pull off. Of course, ideally your wife would be told about your plan in advance, and as a result she'd limit her drinking the night before. But we can't assume everything will work as planned, especially in the beginning. And we haven't discussed whether you'll tell your wife in advance about the plan. But for now, can you tell me what else bothers you about using this situation to try out allowing for natural consequences?

Note: The therapist refers to the drinking episode that was used for the road map (see the discussion of FA, back in Chapter 3), as it already had been established that the episode was occurring frequently. Part of determining whether the CSO's standard response to this episode (i.e., letting his wife sleep in and making excuses for her to the daughter) would be suitable to target entails seeing whether the CSO can picture himself refraining from engaging in that behavior. There is no reason to devote considerable therapy time to planning for the allowance of negative consequences in a particular situation if it is clear from the onset that the CSO is unlikely to follow through.

CSO: I just can't imagine telling Kate's daughter that her mom is sleeping off a hangover and can't get up to take care of her grandchild. I can't do that to my wife, at least not yet.

THERAPIST: I appreciate your honesty. I'd rather know *now* that you can't picture yourself following through with this plan, than to have you report at our next session that you suspected all along you wouldn't be able to follow through. Let's find a different behavior to target. Keep in mind that we're looking for things you do that prevent Kate from experiencing the negative consequences of her drinking.

CSO: Maybe it's so automatic at this point that I don't even think about what I'm doing.

THERAPIST: That's totally understandable. Well, the first thing to decide is whether you want to stick with the common drinking episode we outlined for the road map exercise: your wife's midweek evenings out with her friends.

CSO: Yes, I think that makes the most sense, because they're causing the most problems.

THERAPIST: Maybe it will help if I pull out that road map while we're talking. In the meantime, why don't you walk me through the aftermath of one of those evenings again, and the next morning, too. And this time we'll make sure we pay attention to what *you're* doing at those times.

CSO: Sure. Well, she gets a ride home, usually from a ride service.

THERAPIST: That's very good to hear. As we start to think about which situation to pick, the most important thing to consider is whether changing a specific behavior of yours will put your wife, or anyone else, in harm's way. So at least we don't have to worry about Kate suddenly driving herself home. OK. What do you typically do when she gets home on those evenings?

Note: The therapist is on the alert for safety considerations.

CSO: She likes to talk when she first gets home. Even though she's pretty much "out of it," I sit and listen. After a little while she lies down on the couch and falls asleep. Then I go through this ritual of trying to rally her so that she can get up and go to bed. It's kind of a nuisance, to be honest. Sometimes I have to keep shaking her and pleading with her to get up for about 20 minutes. One night I gave up and left her there and went to bed. But then I felt bad and went back out in the middle of the night to get her up.

THERAPIST: What would happen if you didn't wake her up, if you just let her sleep there on the couch?

CSO: She'd probably still be on the couch in the morning. When she hears me in the kitchen she'd get up and go to the bedroom.

THERAPIST: Interesting. I'm thinking that this might be a good behavior for you to consider changing. What do you think? Can you picture yourself just letting her sleep on the couch once she dozes off there, and leaving her there for the entire night?

CSO: Maybe. It might be hard. But I think I see what you're getting at. Boy, I'm not sure how much it will help.

THERAPIST: I can see why you might be skeptical. We won't really know if it's working until you've given it a try for a while. The key is to be consistent and to do many repetitions over time. And it's also important to keep in mind that this is just one of many changes you're making in your behavior toward Kate. Altogether, these changes will build on one another and should have a powerful effect on her substance use.

Note: The therapist reminds the CSO about the importance of being consistent with the reward withdrawal, and of the fact that these small changes in CSO behavior can accumulate and grow in influence over time.

Make sure the IP will experience the natural consequences as negative and related to the substance use.

Guidelines for the selection of natural consequences to allow are found in Box 8.1, and several examples of natural consequences are in Box 8.2.

THERAPIST: Before we make any final decisions about which behavior of yours to change, I'd like to ask a few more questions about this tentative plan. You said your wife would probably sleep on the couch all night and then get up and go into the bedroom when she hears you in the morning. Would this be experienced by your wife as negative, or wouldn't it matter to her if she slept on the couch all night?

CSO: Oh, she wouldn't like it. She has her nightly "beauty regimen," as she calls it, and she wouldn't be able to do that if she didn't get ready for bed her normal way. Plus, she's complained about our couch being uncomfortable for naps, so I can't imagine

BOX 8.1

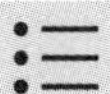

Selection of Natural Consequences to Allow Guidelines

The consequences being allowed to occur naturally should be:

- Experienced by the IP as negative and related to the substance use.
- Relatively easy for the CSO to allow.
- Discussed in terms of how the CSO feels about allowing them.
- Explored in the context of potentially creating other significant problems for the CSO.
- Considered safe to allow.
- Further scrutinized as the CSO practices how and when to communicate the rationale for this change in behavior to the IP.

BOX 8.2

Examples of Natural Consequences to Allow

These are samples of cases in which a therapist *might* work with the CSO to allow for the natural, negative consequences. As noted, many factors need to be considered before stepping back and allowing a consequence to occur. Caution should be exercised!

- A husband (IP) takes a car service home late each Saturday night after drinking heavily with his friends. The inebriated IP routinely heads to the den and starts blasting the TV, while spilling snacks and beer in the process. The wife (CSO) quickly ushers him into the bedroom so that he does not wake up the children and subject them to seeing their father in his loud and out-of-control state. She cleans up the mess in the den the next morning before anyone sees it. The natural consequence would be for the CSO to let her husband stay in the den watching TV until all hours, knowing that the children would come and find him, and to leave the food and beer mess for the IP to deal with in the morning.

- A 16-year-old daughter (IP) regularly heads over to a friend's house on Saturday and Sunday afternoons, supposedly to do homework. When she returns home in the evening she is clearly high. At least once a week she accidentally leaves her cell phone or some schoolwork at the friend's house, and she talks her mother (CSO) into driving her back there to retrieve it. The natural consequence would be for the mother to refuse to drive the daughter back to the friend's house, and as a result, the daughter would spend the evening without her cell phone, and would attend school the next day without some of her homework completed.

- A 24-year-old son (IP) lives with his father (CSO) and younger brother. The IP, who is the coach for his brother's soccer team, started getting high before games and showing up late. The CSO makes excuses for the IP and coaches the beginning of the games until the IP arrives. The natural consequence would be for the CSO to stop making excuses and coaching for the IP, knowing that the IP would be quite upset to find out that his team was left wondering where he was and having to start the game without a coach.

she'd make it through the night on it comfortably. And I know she'd just be embarrassed by the whole thing.

THERAPIST: The fact that your wife would probably experience a number of negative consequences if you did not wake her up on these nights bodes well for it being a good behavior of yours to change. Also, we'll need to be sure she figures out that you left her sleeping on the couch all night because of her substance use. We'll talk about that in a few minutes, but first I want to check on a couple of other things about this plan.

Make sure it will be relatively easy for the CSO to allow for the natural consequences.

THERAPIST: Charlie, can you give me an idea of how difficult it would be for you to pull this off?

CSO: I can't think of any practical problems. I might not feel the greatest at the time, but I can do it.

Discuss how the CSO feels about allowing for the natural consequences.

THERAPIST: I'm glad you brought up your feelings, because our feelings can be bigger barriers than anything else sometimes, right? Can you tell me what you mean when you say you might not feel the greatest at the time you do it?

CSO: I think it's going to be hard to just let her lie there on the couch and go up to bed myself. I feel like I should be taking care of her when she's not up to it. But at the same time, I know it isn't helping.

THERAPIST: Maybe a good way to think of it is that you *will* be taking care of her if you don't help her up to bed, because ultimately you'll be helping her reduce her drinking.

Note: The therapist reframes what it means for the CSO to be "taking care of" his wife.

4. Address potential problems in allowing for the natural consequences.

Explore and address potential problems that might arise when allowing for the natural consequences.

You should spend considerable time discussing the potential fallout for the CSO of allowing the natural consequences. For example, a natural consequence that resulted in the IP getting fired because the CSO stopped calling in "sick" for the IP with a hangover, would likely be an inappropriate natural consequence to allow if the IP was the primary wage earner for the family. If the potential fallout for the CSO is highly problematic, a different behavior should be selected for this exercise.

THERAPIST: Let's assume you go ahead and allow for the natural consequences: You go to bed yourself and let your wife sleep on the couch. What kinds of problems do you anticipate either later that night or the next day?

CSO: Kate will be upset with me and ask why I let her sleep on the couch all night. And then she might act distant for the rest of the day.

THERAPIST: That's understandable, given that it's a change in your normal behavior toward her, and in a way that she won't like. In a few minutes, we'll practice what you could say to her in response, because remember we *do* want her to realize that your new behavior is linked to her substance use. After we do that, you'll have to let me know whether you still want to follow through. What else might happen that could be a problem?

CSO: I guess there's a chance she'll still be asleep on the couch the next morning when her daughter arrives with Tillie.

THERAPIST: How will you handle that if it happens?

CSO: Her daughter is very good about ringing the doorbell, so it would give me time to wake her up before I answer the door. Would that be allowed? Would I wake her up or just let her sleep?

THERAPIST: I'm guessing that the more negative consequence would be to let her be awakened when her daughter and granddaughter arrive. Of course, we'd need to weigh that against your willingness to follow through with it, and any other problems it creates.

CSO: I just don't think I'm ready for that step. Maybe later, if this first plan doesn't work.

THERAPIST: Sounds good. What would you like to do then if Kate is still asleep and it's just about time for her daughter to be ringing the bell?

CSO: I think I'll watch the clock and make sure I get her up at least 20 minutes before her daughter typically arrives.

THERAPIST: Fair enough. We can always revisit that later.

Note: The therapist does not pressure the CSO to agree to the most negative consequence, given his misgivings about carrying it out. It is reasonable to start by allowing for a less negative consequence initially, and then escalating if necessary.

Specifically discuss possible safety/violence concerns and develop a plan if necessary.

THERAPIST: It's important for me to always check about any safety concerns whenever I'm talking with people about changing their behavior at home in a way that might upset their loved one. Is there a chance your wife will get so upset when you let her sleep on the couch that she'll get violent in some way?

CSO (*laughs*): No, she'll be upset, but she'd never be violent.

Remind the CSO to use CRAFT problem-solving skills when needed.

THERAPIST: If you *do* end up running into trouble finding a good solution for addressing your nervousness, keep in mind that you learned a problem-solving procedure. You could turn to that if you feel stuck.

CSO: Oh, I forgot about that. OK. I'll use it if I need it.

Note: The therapist is referring to the Problem Solving procedure we discuss in Chapter 9.

5. Discuss how to explain to the IP the reason for allowing the natural consequences.

One benefit of asking CSOs what they want to tell their IP about the change in behavior is that it makes the planned behavior more "real." As a result, CSOs' concerns about carrying out the behavior tend to come into focus. This is useful clinically, because you can help CSOs sort out their feelings, and can better address whether the planned behavior is reasonable and likely to happen. The CSOs' options for this conversation with their IP (should they decide to have it) essentially are the same as those listed for the Withdrawal of Rewards procedure (Chapter 7, "5. Discuss how to explain to the IP . . . "). And similar to the conversation associated with that procedure, this conversation could occur prior to the CSO allowing for the natural consequences (so as not to surprise the IP *and* to serve as a deterrent to the substance use), or after executing the procedure (in response to the IP's substance use) once the IP is no longer under the influence of alcohol or drugs.

Determine what the CSO will tell the IP about <u>why</u> the natural consequences are being (or were) allowed. This particular procedure, either when enacted by CSOs or just explained to their IP, is the one that most often prompts questions from curious (or annoyed) IPs. For instance, it is common for IPs to ask their CSOs *why* they are acting so differently at the time CSOs share their plans to start allowing the IP to experience the negative consequences of their substance use. You could suggest that CSOs consider disclosing that they are in therapy at these opportune times (see Chapter 11). Although a fair number of CSOs report not being ready to make this disclosure, many find themselves doing so nonetheless once they are in the midst of the actual conversation with their IP.

THERAPIST: Now we have to decide whether you're going to tell Kate *why* you're suddenly letting her sleep all night on the couch. And if you *do* want to tell her why, you need to decide *when* you're going to tell her.

CSO: I guess I was assuming I'd tell her something, but I'm not sure what or when. What do other people do in these situations?

THERAPIST: It varies. Some people feel most comfortable giving their loved one a heads-up so that the individual is forewarned and can possibly even reduce the substance use before any negative consequences are allowed for the first time. Others like to wait and see their loved one's reaction before saying anything.

CSO: It makes me nervous just thinking about telling Kate what I plan to do.

THERAPIST: What do you think your nervousness is about?

CSO: I don't want her to get mad, which she *will*. If I don't say anything in advance, I suppose it will force me to explain after the fact. But then maybe I won't feel pressured to let her sleep there. Help! I think I'd better tell her in advance.

THERAPIST: This is a big step for you, Charlie, so it's understandable that you'd be nervous, even though you are clearly taking this step out of love for your wife. I bet you could get your feelings across to Kate if you use the positive communication skills you've learned already. That should help her to hear your entire message about what you're planning to do and why. And you're probably tired of hearing me say this: You're more likely to get what you want if you use positive communication.

Note: The therapist assumes that this CSO, who is anxiously anticipating a difficult conversation with his wife, is not apt to be automatically thinking about using the positive communications skills he has learned. Therefore, the therapist first reminds the CSO that he has these skills at his disposal, and then provides an incentive to use them.

CSO: That's true. My conversation *will* sound better if I use some of those statements I've already practiced.

THERAPIST: Good. OK. We've established that you want to talk to your wife in advance about your new plan to let her sleep on the couch all night if she comes home from a night of drinking and falls asleep there. Can I assume you'll want to offer her some type of explanation as to *why* you're suddenly not going to wake her up?

CSO: Yes. I guess I have to come right out and tell her that I'm hoping it will make her think twice about drinking so much. Right? And I can remind her how I feel about her, while adding some of the positive communication statements I've learned.

Engage in a role play that incorporates positive communication skills when explaining to the IP why the natural consequences are being (or were) allowed.

Once again, a role play ensures that the CSO will be fully prepared to discuss the change in behavior toward her or his IP, in the event that the CSO decides to have that conversation. Refer to Chapter 4 for Positive Communication Guidelines (Box 4.1) and for Role-Play ("Practicing") Guidelines (Box 4.4).

THERAPIST: Let's practice that conversation with your wife now. I'll start it off.

CSO: Yes, it can't hurt.

THERAPIST (*as Kate*): What did you want to talk about, honey? Oh boy—that's not a happy expression on your face.

Note: As in previous case examples, the therapist jumps in and starts the role play to minimize the amount of time the CSO can devote to becoming anxious about his "performance," and to eliminate the question regarding whether a role play should even be conducted.

CSO (*in role play*): It's my serious expression, I guess. I want to talk with you about the habit we've gotten into on the nights you go out drinking with your friends.

THERAPIST (*as Kate*): Habit?

CSO (*in role play*): Most of those nights you come home and fall asleep on the couch. And then I get you up and help you get to bed. I probably should have mentioned this before; it takes me a *long* time to get you up, like around 20 minutes. If it happened just once in a while I suppose I wouldn't mind, but it's been happening a lot lately.

THERAPIST (*as Kate*): Well, *excuse me* for being an inconvenience (*sarcastic tone*).

CSO (*in role play*): I'm not trying to upset you. I know you need to get out and have fun with your friends. I'm just trying to figure out *my* role in all of this. I want to take good care of you, but I'm wondering if I'm doing this *too much* when you come home clearly "out of it." Maybe it's making it a little easier for you to keep coming home that way. So my plan is to let you sleep on the couch—to *not* wake you up.

THERAPIST (*as Kate*): You're just going to leave me there, even if I sleep there all night?

CSO (*in role play*): Yes. I feel like I need to do something different from what I've *been* doing when you've had a lot to drink. I guess what I'm saying is that I can't keep doing stuff that might be supporting your heavy drinking.

THERAPIST: Let's end the role play now. Terrific! What do you like about how you handled the conversation?

CSO: I think I did OK with sounding positive, and with using some of the communication components.

THERAPIST: Yes, I heard you use several positive communication elements. Do you remember what you used?

Note: The therapist checks to see whether the CSO can identify the specific elements of positive communication he has incorporated into the role play. As noted previously, this makes it more likely that he has learned those skills and will use them once he leaves the therapy session.

CSO: The main one was accepting partial responsibility for the problem. I admitted that I should have spoken up earlier about it bothering me when I had to spend a lot of time trying to wake her up. Oh—but did it come across that the real problem I was having was with her *drinking*? I wonder if it just sounded like I was annoyed to have to spend time trying to wake her up?

THERAPIST: Good question. I'm not sure it was clear when you first started talking about it, but when you made your second set of remarks it was quite obvious. But it wouldn't hurt to try making it clearer from the start, because that's such an important part of your message to Kate. We can practice that in a minute. What were some of the other parts of positive communication that you used?

CSO: I tried to be understanding when I said that I knew she needed time out with her friends.

THERAPIST: Yes, that was a good understanding statement. And you sort of expressed your feelings a few times, too, when you described the struggle you were experiencing. I also liked how you came right out and said you were trying to protect her, but you couldn't continue doing something that might be making it easier for her to keep drinking. It was powerful. What else do you think would enhance your message? Let's give that some thought and then we'll try it again. Oh, and if you think you'll change your mind about telling your wife you're in therapy, we should practice that part of the conversation, too.

Note: The therapist might suggest that the CSO also:

- Use positive wording (Positive Communication Guideline 2; Chapter 4, Box 4.1) by adding what he *likes* about the evenings when she stays home or arrives home early (e.g., they talk during the evening and then go to bed together).
- Offer to help (Positive Communication Guideline 7, Box 4.1), such as by asking what he can do to make it more enticing for her to come home earlier when she is out with her friends (which should have the effect of reducing her drinking time).

Discuss the time or occasion for having the conversation.

THERAPIST: Now that we've practiced the conversation you're planning on having with Kate a few times and are happy with it, we'll just need to figure out when it will take place, and address any possible barriers.

CSO: I think I should go home and talk to her tonight so I don't lose my nerve.

THERAPIST: Sounds good. Is there some particular time tonight that would work best?

CSO: She wasn't sure whether she was going to go out with her friends tonight. But either way, she'll be eating dinner with me. As we're sitting down to eat, I'll tell her that I have something I need to talk to her about. She'll be real curious, so I'll go right into it.

THERAPIST: Sounds good. Now let's think about possible barriers and develop some backup plans for carrying this out.

Note: The therapist would rely on the Homework Assignment Guidelines (Chapter 3, Box 3.1).

COMMON PROBLEMS TO AVOID

Allowing for Natural, Negative Consequences of Use is one of the more challenging procedures for therapists to introduce, in part because many CSOs are hesitant initially to change their behavior in a way that (by design) will *not* be well received by the IP. Fortunately, there are several therapist tips for circumventing the common problems associated with properly implementing this procedure. These are outlined below.

Problem: Clinicians sometimes avoid introducing this procedure because they have experienced "pushback" from CSOs in the past when they have done so. Nonetheless, the procedure is an important component of CRAFT, and consequently should be introduced if/when clinically indicated.

Safeguards:

- You should remind yourself that although certain CRAFT procedures, such as *positive* communication and *positive* reinforcement, tend to be more enjoyable to teach, the CRAFT training will be incomplete for most CSOs if they do not learn the skillful implementation of the *negative* consequences procedures.
- Get into the habit of asking yourself after approximately the fourth session whether it might be time to start planning for the introduction of the Allowing for Natural, Negative Consequences of Use procedure. The answer might be "no," but at least the issue will have been raised to awareness (i.e., not totally avoided).

Problem: Finding the appropriate situation/behavior to target for allowing the natural consequences can prove problematic and frustrating for therapists. This is understandable, since predicting a reduction in an IP's substance use as the result of a behavior change on the part of the CSO is a complicated task.

Safeguards:

- Prepare the CSO (and yourself) for the possibility that trial-and-error may be associated with this task, thereby hopefully enabling both of you to stay motivated and focused.
- Do not necessarily assume that the targeted behavior was a poor choice if the IP does not reduce substance use immediately afterward. As with other CRAFT procedures, it easily could take multiple repetitions of the CSO's planned new behavior before the desired change is seen in the IP.
- If you are spending an inordinate amount of therapy time trying to identify a target behavior or developing the plan for enacting it, step back from the procedure and scale it down. Instead, think in terms of smaller (progressive) steps toward the bigger goal.

Problem: When a CSO repeatedly does not follow through and enact a behavior that appears (in principle) to be the "perfect" one to target, some clinicians automatically simply reassign the same homework, nonetheless.

Safeguards:

- Inquiring about the reasons behind *any* unattempted or incomplete homework assignment is an important part of CRAFT, but even more so if the same assignment has not been completed more than once. In most cases, these assignments will need to be modified or dropped altogether so that they fall in line with the CSO's revised goals.
- Allowing for the Natural, Negative Consequences of Use is a procedure that CSOs would like to believe they can do, but the reality of changing this behavior becomes all too apparent when they leave the therapy session and take steps toward carrying out the behavior at home. As noted, it is worthwhile to have CSOs devote session time to imagining going home and following through with the plan to allow for the natural consequences. Probing for barriers while the CSO is imagining changing the behavior is critical.

Problem: Clinicians might struggle with helping CSOs understand that although they may have engaged in behavior that unintentionally supported the IP's substance use, the CSOs are *not* responsible for the IP's use.

Safeguards:

- Some CSOs need additional time to sort through their own feelings of self-blame. It might be helpful to remind them that they were looking out for their IP the best way they knew how at the time, that they were acting out of love and a sense of wanting to protect their IP throughout, and that they took the important step of coming into CRAFT treatment to learn new skills for dealing with their IP.
- It is possible that you are having difficulty helping CSOs sort through this issue because part of you believes that the CSOs *are* at least somewhat at fault. If this is the case, it might be useful to consider that it will serve no purpose to (indirectly) convey these feelings to CSOs. CSOs who feel judged about their past behavior are more apt to drop out of treatment.

Problem: It is fairly common for new CRAFT clinicians to back away immediately when CSOs state that they do not want to tell their IP *why* they are suddenly no longer blocking the negative consequences of the IP's use. These CSOs report that they simply want to try out the behavior without any explanation. However, given that IPs frequently ask their CSOs why they are acting differently at times such as these, it is worthwhile to have CSOs prepared for such a conversation.

Safeguards:

- Go into the procedure of Allowing for Natural, Negative Consequences of Use with the assumption that you will be teaching each CSO how to have this conversation with her or his IP, regardless of when (or whether) the conversation takes place. Let CSOs know the rationale for doing this and remind them that it never hurts to devote more time to practicing communication skills, especially for possible interactions with their IP.
- Help CSOs sort out their reasons regarding why they do not want to tell their IP about the planned behavior change. Always check about safety concerns.

SUMMARY

This chapter presents step-by-step instructions for teaching CSOs the second "negative consequences" procedure and includes suggestions for addressing their concerns (and therapists') about carrying it out. Therapist support is of paramount importance for this procedure, given that CSOs can become quite upset when discussing and targeting their behavior that has unintentionally facilitated IP substance use. The next chapter introduces Problem Solving, which is a technique that is often used in conjunction with the two negative consequences procedures.

FORM 8.1

Allowing for Natural, Negative Consequences of Use: Checklist

1. Offer common examples of CSOs' unintentional support of substance use and the resulting consequences.

- ☐ a. Explain how it is common for CSOs to support their IP's substance use unintentionally.
- ☐ b. Describe one or two examples of unintentional support of an IP's substance use that result from blocking the negative consequences of the use.

2. Explore the CSO's unintentional support of the IP's substance-using behavior.

- ☐ a. Ask whether the CSO may sometimes be supporting the IP's substance use unintentionally.
- ☐ b. Ask the CSO to describe in some detail an example of her or his own behavior that might result in unintentional support of the IP's substance use.
- ☐ c. Reassure the CSO that she or he is not at fault for engaging in this type of behavior.

3. Discuss how to change a particular CSO behavior in order to allow for the natural, negative consequences of substance use.

- ☐ a. Help select a CSO behavior to change in order to allow for the natural consequences.
- ☐ b. Make sure the IP will experience the natural consequences as negative and related to the substance use.
- ☐ c. Make sure it will be relatively easy for the CSO to allow for the natural consequences.
- ☐ d. Discuss how the CSO feels about allowing for the natural consequences.

4. Address potential problems in allowing for the natural consequences.

- ☐ a. Explore and address potential problems that might arise when allowing for the natural consequences.
- ☐ b. Specifically discuss possible safety/violence concerns and develop a plan if necessary.
- ☐ c. Remind the CSO to use CRAFT problem-solving skills when needed.

(continued)

5. Discuss how to explain to the IP the reason for allowing the natural consequences.

- ☐ a. Determine what the CSO will tell the IP about *why* the natural consequences are being (or were) allowed.
- ☐ b. Engage in a role play that incorporates positive communication skills when explaining to the IP why the natural consequences are being (or were) allowed.
- ☐ c. Discuss the time or occasion for having the conversation.

Chapter 9

Problem Solving

The Problem Solving procedure presented in this chapter teaches a basic skill that is useful for a large variety of problems. The ultimate objective is for CSOs to take this new skill and apply it to future problems they encounter. This comprehensive exercise is generally well received by CSOs who feel overwhelmed by their problems and are appreciative of a step-by-step guide to approaching them.

THE BASICS

General Description

Many variations of problem-solving exercises exist. CRAFT's version is the one found in the scientifically supported Community Reinforcement Approach (CRA), the treatment designed to be used directly with an individual with a substance use problem (Hunt & Azrin, 1973; Meyers & Smith, 1995). The procedure begins with you providing a rationale for conducting Problem Solving at that particular time, and giving an overview of the process. It is then a simple matter of introducing the step-by-step structured exercise, while making sure to *teach* it to CSOs as opposed to doing it for them. The procedure ends with a specific assignment for the week.

Procedure Timing

The formal Problem Solving procedure is introduced when clinically indicated—when CSOs talk about a problem that appears difficult for them to solve on their own. Within the context of the CRAFT program, Problem Solving frequently is needed either in conjunction with or after one of these procedures: Allowing for Natural, Negative Consequences of Use (Chapter 8), or Withdrawing Rewards for Using Behavior (Chapter 7). However, it certainly can be introduced in earlier CRAFT sessions.

Forms

- Problem Solving: Checklist (Form 9.1)
- Problem Solving Worksheet (Form 9.2)

CLINICIAN GUIDANCE AND SAMPLE DIALOGUE

The components for the CRAFT Problem Solving procedure are presented below. A sample case that illustrates clinician–CSO dialogue is included. The components for conducting this exercise are outlined in Form 9.1, Problem Solving: Checklist, found at the end of this chapter.

Case Description

The same CSO and IP case from Chapter 8 that was used to illustrate the Allowing for Natural, Negative Consequences of Use procedure is used here to illustrate Problem Solving because, as noted, the latter procedure is often conducted after or in conjunction with the former. As a reminder, the CSO (Charlie) is the 66-year-old husband of the IP (Kate). The IP significantly increased her drinking after retiring. She goes out with friends several nights a week, and then has difficulty getting up on time the next morning to babysit her granddaughter. The plan determined during the Allowing for Natural, Negative Consequences of Use procedure (Chapter 8) was for Charlie to refrain from waking his wife and getting her to bed when she fell asleep on the couch upon returning home late from her nights out. As a result, the IP likely would find herself on the couch the next morning. The CSO planned to wake her up in the morning (if necessary) such that she would have just enough time to scramble out of sight before the IP's daughter arrived with her granddaughter. Assume this plan has been in place for 2 weeks now.

As always, you would start the session by inquiring about the assignment from the previous week. In this case, it entailed checking on Charlie's progress toward allowing for the natural, negative consequences, including whether he was following the plan and whether it was having the desired impact on the IP's drinking. Note that when the CSO reports wanting to move forward but is uncertain how to navigate around an obstacle, the therapist uses the opportunity to introduce the Problem Solving procedure.

1. Introduce the Problem Solving procedure and explain its purpose.

As noted, it is important to *teach* the Problem Solving procedure to CSOs instead of just *doing it* for them. Once CSOs learn the procedure, they can apply it to other problems in their lives on their own.

Identify a problem that seems appropriate for teaching the Problem Solving procedure.

THERAPIST: So you're saying, Charlie, that you've seen a little improvement in your wife's drinking since you started to allow for the natural consequences 2 weeks ago? I know you weren't sure after just the first week.

CSO: Yes, lately she's been coming home about an hour earlier whenever she goes out. So that's good. But she's still had plenty to drink and flops on the couch and falls asleep. I still find her on the couch most mornings after those nights out; I think she got up on her own in the middle of the night twice. I guess that's a good sign. But like I said, she's asleep on the couch most mornings and I have to wake her up before her daughter arrives. At least she's been easier to wake up this week.

THERAPIST: I'm guessing you're probably right about Kate doing a bit better, given that she's drinking for shorter periods of time and is easier to wake up in the morning. I know you spoke to her about what you were doing and why. Has that come up again? Has she said anything about it?

CSO: No. She hasn't brought it up. I get the feeling she's annoyed with me, but she's trying harder in spite of it. I'm just not sure it's going to get that much better though. She could keep this up for a long time.

THERAPIST: She's doing better, but you're hoping for more. What would you like to do?

CSO: I've been thinking about how you'd originally asked what would happen if I just let her sleep on the couch in the morning—if I didn't wake her up. I wasn't ready for that because I kept picturing her on the couch when my stepdaughter brought over Tillie. I know it's a natural consequence for her like we talked about, but I wasn't prepared to deal with all of the uncomfortable questions.

THERAPIST: How are you feeling about that now? Are you thinking you might want to give it a try?

CSO: Yes and no. I agree that it might help her in the long run, but I'm worried about how to deal with the fallout.

THERAPIST: What's the fallout you're worried about dealing with?

CSO: I guess I picture my wife waking up as the door opens and my stepdaughter and granddaughter come in. Kate would be surprised and embarrassed. She'd excuse herself and rush away to the bedroom. I'd be left explaining what was going on. I don't know what I'd say, and I really don't want to be in that position.

THERAPIST: And yet you're considering this new bold plan. If you *do* want to go ahead with it, I can help you sort through the main problem that is standing in your way. What would you say that is?

CSO: Not knowing what to do if my stepdaughter comes in and finds her mom just waking up on the couch.

THERAPIST: This seems like a good time for me to introduce another CRAFT procedure: Problem Solving.

Note: The Problem Solving procedure was introduced here because the CSO was facing a barrier that clearly was interfering with him taking the next step in treatment. If CSOs have already learned the procedure to deal with a different problem, you would ask them if the problem at hand might be suitable for the Problem Solving procedure. For the current case, if the issue had been one of the CSO simply not knowing what to *say* to the stepdaughter, then CRAFT's communication skills (Chapter 4) could have been revisited here instead.

Give a rationale for doing Problem Solving.

THERAPIST: You've identified a real problem that is interfering with your continued efforts to help reduce your wife's drinking. Problem Solving is a procedure designed to help someone take a highly structured, step-by-step approach to addressing a problem, making problems feel more manageable. Once I teach you how to do Problem

Solving, you'll be able to use this skill to solve a variety of problems on your own. Are you up for learning Problem Solving?

CSO: Why not, right?

Briefly describe the Problem Solving procedure.

THERAPIST: Excellent. I'll start by showing you the Problem Solving Worksheet that contains all of the steps for the procedure (*shows Form 9.2*). Notice that there are eight specific steps. Seven of these steps we'll do here today, and the last one will be part of your assignment. As I explain each step, we'll apply it to the current problem you've brought up. Then I'll send you home with a copy of this worksheet so you can refer to it.

Note: You can use a variety of methods for recording the responses to the problem-solving steps. Common ones include writing on a whiteboard or on a large pad atop an easel, or simply filling out the paper worksheet. Regardless, you should give the CSO a copy of the completed worksheet to take home. If you use a whiteboard, take a photo of the completed board and send it to the CSO, or have the CSO fill in a worksheet with the main responses before leaving the session. If the procedure is being done remotely, virtual whiteboards work well, too.

2. Describe the steps of the Problem Solving procedure and conduct it using the CSO's problem as the example.

If the Problem Solving procedure has already been introduced/taught for a different problem, it is best to have the CSO take the lead in conducting the procedure for subsequent problems that arise in session. For example, the CSO could be handed the Problem Solving Worksheet (Form 9.2) and asked to walk you through the procedure as it applies to the new problem. You would assist as needed. (See Box 9.1 for the Problem Solving Guidelines.)

Explain "define the problem narrowly" and apply it to the current problem.

You should explain that complex problems can seem overwhelming, and so this first step breaks down complex problems into very specific, manageable ones. CSOs generally

BOX 9.1

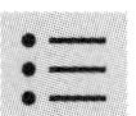

Problem Solving Guidelines

1. Define the problem narrowly.
2. Brainstorm possible solutions.
3. Eliminate unwanted suggestions.
4. Select one potential solution.
5. Identify possible obstacles.
6. Address each obstacle.
7. Make the selected solution into the assignment.
8. Evaluate the outcome after doing the assignment.

begin by defining the problem in quite vague terms. It is worthwhile to assist in narrowing down the problem description from the start, as it helps constrain the potential solutions generated during brainstorming (Step 2) such that they are highly relevant to the specific problem at hand.

THERAPIST: Step 1 on the worksheet (*refers to Form 9.2*), "Define the problem narrowly," is asking us to break down a problem that seems *overwhelming* into smaller pieces so that you can tackle it more easily. You were pretty specific a minute ago when you described the problem that you were telling me about. Do you remember what you said?

CSO: I think I said something like "I'd be upset when my wife is discovered asleep on the couch by her daughter after a night out."

THERAPIST: That's a great start. And I bet you can be even more specific in terms of what the problem is. The more we can pinpoint exactly what the issue is, the better we can generate relevant solutions. For example, can you explain what you mean when you say that the problem is you being "upset" when your wife is found asleep on the couch?

CSO: I just wouldn't know what to do (*exasperated*). I'd feel stuck in the middle with no good way out. Would I say something to my stepdaughter about the situation? What about my wife?

THERAPIST: It sounds like you're saying that you'd be upset, at least in part, because you wouldn't know what to do in that situation.

CSO: Exactly.

THERAPIST: That's very helpful, because we've now narrowed down the problem to one in which you'd be *unsure what to do* in this situation. OK. And I assume we're talking about the mornings in which your stepdaughter brings Tillie over, right?

CSO: Yes, that's right. Oh, and I should probably say that Kate would be groggy when waking up, because she'd wake up as they knocked and came through the front door.

THERAPIST: Very good. Here's what I have now (*reads*): "Not knowing what to do if my stepdaughter and Tillie walk in and discover my wife groggy and just waking up on the couch after a night out." Does that capture it?

CSO: Yes, that's good.

THERAPIST: I'm going to add this to Step 1 on the worksheet (*refers to Form 9.2* [see Figure 9.1]).

Note: If the therapist had not inquired as to what the CSO meant by being "upset," the upcoming brainstorming step might have incorrectly focused instead on methods for helping the CSO deal with his feelings in the situation, as opposed to generating ideas regarding how to respond. The CSO already had been specific as far as the exact event, including the time it would occur and the relevant individuals, so the therapist did not need to probe those factors.

Explain "brainstorm possible solutions" and apply it to the current problem.

Encourage the CSO to be creative and to offer possible solutions that normally would not be considered. These potential solutions should not be judged. As far as how many

1. **Define the problem narrowly.** [Just one. Keep it real specific. Write it below.]

   Not knowing what to do if my stepdaughter and Tillie walk in and discover my wife groggy and just waking up on the couch after a night out.

2. **Brainstorm possible solutions.** [The more the better! List below.]
   [*Note that Step 3, "eliminate unwanted suggestions," is illustrated here as well.*]

   - ~~Leave the room without saying anything.~~
   - ~~Ask Kate to tell her daughter what's going on, and then leave.~~
   - ~~Join Kate on the couch and encourage her to tell her daughter what's happening.~~
   - ~~Tell my stepdaughter that her mom isn't feeling well again.~~
   - ~~Tell my stepdaughter that her mom has a drinking problem.~~
   - ~~Help Kate up and get her into the bedroom. Go back out to the living room and encourage my stepdaughter to ask her mom what's going on.~~
   - Help Kate up and get her into the bedroom. Go back out to the living room and ask my stepdaughter to invite her mom to lunch so they can talk about what's going on.
   - ~~Let Kate know in advance that I can't keep covering for her, and ask her what options she'd suggest for me handling it differently.~~
   - Speak to Kate in advance about CRAFT and invite her to sample treatment.

3. **Eliminate unwanted suggestions.** [Cross out any that you can't imagine yourself doing.]
   [*Note that this is illustrated above in Step 2.*]

4. **Select one potential solution.** [Which one can you imagine yourself doing this week? Describe exactly how you'd carry it out.]

   Help Kate into the bedroom; then ask my stepdaughter to invite her mom to lunch so they can talk. If my stepdaughter is standing around wondering what's going on and asking lots of questions, leave the house with Tillie and take a walk.

5. **Identify possible obstacles.** [What might get in the way of this working? List below.]
   [*Note that Step 6, "address each obstacle," is illustrated here as well.*]

   - Stepdaughter might start firing questions at me about her mom.
     Solution: Tell her to talk directly with her mom.
   - Stepdaughter might go right into the bedroom and confront Kate.
     Solution: Follow her, and suggest they pick another time that might work better.
   - The lunch might never happen because Kate keeps making excuses.
     Solution: Ask my stepdaughter to let me know if she can't get her mom to schedule lunch. Talk to Kate about it if that occurs.
   - Leaving the house with Tillie might infuriate Kate, resulting in her not speaking to me.
     Solution: Tell Kate in advance that I plan to leave the house with Tillie under these circumstances as a way to encourage her to reduce her drinking.

(continued)

FIGURE 9.1. Completed version of Form 9.2, Problem Solving Worksheet, expanded for readability.

- It will be hard to walk out of the house while my wife is in her room getting ready and my stepdaughter is standing there asking questions.

  Solution: Tell my wife and stepdaughter that Tillie and I are heading out for a walk. Ask my stepdaughter again to take her mom to lunch so they can talk. Then leave with my granddaughter.

- If Tillie is sick I won't be able to leave the house with her.

  Solution: Head into the playroom with Tillie and start reading to her. If my wife follows, tell her I'd like some time alone with Tillie.

6. **Address each obstacle.** [What solution would you use to address each obstacle? Indicate above. Can't solve each obstacle? Pick a new solution and go through the steps again.]
   [*Note that solutions are illustrated above in Step 5.*]

7. **Make the selected solution into the assignment.** [List below exactly when/how you'll do it.]
   - Do <u>not</u> wake Kate up if she's still sleeping on the couch when it's time for my stepdaughter to arrive with Tillie.
   - Help Kate get back to the bedroom once my stepdaughter arrives. Encourage stepdaughter to take her mom to lunch that week so they can talk. If she keeps asking what's wrong, say I'm uncomfortable speaking for her mom. If she goes into the bedroom to confront Kate, suggest they pick another time for the conversation.
   - Ask my stepdaughter to let me know if she has trouble scheduling a lunch with her mom; talk to Kate about it if necessary.
   - Tell Kate in advance about my plans to leave the house with Tillie for a walk under these circumstances, and tell her this is to help her reduce her drinking. When the time comes, tell Kate and my stepdaughter that Tillie and I are going for a walk. Again encourage stepdaughter to take her mom to lunch so they can talk. Leave with Tillie. If Tillie is sick, go to the playroom and read to her alone.

8. **Evaluate the outcome after doing the assignment.** [Did it work? If it's worth trying again but some changes are needed, list them below.]
   - Stepdaughter kept asking what was wrong; told her that her mom was feeling "down" instead of telling her to speak directly to her mom. Did this let Kate off the hook?

     New plan: Keep rehearsing the conversation of encouraging stepdaughter to speak directly to her mom so it feels natural.
   - Forgot to tell stepdaughter to let me know if she had trouble scheduling the lunch, and now not sure if the lunch is planned.

     New plan: Ask Kate if her daughter has contacted her about lunch. Mention to Kate having encouraged her daughter to ask her to lunch so they can talk about what's going on. Urge Kate to go as a way to get support. Follow up with stepdaughter if the lunch still isn't scheduled.

FIGURE 9.1 *(continued)*

solutions should be generated, there is no magic number, and yet five seems like an absolute minimum. Jumping in and offering a few solutions as part of this process (even if it is unlikely that the CSO will select the proposed solution) is worthwhile because it encourages CSOs to consider novel solutions and prompts them to generate fresh ideas themselves.

THERAPIST: On to Step 2 now: "Brainstorm possible solutions." Charlie, this is where we have fun and just come up with a variety of *possible* solutions to this problem. Don't worry about whether you think they'll work, or if you can even picture yourself doing them. Just get your creative juices flowing and don't judge yourself. I promise I won't judge you either. I'll help out if you get stuck. As a bare minimum we need five ideas, but I bet we can come up with more than that.

Note: Together the CSO and therapist came up with the following possible solutions regarding what the CSO could do if his stepdaughter and granddaughter walked in on his wife as she was just waking up on the couch after a night out:

- Leave the room without saying anything.
- Ask Kate to tell her daughter what's going on, and then leave.
- Join Kate on the couch and encourage her to tell her daughter what's happening.
- Tell my stepdaughter that her mom isn't feeling well again.
- Tell my stepdaughter that her mom has a drinking problem.
- Help Kate up and get her into the bedroom. Go back out to the living room and encourage my stepdaughter to ask her mom what's going on.
- Help Kate up and get her into the bedroom. Go back out to the living room and ask my stepdaughter to invite her mom to lunch so they can talk about what's going on.
- Let Kate know in advance that I can't keep covering for her, and ask her what options she'd suggest for me handling it differently.
- Speak to Kate in advance about CRAFT and invite her to sample treatment.

Explain "eliminate unwanted suggestions" and apply it to the current problem.
Have the CSO read each potential solution one at a time, while imagining *doing* that solution in the upcoming week. If the CSO cannot imagine carrying out the solution (for any reason), it should be deleted. Despite being told it is unnecessary to explain *why* they are crossing out a particular solution that they cannot imagine themselves doing, many CSOs proceed to share their reasons, nonetheless. This is not problematic, other than lengthening the time to complete the procedure. If *all* solutions are crossed out, the brainstorm step is repeated.

THERAPIST: For Step 3, "Eliminate unwanted suggestions," we should go down this list one solution at a time. Try to picture yourself doing each solution in the upcoming week. If for any reason you can't see yourself doing it, just cross it out. There's no need to explain it to me—just cross it out.

Note: Common reasons for crossing out potential solutions in a case such as this would include the CSO being uncomfortable at the thought of engaging in the behavior, being quite certain that the behavior would not have the intended consequences of decreasing his wife's drinking, and being skeptical because he had unsuccessfully tried something similar in the past.

Explain "select one potential solution" and apply it to the current problem.

From the potential solutions that remain, have the CSO select one and describe *exactly* how it will be carried out. This makes the assignment *real* and offers the CSO (and you) a first glimpse into possible obstacles. Determine whether the chosen solution is worth pursuing, or whether it is too complex, vague, or out of the CSO's control. Also listen for obstacles for the chosen solution. Keep in mind that it might be reasonable for the CSO to select two solutions if they are small and easy to implement.

THERAPIST: Excellent job. Now, on to Step 4, "Select one potential solution." Of the remaining solutions, which is the main one you can imagine yourself doing this week?

CSO: I think I'll help Kate into the bedroom; then I'll ask my stepdaughter to invite her mom to lunch so they can talk. My stepdaughter will ask a lot of questions at lunch, so Kate won't be able to avoid the topic altogether.

THERAPIST: Good. Take your time now—let's think this through a little bit more. Imagine yourself actually carrying this out.

CSO: I'll need something to do if my stepdaughter is standing around wondering what's going on and asking questions. I think I'll leave the house with Tillie and take a walk if that happens. I'm not sure what will happen at home when I leave, but at least I won't be in the middle of it.

Note: This CSO decided to use a two-part solution, with the essential second half being added only when the therapist encouraged the CSO to imagine the scenario unfolding.

Explain "identify possible obstacles" and apply it to the current problem.

Ask the CSO to describe what might get in the way of completing the task. CSOs tend to need assistance with this process, so once they have seemingly identified all barriers, feel free to jump in with additional ones that appear relevant to their case.

THERAPIST: What do you see here for Step 5 (*refers to Form 9.2*)?

CSO (*reads from the form*): Identify possible obstacles. OK. Well, I know you always ask me about obstacles when we're coming up with homework assignments. Is that what this means?

THERAPIST: Yes! Wow, good for you for seeing this connection. Yes, the solution we come up with at the end of this problem-solving exercise will be your assignment for the week. And so like we always do, we'll be looking for things that might get in the way of you successfully completing the assignment. It might help to take a moment and again picture yourself trying to carry out this plan at home. What might get in the way?

CSO: A few things come to mind right away. My stepdaughter might start firing questions at me about her mom. Or she might go right into the bedroom and confront Kate.

THERAPIST: These are important. I'm writing them on our form (*refers to Form 9.2* [see Figure 9.1]). We'll come up with ways to tackle these obstacles in a minute. For now: What else might get in the way?

CSO: I'm not sure. Hmm. I bet there's a chance the lunch never happens because Kate keeps making excuses.

THERAPIST: You could be right. This gets a little bit away from the main problem we're working on right now, which is to help you to know what to do if your stepdaughter walks in on her mom asleep on the couch after a night of drinking. But since you're so good at this, I think it's fine for us to see if we can add something pretty straightforward to your plan so that it's more likely that the lunch happens. Otherwise, we might find ourselves using the Problem Solving procedure to address that specific problem in a week or so. Should we add it to the list of obstacles to address?

CSO: I'd definitely like to put that on the list.

Note: The therapist decided to include the obstacle raised by the CSO despite it not being strictly related to the initial problem, given that it *was* a secondary problem that could readily arise, and it possibly could be prevented by adding a simple element to the current plan.

THERAPIST: Done then. And what about the second part of your plan; leaving the house with Tillie if your stepdaughter is standing around waiting for answers?

CSO: Leaving the house with Tillie might infuriate Kate, which could end up with her not speaking to me. I think I could deal with that. But it will be hard to just walk out with Tillie while my wife is in her room getting ready and my stepdaughter is standing there asking me questions. We should talk about that one for sure. And I guess if Tillie is sick, I wouldn't be able to leave the house with her. Wow, this seems like a lot of obstacles.

THERAPIST: Yes, but you're generating the obstacles *now*, which is good because we can figure out how to deal with them. This is much better than having them sneak up on you when you're not prepared. I'm adding them to our worksheet (*refers to Form 9.2* [see Figure 9.1]).

Explain "address each obstacle" and apply it to the current problem.

It is not necessary for CSOs to list out all the ways in which the obstacles could be addressed, but it *is* safer to have them do so if there is concern that they might forget the plans. Importantly, if CSOs cannot satisfactorily address each obstacle, have them pick a new solution and go through the steps again.

THERAPIST: Charlie, I imagine it *does* seem like a lot of obstacles. But let's see if the whole thing can be made to feel manageable. Can you tell me what Step 6 says (*refers to Form 9.2*)?

CSO (*reads*): Address each obstacle. I guess I might as well start with the first one here: "Stepdaughter might start firing questions at me about her mom."

THERAPIST: What do you think? What can you do to address that obstacle if it happens?

CSO: I don't know. I mean, I might be able to just say that she should talk directly with her mom. Is that enough?

THERAPIST: I guess it depends on how you deliver the message. Will you be able to convince her that it's what she needs to do? I bet you will if we practice communication skills.

CSO: I think you're right.

THERAPIST: Then I'm going to make a note about this planned solution to this potential obstacle on this Problem Solving Worksheet *(refers to Form 9.2* [see Figure 9.1]). What was the next obstacle, and what could you do to address it?

CSO: She might go right into the bedroom and confront Kate. Let's see (*pauses*). I might need to practice this conversation, too, but I'm thinking I could follow her, and suggest they pick another time that might work better for the conversation.

THERAPIST: Sounds like a great idea because Kate will be hungover and not in the best mood for such an intense conversation. As a result, we can pretty much predict it wouldn't go well. And yes, we can practice this conversation, too, so you're all set. We have a few more obstacles to address.

Note: Several solutions for this particular problem entail the CSO communicating with either the IP or the stepdaughter. Consequently, the therapist would make sure the CSO was prepared for these conversations by briefly referring to the CRAFT communication skills (Chapter 4), and by doing role plays if considered necessary. The proposed solutions to the remaining four obstacles (should they arise) are included on Figure 9.1 under Step 5.

Explain "make the selected solution into the assignment" and apply it to the current problem.

Follow the guidelines for developing homework assignments (See Homework Assignment Guidelines in Chapter 3, Box 3.1). Have the CSO verbalize the selected solution and the plans for addressing obstacles, so that any confusion is apparent and can be clarified. Be sure the CSO knows that the planned solution *is* the homework assignment (for the upcoming week).

THERAPIST: Charlie, in a minute we'll practice those conversations we mentioned. Other than that, I think you're almost set as far as being ready to address the problem you raised for our problem-solving exercise—namely, knowing what to do when you let Kate stay asleep on the couch after a night out with her friends, and she's still there when her daughter and granddaughter arrive in the morning. But first, Step 7 says, "Make the selected solution into the assignment." Basically, it means we should go over all the parts of your assignment, including the plans for addressing any obstacles that might get in your way. Can you start it off?

CSO: Absolutely. First, I'll help Kate get back to the bedroom once my stepdaughter arrives. When back in the living room I'll encourage my stepdaughter to take her mom to lunch that week so they can talk. If she keeps asking me what's wrong, I'll say I'm uncomfortable speaking for her mom and she should talk to her directly.

THERAPIST: Excellent. That's exactly how our problem-solving exercise started off. But as a quick reminder, you want to be sure that you don't wake Kate up if she's still sleeping on the couch when it's time for your stepdaughter to arrive with Tillie.

CSO: Oh right! A very important step!

THERAPIST: Wonderful. What comes next?

Note: See Figure 9.1, Step 7 for the remaining parts of the assignment.

Explain "evaluate the outcome after doing the assignment" and apply it to the current problem.

CSOs should be told that the final step of the Problem Solving procedure occurs at the start of the *next* session, given that it entails following up on the status of the (hopefully) attempted solution to the problem (i.e., the homework assignment for the week). At this follow-up session (illustrated below), you should determine the extent to which the selected solution worked, and whether it needs to be modified, reassigned, or replaced altogether.

THERAPIST: Charlie, as always, we'll start the session today by seeing how the assignment went. We did problem solving last week to develop a plan for how you'd deal with the uncomfortable situation if your stepdaughter found her mom asleep on the couch in the morning. I see that you brought the problem-solving handout we'd been working on, and you filled out Step 8 (*refers to Figure 9.1*). Great! Let's take a look at and talk about what you did, what worked or didn't work, and what you want to do differently next time.

CSO: I'd say it was partly successful. I didn't wake Kate up on Tuesday morning, and her daughter found her asleep on the couch. Kate hopped up and went into the bedroom. So that part was OK. I could tell that my stepdaughter didn't quite know what was going on, but she didn't say anything right away because she was preoccupied with getting the new stroller set up.

THERAPIST: That sounds *really* good to me, because you said it was going to be hard for you to let Kate sleep on those mornings when your stepdaughter was coming over.

CSO: I guess you're right. That part was good. And I asked my stepdaughter to take her mom to lunch so they could talk over what was going on. But when she asked me a few times what was wrong, I didn't follow my plan to say she should talk to her mom. Instead, I said something like "Your mom is feeling down." So now I'm wondering if I let Kate off the hook by saying she was just feeling "down"? Do I need to fix this? Oh, and to top it off, I forgot to tell my stepdaughter to let me know if she had trouble scheduling the lunch, and now I don't even know if it's been scheduled, but I doubt it. I'm not sure what to do, because it would seem strange to call my stepdaughter now, like I was going behind Kate's back. I could talk to Kate about it, but she's not going to rush to schedule it.

THERAPIST: Well, first of all, good for you for following through and suggesting that your stepdaughter take her mom to lunch to talk! I wouldn't worry about needing to "fix" what you said about Kate feeling down, because I'm guessing that the real story, Kate's drinking, will come up during the lunch. But we'll rehearse a conversation in which you stick with your overall plan to have your stepdaughter speak directly to her mother, and then you can practice it on your own so it feels natural if you need to use it. Now, it might help for me to first hear about Kate's reaction to being found asleep on the couch before we come up with our next step. For instance, what did Kate say to you afterward? And what about her drinking?

Note: The therapist praised the CSO for completing several parts of his assignment, particularly since the CSO seemed focused on the elements of the homework he had *not* completed. The therapist also checked to determine whether the assignment had "worked" as far as decreasing the IP's drinking.

CSO: I could tell Kate was annoyed with me, but she didn't say anything. And she definitely got home much earlier Wednesday night. Maybe she found a loophole though, because she went straight to the bedroom instead of heading for the couch. But she *was* up on time when her daughter arrived Thursday morning.

THERAPIST: This sounds great, Charlie! Even if she's found a loophole so that she won't get discovered asleep on the couch again, your behavior seems to have had an effect, because she came home earlier and was able to get up on time. This certainly suggests she is drinking less.

CSO: Yes, I agree. But I really want her to have a talk with her daughter.

THERAPIST: What would you be willing to do at this point to make that happen?

CSO: Like I said, I don't even know if my stepdaughter has contacted Kate about having lunch. I guess I'll start by asking Kate if she has. Either way, I could tell Kate that I'd encouraged her daughter to set up a lunch so the two of them could talk about what's going on. If Kate *has* been contacted about the lunch already, I'll urge her to go and use it as a chance to get some support from her daughter. Of course, I'll use my communication skills (*smiles*). I could say, "I understand it might be hard to talk about what's been going on, but I bet you'll end up getting lots of support." And I'd feel OK about following up with my stepdaughter about scheduling the lunch then, if necessary.

THERAPIST: Listen to you (*smiles back*)! Sounds like a good plan. And before you leave today, let's rehearse using more of those positive communication skills, in addition to the understanding statement you just demonstrated. But let me go back a minute to the recent, important change in your behavior: not waking Kate up when she's asleep on the couch. Are you willing to keep doing that if Kate *does* go back to sleeping on the couch?

Note: The therapist reminds the CSO of the need to be *consistent* in using the new behavior.

CSO: Yes. I think it's helping.

THERAPIST: Excellent. Then in a minute we can talk about whether you might handle the conversation differently with your stepdaughter if she finds her mom asleep on the couch again. Since you've already had an encounter with her in this exact situation, you might have some insight into what might work better.

CSO: Sure, makes sense.

THERAPIST: But I also want to check on your plan to leave the house with Tillie and go for a walk. Sounds like Kate was only discovered by her daughter on the couch once so far. Did you head out on the walk with Tillie then? And I know you wanted to tell Kate in advance about this plan.

CSO: You're right. Kate only had to scramble off the couch once so far, and she got herself ready in such record time that morning that I didn't have the chance to say goodbye and leave with Tillie. Like I said, my stepdaughter was working on setting up the new stroller, so that took awhile. But that's when I talked to her about inviting her mom to lunch. Anyway, I'm hoping Kate will continue to be up and ready to help with Tillie, but if she's not, I've decided that I'll take my granddaughter on a walk to the park. If it's too cold, I'll take her to the aquarium. And I already have a plan in case Tillie is sick.

THERAPIST: Look at you; you're coming up with backup plans! I was going to suggest that you could rely on problem solving to generate more ideas as to where you could take Tillie, but you've already figured it out. And what about as far as telling Kate in *advance* about this plan to leave with Tillie?

CSO: Yes. I told her about the plan and the reason for it right after our last session. You would have been proud of my communication skills (*smiles*). She didn't act upset at the time, but like I said, I can tell she's been annoyed with me. But I'm OK with that because this is important.

THERAPIST: Bravo!

Note: The therapist would conduct role plays of the noted conversations, and then ask the CSO to specify each step of the new homework assignment. A discussion of potential barriers would need to be addressed yet (see Homework Assignment Guidelines in Chapter 3, Box 3.1).

COMMON PROBLEMS TO AVOID

Problem Solving is a highly structured, straightforward procedure that appeals to CSOs and is easy for clinicians to administer. A few pitfalls can be avoided by following the safeguards below.

Problem: The most common error entails therapists doing the Problem Solving procedure *for* CSOs, as opposed to *teaching* CSOs how to do it.

Safeguards:

- Be sure to show the Problem Solving Worksheet (Form 9.2) to CSOs while working through the procedure, and send them home with a copy to use as needed.
- Make a point of announcing the various steps as you conduct Problem Solving, such as by saying, "Step 1 is to define the problem narrowly."
- Keep in mind that it will be up to CSOs to lead the Problem Solving procedure the second time it is needed in session.

Problem: Some therapists simply use the wording of the problem as initially stated by the CSO to satisfy Step 1, as opposed to narrowing it down into a more manageable problem. Such broadly stated problems lead to an unwieldy brainstorming step (2) that generates potential solutions to many different (unrelated) aspects of the initial problem. It is difficult to move forward with these suggestions, since they pull the CSO in multiple directions as opposed to allowing for a focus on one specific problem.

Safeguards:

- Do not automatically accept the CSO's wording of the problem—assume it can be made more specific.
- Ask the CSO (and yourself) whether just one problem is being described, or whether it can be broken down into several smaller problems that will be addressed separately.
- Assume that if you cannot think of any *measurable* potential solutions to the problem as stated, then it probably is not narrowly defined.

Problem: At times clinicians have been reluctant to step in and assist CSOs who are struggling to generate potential solutions during brainstorming (Step 2). Although it is important for CSOs to tackle this task the best they can, you are encouraged to help CSOs generate new, creative ideas, particularly if they become stuck.

Safeguards:

- Begin Step 2 with the assumption that you *will* be assisting with the generation of potential solutions.
- Offer one potential solution early in the process so that you do not later find yourself in the position of debating whether to assist.

Problem: Therapists have been known to refrain from offering guidance on those occasions when a CSO selects a potential solution (Step 4) that appears likely to fail (for example, because it is too complex or vague, or is outside of the CSO's control).

Safeguards:

- If you are saying to yourself, "This is never going to work" while a CSO is describing the plan for carrying out the selected solution, then it is definitely time to step in and assist. With your help it should become apparent that the plan has too many complications or barriers, or it is not under the CSO's control. When revising the plan, simplify and specify!
- If you are confused or cannot follow the CSO's proposed plan, then the selected solution is too vague. Assist with making the plan clearer and more measurable.

Problem: Clinicians sometimes accept a CSO's declaration that there are no obstacles to a proposed solution (Step 5).

Safeguards:

- Assume there are obstacles associated with *any* solution, and that the CSO just needs help identifying them.

Problem: Occasionally clinicians are so pleased when CSOs are able to identify obstacles to a planned solution (Step 5) that they accidentally skip the step that *addresses* the obstacles (Step 6).

Safeguards:

- Keep a close eye on the Problem Solving Worksheet (Form 9.2) so that steps are not skipped.
- As with any homework assignment (see Homework Assignment Guidelines in Chapter 3, Box 3.1), automatically check to see whether a plan is in place for addressing potential obstacles when converting the selected solution into a specific assignment (Step 7).

Problem: Although Step 7 already explicitly says to make the selected solution into an assignment, it is still important to be sure CSOs know that the assignment is to be done *in the upcoming week*. Clinicians assume that CSOs understand this, but unfortunately this is not always the case.

Safeguards:

- Again, as with other homework assignments, let CSOs know at the end of the session that the assignment (generated by the Problem Solving exercise; see Form 9.2) is the first thing you will ask them about at the next session.
- When CSOs are describing how they will carry out the selected solution/assignment, make sure they are referring to a day/time that occurs in the upcoming week.

SUMMARY

This chapter describes a step-by-step Problem Solving procedure that is introduced when CSOs bump up against major obstacles toward reaching a goal. The key is to teach CSOs how to do the procedure themselves so that they have a handy tool for addressing a wide variety of problems.

FORM 9.1

Problem Solving: Checklist

1. Introduce the Problem Solving procedure and explain its purpose.

- ☐ a. Identify a problem that seems appropriate for teaching the Problem Solving procedure.
- ☐ b. Give a rationale for doing Problem Solving.
- ☐ c. Briefly describe the Problem Solving procedure.

2. Describe the steps of the Problem Solving procedure and conduct it using the CSO's problem as the example.

- ☐ a. Explain "define the problem narrowly" and apply it to the current problem.
- ☐ b. Explain "brainstorm possible solutions" and apply it to the current problem.
- ☐ c. Explain "eliminate unwanted suggestions" and apply it to the current problem.
- ☐ d. Explain "select one potential solution" and apply it to the current problem.
- ☐ e. Explain "identify possible obstacles" and apply it to the current problem.
- ☐ f. Explain "address each obstacle" and apply it to the current problem.
- ☐ g. Explain "make the selected solution into the assignment" and apply it to the current problem.
- ☐ h. Explain "evaluate the outcome after doing the assignment" and apply it to the current problem.

FORM 9.2

Problem Solving Worksheet

1. **Define the problem narrowly.** [Just one. Keep it real specific. Write it below.]

2. **Brainstorm possible solutions.** [The more the better! List below.]

3. **Eliminate unwanted suggestions.** [Cross out any that you can't imagine yourself doing.]

4. **Select one potential solution.** [Which one can you imagine yourself doing this week? Describe exactly how you'd carry it out.]

5. **Identify possible obstacles.** [What might get in the way of this working? List below.]

6. **Address each obstacle.** [What solution would you use to address each obstacle? Indicate above. Can't solve each obstacle? Pick a new solution and go through the steps again.]

7. **Make the selected solution into the assignment.** [List below exactly when/how you'll do it.]

8. **Evaluate the outcome after doing the assignment.** [Did it work? If it's worth trying again but some changes are needed, list them below.]

Chapter 10

Helping Concerned Significant Others Enrich Their Own Lives

Most of the procedures in this manual thus far have focused on influencing the IP's behavior through changes in the CSO's behavior. As the IP's behavior changes for the better, the CSO typically benefits as well, such as from an improved CSO–IP relationship and decreased stress. Still, CSOs frequently struggle in several life areas, in part because they have had to put their own needs on hold in the context of a chaotic home environment affected by alcohol and/or drugs. This chapter directly works to enrich the CSOs' own functioning and quality of life, regardless of whether their IPs ever enter treatment. This third goal of CRAFT is addressed by procedures that are taken from CRA, the program that is used with the individuals who have the substance use problem (see Chapter 12). The main exercises in this chapter are the Happiness Scale and the Goal Setting worksheet (see checklist, Form 10.1, and Forms 10.2 and 10.3, each found at the end of this chapter).

THE BASICS

General Description

The Happiness Scale (Form 10.2) is a clinician-friendly assessment tool that CSOs complete after a brief rationale and instructions. This scale examines CSOs' happiness across a variety of life categories. The ratings on this scale form the foundation for setting goals, which is a comprehensive behavioral exercise that results in highly specific goals and the strategies (weekly assignments) for achieving them. This information is recorded on the Goal Setting form (Form 10.3), an instrument that is used by many therapists and agencies as a treatment plan.

The Happiness Scale is administered relatively easily, while the Goal Setting exercise is more labor intensive, particularly if you do not routinely set goals in behavioral (objective/measurable) terms. Still, this precise style of goal setting is a learnable, valuable skill that improves greatly with practice. As far as actually filling in the Goal Setting form, it is acceptable to have CSOs (as opposed to you) write the goals/strategies on the form during the session discussion if it helps to further engage the CSOs in the process. Many CSOs appreciate having a copy of the form to take home, given that it lists their weekly assignments.

Procedure Timing

The Happiness Scale is often introduced in one of the earlier CRAFT sessions, partially as a means to enhance rapport and motivate the CSO. On these occasions, the Goal Setting exercise is usually started as well. However, since a fair number of CSOs are eager to work exclusively on their IP's problems first, both the Happiness Scale and the Goal Setting exercises can be delayed and introduced later when clinically indicated. The Happiness Scale is commonly repeated every few sessions once it has been introduced, so that progress toward goals can be monitored. The Goal Setting form should be referred to weekly once it has been started, as strategies/assignments are reviewed and updated regularly.

Forms

- Helping CSOs Enrich Their Own Lives: Checklist (Form 10.1)
- Happiness Scale (Form 10.2)
- Goal Setting (Form 10.3)

CLINICIAN GUIDANCE AND SAMPLE DIALOGUE

The components for conducting the Happiness Scale and the Goal Setting exercises are presented below, and a sample clinician dialogue for a case is included. The Helping CSOs Enrich Their Own Lives: Checklist (Form 10.1) contains all of the components for the administration of these two instruments as well.

Case Description

The case is that of a 45-year-old non-Hispanic white married woman (CSO; Stella) who is seeking treatment for her husband (IP; Arthur) of 22 years. Arthur, who also identifies as non-Hispanic white, was injured on the job 2 years prior and was prescribed oxycodone for pain. His reliance on the drug increased rapidly, so he turned to buying it from acquaintances through work. His alcoholic beverage consumption increased in conjunction with the oxycodone use. Stella works as a receptionist at a health care office. She reports having lost contact with most friends due to embarrassment over her husband's drug and alcohol problems. Their 20-year-old daughter lives in her own apartment nearby, but rarely visits due to her father's issues.

1. Give the rationale for focusing on the CSO's own happiness.

State that CSOs' own happiness and health is an important part of CRAFT.

THERAPIST: Stella, I'm not sure if you remember us talking about this during your first session, but I'd mentioned that one of the main goals of CRAFT was to help loving family members, like you, make their own happiness and health a priority. So yes, you are here to help Arthur get into treatment, but part of my job is to help you focus on yourself, too.

Explain that CSOs often are isolated and suffering emotionally as a result of their IP's problem.

THERAPIST: One of the things we've noticed is that loving family members get pretty isolated and distant from their friends and extended family, as a result of feeling embarrassed or ashamed about the ongoing drinking or drug use in the home. And often they're depressed, too, or maybe they feel really stressed. In your case, I bet we can identify some ways in which you've isolated yourself, or can pinpoint signs of being sad or anxious because of the substance-related chaos in your home.

Explain how CSOs are better able to take care of their IPs if the CSOs are taking better care of themselves, and as a result feel better (e.g., less anxious and depressed).

THERAPIST: We've found that when people take better care of themselves, they're usually in a better frame of mind emotionally to attend to all sorts of family issues, including dealing with the person who drinks or uses drugs at home. As an example, imagine what it would be like to deal with Arthur if you were feeling your best; if you weren't feeling sad or stressed.

2. Introduce and provide the rationale for the Happiness Scale.

State that the Happiness Scale is a tool that will allow the CSO to rate her or his happiness in different life areas.

THERAPIST: I'd like to show you the Happiness Scale, which I think you'll find to be a fun tool (*shows Form 10.2*). It's exactly what the name says: It's a scale for rating how happy you are with lots of different areas of your life.

Explain that the information helps the CSO set goals for areas in which the CSO would like to see changes.

THERAPIST: Stella, once we see how you rate different areas of your life, you can decide which areas you'd like to see some changes in. Then I'll help you set goals in those areas and specific plans for achieving them.

Explain that the Happiness Scale will also be used to monitor progress in achieving goals over time.

THERAPIST: I'll ask you to complete the Happiness Scale periodically so that we can see the progress you've made toward your goals. We'll also be watching to see if you'd like to change some of your goals altogether.

3. Give instructions for the Happiness Scale.

Explain that the CSO should rate her or his current happiness in each of the categories using the 1–10 scale.

THERAPIST: I'd like you to go ahead and rate how happy you are in each of these categories using the 1–10 scale you see here (*points to Form 10.2*). Notice that a "1" means you're totally *un*happy with that part of your life, and a "10" means you're totally happy. Just do the best you can here; you don't need to spend a lot of time on each one.

Ask the CSO to rate each category independent of the others, and to focus on how she or he is feeling today.

THERAPIST: Try not to let the rating you give for one category influence how you rate the others. In other words, try to rate them all independently. Sometimes a person comes in feeling really down and so automatically rates pretty much every category low. It's more helpful if you can sort out your feelings for each of them on their own. Oh—and don't forget to rate these feelings for *today*.

Encourage the CSO to ask questions at any point.

THERAPIST: Don't hesitate to ask questions. For example, some people aren't quite sure what some of the categories mean. I'm here to help!

4. Review some of the ratings on the Happiness Scale.

Discuss the ratings of at least several categories by asking why a particular rating was given.

If it is the first time the Happiness Scale is being administered, you should review a CSO's response to each category briefly as a way of getting to know a bit more about the CSO. If there are time constraints, it is recommended that you start with one or two of the highest-rated (happiest) categories. This allows you to ease into the often difficult conversation by first showing that there are some positive aspects to the CSO's life. Then finish with one or two of the lowest-rated items. Additionally, in the absence of very high (happy) ratings (e.g., 8–10) for substance use (i.e., the CSO's own substance use), you should check with the CSO about it. Although it is unlikely that a CSO's own substance use problem would have gone undetected to this point, it never hurts to ask.

As part of reviewing each of the CSO's ratings, you should ask *why* a particular rating was given, as it allows you to (1) determine whether the CSO is using the scale appropriately, and (2) gather specifics regarding the factors associated with the CSO's happiness in various life areas (see Figure 10.1 for a completed Happiness Scale sample). When administering the Happiness Scale in subsequent sessions as a means of monitoring progress, you would primarily inquire about the categories with notable changes from previous ratings.

THERAPIST: Looks like your ratings overall max out at a 7. You gave a 7 to legal issues. Can you say a bit about why you gave legal issues a 7?

CSO: We haven't had any legal problems . . . yet. But it's always on my mind. I assume it's just a matter of time before Arthur gets caught, and it will probably happen at work.

	Completely unhappy									Completely happy
Social life	1	(2)	3	4	5	6	7	8	9	10
Job or education	1	2	3	(4)	5	6	7	8	9	10
Money management	1	2	3	4	5	6	(7)	8	9	10
Substance use	1	2	3	4	5	(6)	7	8	9	10
Health and wellness	1	2	3	4	(5)	6	7	8	9	10
Family relationships	1	2	3	4	(5)	6	7	8	9	10
Legal issues	1	2	3	4	5	6	(7)	8	9	10
Emotional life	1	2	3	(4)	5	6	7	8	9	10
Communication	1	2	3	(4)	5	6	7	8	9	10
Spirituality	1	2	3	4	5	(6)	7	8	9	10
Other: ________________	1	2	3	4	5	6	7	8	9	10
General happiness	1	2	3	4	(5)	6	7	8	9	10

FIGURE 10.1. Completed version of Form 10.2, Happiness Scale.

Ask what would have to change in order for the rating to improve by a point or two. By phrasing the question in this manner, it gives you (1) quick insight into what the CSO thinks needs to change *and* the role (if any) played by her or him in the process, (2) the opportunity to start shaping the CSO's goals and change strategies so that they are specific and measurable, and (3) ideas regarding which categories might be good candidates for goal setting.

THERAPIST: I can understand why worrying like that would affect your happiness. So let me ask you, What would have to change in order for your happiness rating in legal issues to go up to an 8? In other words, let's say that in a few weeks when we do this scale again, you're able to give legal issues an 8. What would have changed?

CSO: That's an interesting question. I've got to think about it a minute. Hmm. Well, obviously he still wouldn't be caught for doing anything illegal.

THERAPIST: Right, but that's what prompted you to give legal issues a 7 this time. What would have to be *different* in order to rate that category a little higher? It's a tough question, because it sounds like your fear—about him getting caught—is a large part of that rating. So what would make your fear go down? For example, is there anything that *you* could do to improve the rating?

Note: The therapist is attempting to get the CSO to think about positive change in terms of specific and measurable steps. As will be outlined in detail later, the best short-term goals (and the strategies for achieving them) are ones that directly involve the *CSO's* behavior (as opposed to the IP's) and can be set up to show measurable signs of progress in small steps.

CSO: The only thing that would help is if he got into treatment.

Note: Although the therapist does not need to have the CSO select a category for goal setting quite yet, information is being gathered for possible candidates based on this review of her ratings. In this case, the legal issues category is an example of a poor candidate for setting a goal, given that an improvement in the CSO's rating in that category is dependent upon the IP getting into treatment. Thus, the change involves the *IP's* behavior (not the CSO's), and the step is not a small one, but instead a longer-term and more complex focus of treatment. Still, if the CSO was determined to work on the legal issues category, the therapist would help her first develop a more objective/measurable goal and the strategy for achieving it.

THERAPIST: You also gave a 7 to money management. Can you tell me why you decided to give that a 7?

CSO: On a daily basis we're OK financially, but we can never save any money. I've been wanting to go back to school to finish up my degree so that I can get a better job, but it just hasn't been a priority with everything else going on.

THERAPIST: Is that what you had in mind when you gave job or education a 4?

Note: The first part of the review is the inquiry about several of the top-rated categories on the Happiness Scale. The therapist also makes a connection between the theme/content behind the ratings of two different categories. It is fairly common for the goals in several categories to be related, and for the resulting assignments to overlap as well.

CSO: Yes. I'm not happy with my job, but I can't do much better without getting my bachelor's degree.

THERAPIST: We can certainly focus on that if you decide it's a priority. But let me first get an idea as to what it would take to get just a small boost in your happiness in each of those areas. Let's do money management first. Can you think of something specific that would have to change in order for you to come back in a few weeks and give money management an 8?

CSO: I'd feel better if we started to save even $20 a week. I bet we could do it if Arthur and I sat down and took a good look at our spending.

THERAPIST: Great! You'll see in a few minutes when we actually start setting some goals that coming up with specific ones are important—and you're already doing that. Now, what would make you rate job or education a 5 in the next few weeks? More specifically, What's something that *you* could do to improve your own happiness in that area?

CSO: I think I'd be happier with myself if I found out what requirements I have left to finish up my bachelor's degree.

THERAPIST: Excellent. And again—we'll get back to that in a few minutes. Let me just finish up this quick review by asking you about one of the lowest-rated categories: You gave social life a 2. Can you say more about that?

CSO: It's pretty simple: I don't have a social life, with or without my husband. Even my daughter stays away lately. It sucks.

THERAPIST: And can you think of something that would have to change in the next few weeks in order for you to give it a 3 or 4?

CSO: I don't really know. It's hard to imagine that getting better any time soon.

Note: The therapist still is not helping the CSO settle on a goal, but instead is continuing to gather information that will, in all probability, rule out certain categories. For instance, in addition to avoiding the legal issues category (explained above) for now, the therapist would likely encourage the CSO to select a category other than the social life one as well. Not only did the CSO give social life one of her lowest ratings, but she sounded pessimistic about it improving and offered no specific ideas regarding how to change it.

THERAPIST: Actually, let me ask you about your substance use rating, too. You gave it a 6. Can you say more about that?

CSO: Oh, I've just been wondering if my own drinking is making things worse at home. I enjoy a glass of wine with dinner each night, but maybe that's not helping Arthur. I guess it's mostly about me worrying again. I don't think I drink too much.

THERAPIST: I understand. Well, let's hold off on further exploring that for now. We'll come back to it though.

Note: As indicated earlier, a situation such as this in which the CSO gave herself a less than stellar happiness rating for her own substance use is one worth following up on.

5. Select a category from the Happiness Scale for setting a goal.

When it is time for a CSO to select a category from the Happiness Scale for setting a goal, take note of whether the selected category is one that you have reviewed already in terms of *why* the CSO assigned the particular rating and *what would have to change* in order for the rating to improve. If you have not reviewed it, ask those questions before deciding whether it is a good idea to proceed with setting a goal in that category.

Encourage the CSO to select a category on which she or he wants to work in the upcoming week, ideally one rated in the 4–7 range.

Since early success with homework assignments is highly motivating, efforts are made to increase the likelihood of CSO success. Categories with moderate ratings (4–7) are considered good choices for initial goal setting, as they often result in challenging but achievable homework assignments. For those CSOs who insist on choosing a less than ideal category as a starting point (see Box 10.1), you should take great care to ensure that the goal and strategy (assignment) are broken down into very small steps that are likely to be achievable.

THERAPIST: The next step is for you to pick one of these categories so that we can set a goal or two for you to work on this week. It's important to pick one that you can picture

BOX 10.1

Low-Rated Goal Categories Made Acceptable for Assignments

Assume a CSO insists upon selecting the family relationships category, despite rating it a 1. She then states that it will improve to a 2 once her cocaine-using husband (the IP) starts to approach her sexually again *after* he has been completely substance-free for 3 months. You would work with the CSO to identify a "first step" in the direction of this longer-term goal. One example might be to have the CSO focus on romantic precursors that are under her own control, and which she would use only when her husband was substance-free for 24 hours (see Chapter 5). Subsequent assignments would build on any success.

yourself working hard to make some changes in *now*. I'd also like to suggest that you focus on the categories you rated between a 4 and a 7. These tend to represent good categories to start with, because although they can result in challenging assignments, they will likely still be achievable. In other words, they won't be too hard and they won't be too easy.

CSO: So, I shouldn't pick social life because I only gave that a 2. Fine by me. I didn't want to start with that anyway.

THERAPIST: Right, social life might be too much of a challenge as far as our first goal area to work on. But it doesn't mean we won't work up to it eventually. Also, we could possibly help you increase the time you spend with your daughter; social life doesn't have to only be about doing things with your husband. Anyway, you had some good ideas about a few of the other categories. We talked about money management and job/education, but you have quite a few more in the 4–7 ratings. Shall we talk about some of them before you decide where to start this week?

Note: The therapist lets the CSO know that eventually it will be important to focus on improving her social life, and that this would not necessarily be restricted to increasing pleasant activities with her IP (see Box 10.2).

BOX 10.2

Social Activities as CSO Goals

Addressing a CSO's social life, including one that is partly independent of the IP, is a critical part of CRAFT. Although a very low rating for a CSO's social life category would be a deterrent for selecting it early in the goal-setting process, it would be targeted later in treatment, since social activities are a great source of support.

For cases in which the IPs are the romantic partner of the CSOs, the CSOs often feel guilty about planning social activities that do not involve their IP. Be prepared to discuss the need for these CSOs to take care of themselves in multiple ways as part of CRAFT. At the same time, the potential for CSOs to put themselves at risk for violence (from the IP) with an independent social activity assignment is reviewed. In high-risk cases, you might suggest including the IP in the new social activities, but only if he or she is substance-free.

CSO: I noticed myself getting kind of excited when you asked me about what steps I might take to work toward my bachelor's degree. I'd like to start with the job/education category.

THERAPIST: Excellent choice, Stella. And if you decide that the plan for the week ends up sounding too easy, you can always pick a second category.

6. Establish a goal and a strategy for attaining it.

CRAFT offers therapists a set of guidelines for developing specific goals *and* the strategies for achieving them (see Box 10.3). These same guidelines are listed at the top of the Goal Setting form (Form 10.3) that is shared with CSOs and are referred to throughout the therapist–CSO dialogue.

Set a goal that meets the goal and strategy guidelines.

THERAPIST: Stella, we've found that it helps to follow a few basic guidelines when setting up goals and the weekly plan for working on them. As we get specific about what you plan to do in the job/education area, I'll be introducing them to help shape your plan. Does that sound OK?

CSO: Sure. Whatever you think will help.

THERAPIST: Wonderful. Let's go back to the goal you've already mentioned for this category. You said that in order to raise your Happiness Scale rating from a 4 to a 5 you'd need to find out what the requirements are for finishing up your bachelor's degree. I'm guessing you could probably accomplish this goal rather quickly, probably even this week. And so I'm going to suggest we come up with a bigger goal in the job/education area, one that will take a little longer but which you should be able to achieve during our remaining time together in treatment.

CSO: My dream is to finish the degree. But I think that's going to take about 2 years if I work really hard at it part-time. I know I have almost 2 months left in therapy.

THERAPIST: Yes, finishing your degree is a great long-term goal. And you're right, you have almost 2 months left in treatment. What would you like to accomplish by the time we're done?

CSO: I'd like to start taking a course toward my degree requirements.

BOX 10.3

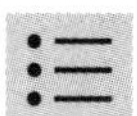

Goal and Strategy Guidelines

1. State goals/strategies that are concise and uncomplicated.
2. Use positive/action-oriented wording, indicating what *will* be done.
3. Use specific, measurable behaviors.
4. Design goals/strategies that are reasonable.
5. Select goals/strategies that are under the CSO's control.

Note: The first three guidelines are essentially the same ones used in positive communication training.

THERAPIST: Excellent. As I mentioned a few minutes ago, I'd like us to make sure this is a goal that meets the goal-setting guidelines. Here's a list of them at the top of this Goal Setting form (*hands CSO Form 10.3*). What does the first guideline say?

CSO (*reads off the list*): "State goals/strategies that are concise and uncomplicated." I think I've done that, haven't I?

THERAPIST: I totally agree. Your goal is clear and straightforward. We won't need to break it up into smaller goals. What's next?

CSO (*reads*): "Use positive/action-oriented wording, indicating what *will* be done." I'm not sure what that means. Wait—this sounds vaguely familiar. . . .

THERAPIST: Good for you! Yes, we spoke about this guideline, and several others, when we worked on communication skills. That should make it easier to remember and use. And you're definitely already using positive wording. As a reminder, it means that we like people to say what they're going to do, as opposed to what they're *not* going to do anymore. It mostly comes up when people are planning to change an unhealthy habit. Like someone might say, "I'm not going to sit and watch TV or play computer games all night anymore." But since it doesn't say what they *are* going to do instead, we'd rather have them say something like "I'm going to take the dog for a 30-minute walk every night after dinner." By the way, I wouldn't bother going into this much of an explanation right now if I didn't think this could be helpful as we set more goals down the road.

CSO: It makes good sense to me. I get it now.

THERAPIST: Great. What's the third one?

CSO (*reads*): "Use specific, measurable behaviors." I said that I'm taking a course. Is that specific enough? I don't know what they're offering yet.

THERAPIST: Your goal is pretty specific: one course that's required to complete your degree. And it's measurable because we'll know for sure once you've done it. The only thing I might add is the semester you're talking about. I'm assuming it's for this fall, since you said you'd be starting it soon?

CSO: Yes. I'll have to find out when the semester starts.

THERAPIST: That can be part of your assignment for this week, one of the steps I mentioned toward reaching your goal of starting the class. What's the fourth guideline?

CSO (*reads*): "Design goals/strategies that are reasonable." It sounds reasonable to me. Am I missing something though?

THERAPIST: Probably not, but it's always good to stop and ask yourself that question. Can you think of any reasons why you might not be able to start your course in the next 2 months? What might get in the way?

CSO: We have enough money for the tuition for one course, so that won't be a problem. Arthur knows I've been talking about doing this for some time, so he'll be OK with it. I guess the only thing would be if they didn't offer a course that I need yet, but that's really unlikely. Or maybe the course will be closed if I wait too long to register.

THERAPIST: Good job thinking this through, Stella. Seems like the main obstacle would be missing out on a course you want if you wait too long and it's closed.

CSO: I better get moving on this then! OK. I see that the final guideline is to "Select goals/

strategies that are under the CSO's control." I think I'm good with this, too. I can use my own money that I've set aside, if necessary, for the tuition.

THERAPIST: Let's take another look at the form I just showed you with the Goal and Strategy Guidelines listed on the top (*refers to Form 10.3 again*). The categories are set up to match the ones on the Happiness Scale. I'm going to write your goal on the form under Category 2.

Note: See Figure 10.2 for a completed Goal Setting sample for this CSO and Box 10.4 for samples of problematic and improved goals for other CSOs.

Create a strategy for achieving the goal that meets the goal and strategy guidelines. CSOs sometimes have a clear idea of a goal, but they struggle when it comes to laying out a plan (strategy) for reaching it. Under these circumstances it can be worthwhile to introduce the Problem Solving procedure (Chapter 9). Additionally, at times CSOs (*and* therapists) experience some confusion about the difference between a goal and a strategy:

- **Goal:** more long term, such as within the next month. Although it is *not* something that typically will be accomplished in the upcoming week (like a strategy), it is still scheduled so that the CSO will have the opportunity to work toward it and achieve it while in treatment. Achieving the goal should result in a CSO increasing the rating by several points for that category on the Happiness Scale.
- **Strategy:** essentially the weekly (homework) assignment. Strategies are small steps on the path toward a goal.

THERAPIST: Now that you've got a clear goal, we need to line up the first steps toward achieving it. These steps or "strategies" are really the same as a homework assignment. And we'll be following the five guidelines we used when finalizing your goal. As you know, your goal is to start taking a course toward your degree requirements this fall. What are you willing to do *this week* to work toward that goal?

CSO: I need to find out what requirements I have left for my degree. I'm not sure who I need to ask about that though. Maybe that should be part of the assignment?

THERAPIST: Yes, let's make that one of the steps this week. How should we word it? I bet you can make it meet most of the five guidelines by just trying to be very specific about what you want to do.

CSO: I really prefer talking to someone, so I'm going to call the Sociology Department at the university and ask who I need to speak to about my remaining requirements. Then I'll contact that person, I guess through email if I need to.

THERAPIST: You're off to a good start. I'll just run down the guidelines for these first two steps quickly. They are both stated concisely and clearly, they spell out what you *are* going to do, they're reasonable, and they're under your control. I skipped over the third guideline, the one about being specific, because I think you can make them even more specific if we nail down *when* you're going to contact these two people.

CSO: I'd better say that I'm going to do it tomorrow morning, because otherwise I might forget.

THERAPIST: I'll put tomorrow's date under "Time Frame" for them both then.

Problem areas/goals	Step-by-step strategy (weekly assignment)	Time frame
1. In the area of **social life,** I will:		
Contact 2 former good friends (Dolores, Paul) and invite them each out for coffee.	a. Write out what I want to say to these friends before contacting them.	Thurs. (6/14)
	b. Contact both friends electronically.	Fri. (6/15)
	c. Follow up electronically a week later with a brief, casual conversation.	Fri. (6/22)
	d. Invite these friends to coffee individually.	Thurs. (7/5)
2. In the area of **job or education,** I will:		
Start taking a course toward degree requirements this fall.	a. Call the Sociology Department or check website to get contact information.	Tues. (6/5)
	b. Contact the person who advises about degree requirements.	Tues. (6/5)
	c. Inquire about remaining degree requirements and see which courses are being offered this fall.	Fri. (6/8)
	d. Find out how to register and how to pay.	Fri. (6/8)
3. In the area of **money management,** I will:		
Save $80 this month.	a. Record my expenses in an online budget planner.	Mon. (6/11)
	b. Ask husband to tell me what he spends or show him how to record it online himself.	Mon. (6/11)
	c. Decide what needs to change in order for me to set aside $20/week.	Mon. (6/18)
	d. Try saving the $20; if not successful, do problem solving.	Mon. (6/25)
4. In the area of **substance use,** I will:		
Limit wine drinking to dinners out with friends.	a. Buy my favorite flavored water to drink at home with dinner.	Thurs. (6/14)
	b. Check before leaving house each morning to be sure there's flavored water chilling in fridge.	
5. In the area of **health and wellness,** I will:		
Join a Zumba class.	a. Check YWCA's website to see when Zumba classes are offered and the cost.	Thurs. (6/21)
	b. Sample at least two Zumba classes before making a commitment to one.	Thurs. (7/12)
6. In the area of **family relationships,** I will:		
Start inviting my daughter to lunch every other week.	a. Plan and practice a conversation to have with my daughter about me being in CRAFT.	Wed. (6/27)
	b. Ask daughter if she is willing to meet privately to talk.	Mon. (7/2)
	c. Try to schedule a time to meet daughter for coffee.	Mon. (7/9)

(continued)

FIGURE 10.2. Completed version of Form 10.3, Goal Setting.

Problem areas/goals	Step-by-step strategy (weekly assignment)	Time frame
7. In the area of **legal issues,** I will:		
[See number 9, Communication.]		
8. In the area of **emotional life,** I will:		
Take a 20-minute walk each weekday to unwind upon arriving home from work.	a. Buy some good walking shoes.	Sun. (7/29)
	b. Map out a safe route that appears to have many other walkers.	Mon. (7/30)
	c. Start by walking 10 minutes for 3 weekdays.	Mon. (8/6)
	d. Increase to 15 minutes for 4 weekdays.	Mon. (8/13)
9. In the area of **communication,** I will:		
Use positive communication skills to tell my husband my fears about him getting caught at work buying and using oxycodone illegally.	a. Review the components of positive communication skills.	Tues. (7/17)
	b. Plan out what I will say to my husband about the Oxycodone use.	Fri. (7/20)
	c. Practice the conversation and get feedback from therapist.	Mon. (7/23)
	d. Decide on the best time/place for the conversation.	Wed. (7/25)
10. In the area of **spirituality,** I will:		
Read one spiritual or inspirational book each month.	a. Go to a used book store and buy a spiritual book.	Mon. (7/9)
	b. Read the book and ask myself how I can apply it to my own life.	Mon. (7/16)
11. In the area of ______________________, I will:		

FIGURE 10.2 *(continued)*

Note: The therapist opted to move quickly through the review of the guidelines here (see Box 10.3), given that the CSO was quite skilled at specifying a solid strategy. As an example, the CSO automatically stated her strategy in positive terms (i.e., what she wanted to do as opposed to what she wanted to *stop* doing), and thus satisfied the second guideline. This is noteworthy because many CSOs instead stay focused on the things they want to stop doing (see Box 10.5).

Discuss potential obstacles to completing the assignment, and generate solutions when necessary.

THERAPIST: It's smart to be thinking about potential obstacles to getting the assignment done, like simply forgetting! And sounds like you have a solution to that already planned—you're jumping right on it tomorrow morning. Can you think of anything else that might get in the way of you contacting those two people tomorrow?

BOX 10.4

Problematic and Improved Goals

Below are examples of commonly seen goals that are first presented as "problematic"—namely, they do not adhere to several of the Goal and Strategy Guidelines. The specific violations of these guidelines are spelled out next, and improved goals that adhere to the guidelines follow. Although the strategies for accomplishing these goals are mentioned briefly, only the *goals* strictly meet the guidelines. A 1-month time frame for achieving each goal is implied throughout.

Problematic goal (*family relationships category*): "Improve my relationship with my sister."

- Does not adhere to guidelines 1 (too complicated, involves many steps), 3 (not a specific behavior), and 5 (not entirely under CSO's control).
- **Improved goal:** "Spend 2 hours each week doing something pleasant with or for my sister."
- (Weekly strategies focus on experimenting with different activities [e.g., Coffee with sister? Babysit her kids?] to see which ones are well received and which days work best.)

Problematic goal (*emotional life category*): "Stop getting upset over stuff that doesn't really matter."

- Does not adhere to guidelines 2 (does not say what *will* be done), 3 (not a specific behavior), 4 (not reasonable), and 5 (not entirely under CSO's control).
- **Improved goal:** "Read a self-help relaxation or meditation book."
- (Weekly strategies focus on researching which book the CSO wants to purchase, purchasing it, and setting aside time daily to read it and start practicing the exercises.)

Problematic goal (*health and wellness category*): "Get more sleep."

- Does not adhere to guidelines 1 (too complicated), 3 (not specific), and 5 (not entirely under CSO's control).
- **Improved goal:** "Get into bed at 11:00 P.M. every night and turn off the TV and phone."
- (Weekly strategies focus on finding ways to get work and other activities done earlier in the evening, and experimenting with ways to "wind down.")

BOX 10.5

What CSOs Plan to *Start* Doing

The use of "negative" wording (what CSOs plan to *stop* doing) appears to occur naturally to many people when they are thinking about ways to change problematic behavior. Thus, the second Goal and Strategy Guideline (use positive/action-oriented wording, indicating what *will* be done) typically requires both an explanation and an example. But it is time well spent, since positive statements tend to spell out specific ways in which the CSOs are going to start behaving, as opposed to simply reporting what they are not going to do anymore. The latter begs the question "If you're not going to do *X*, *Y*, or *Z* anymore, what *are* you going to do instead?"

CSO: Maybe it's one of those places where you only get voicemail. If I don't get the information from the first person pretty quickly, I won't be able to contact the second.

THERAPIST: Good point. So you'll need a backup plan. Can you think of another way to get contact information for the person who can check on your degree requirements?

CSO: I bet I can find it on the department's website. I'll look there if nobody answers the phone when I call the department.

THERAPIST: Good. Let me just stick with this question about obstacles for another minute. Imagine yourself getting up tomorrow morning with the intention of making the first call. What might get in the way?

CSO: Myself! I have thought about doing these calls many times, and I always manage to talk myself out of them. I guess I just figure there's no point, because I won't actually take the classes anyway. I mean, I don't feel like that now, but who knows by tomorrow. . . .

Note: The therapist asks the CSO to picture herself preparing to attempt a strategy (assignment) because it is helpful in bringing to mind potential obstacles she otherwise might not have imagined. This allows time to address the anticipated problems in advance, or to decide that the obstacles render the planned assignment too risky. In the latter case, the therapist would propose that the CSO selects a different strategy.

THERAPIST: I really admire your honesty and insight. How will you tackle those thoughts if they do appear tomorrow?

CSO: I'll tell myself that I made a commitment to do the assignment, and that it doesn't hurt to just gather information.

THERAPIST: Very good. And it might also help to remind yourself that you're working toward a long-term goal that you described as a dream of yours: to get your bachelor's degree. Sometimes that can provide extra motivation.

Note: The therapist suggests that the CSO remind herself of a major reinforcer, finishing her degree, if she faces an obstacle to completing her assignment. Often it is helpful to link the completion of an assignment back to the achievement of an important goal.

Decide whether to add more strategies for the week to the current goal.

THERAPIST: Stella, should we add another strategy or two for this week? You plan to contact these two people tomorrow, and I'm guessing the phone calls, and maybe an email, won't take that long. What do you think?

CSO: Yes, because not only do I need to find out what my remaining requirements are, I also need to know what courses are being offered this fall that I can take, and how I go about registering and paying. I haven't done this in a long time, so I'm sure things have changed.

THERAPIST: Listen to you—very impressive! So tell me, are you up for all of these? I bet the main contact person or the advisor can tell you how to get this information.

CSO: You're probably right. And yes, put me down for all of these things.

Note: The therapist believed that this CSO could tackle additional steps that week toward the ultimate goal without overwhelming her, and so encouraged her to add assignments to her list. The therapist next checks on the wording of the strategies and addresses potential barriers.

THERAPIST: Let's just check on the wording first to make sure we've satisfied the guidelines. What do you think?

CSO: The only one I'm not sure about is whether it's totally under my control. What if the advisor is on vacation for the week, or out sick, and I can't get the information?

THERAPIST: You're already anticipating obstacles to successfully doing the assignment. Good for you! Yes, we'll need a backup plan. But first, maybe we just need to change the wording a little so that the assignment is definitely under your control. Maybe there *is* only one person who can get you the information about your remaining requirements, and like you said, that person might be unavailable. Since we can't guarantee that you'll be able to find out what you need to take, how about we instead say that you'll *inquire* about it? This allows you control, because you can at least email the person or leave a phone message with your question in the event that he or she is out of the office all week.

CSO: That makes sense.

Note: The therapist wants to be sure the CSO has every chance of succeeding with the assignment, and thus modifies the wording so that it is, in fact, under the CSO's control.

THERAPIST: But what do you think about the other parts of the assignment? Do you think you might be able to find other ways to get information about fall course offerings, and both registration and payment?

CSO: Nowadays that information should be online.

THERAPIST: I'll add these strategies to your Goal Setting form then. How about we put Friday as the due date in case you run into a few roadblocks?

CSO: Good idea.

THERAPIST: What other barriers might get in the way of you getting this information?

CSO: I really can't think of any.

THERAPIST: The only thing I can think of is the Internet being down if you're trying to get some of this information from the university's website.

CSO: I better not wait until the last possible day to do this then!

7. Set additional goal/strategies if indicated.

Decide whether to add another goal (and strategies)—if so, follow guidelines.

Whether to assign another goal and its corresponding strategy depends on your perception of the CSO's ability to tackle additional assignments in the upcoming week. The primary factors to consider include the amount of time and effort required to address the homework already assigned, and the CSO's track record for completing multicomponent assignments.

THERAPIST: You're doing a great job today, and I think you're going to feel really good when you tackle these assignments this week. Now it's time to decide if the one goal and its multistep assignments are enough for the upcoming week, or whether you want to do more. If you decide you want to do more, we could either make another goal in the job/education area, or we could pick a different category. You know yourself best—What do you think?

CSO: I don't think it's going to take long to do these other things. Oh heck—let's do another category!

THERAPIST: I agree. So which of these other categories looks appealing? And again, it's best if we stay in the 4–7 range, as far as your ratings. That leaves us with money management, substance use, health and wellness, family relationships, emotional life, communication, and spirituality.

CSO: I want to try to save some money, so let's go with money management. I think I said that I wanted to start saving $20 a week. Can that be my goal? Oh wait; that sounds more like my strategy for the week. Can it be both?

THERAPIST: It can be confusing, can't it? But don't let it bog you down; it will all work out regardless. Let's think of it this way: Saving $20 a week is a good goal, but it doesn't spell out *how* you're going to do it, so there's no "strategy." In other words, where is the money going to come from? Also, I think it's good to make the goal a little more long term, like something at least a month away. It gives you a little more flexibility to work step-by-step toward the goal. And ideally if you reach your goal, you'll be able to rate that category on the Happiness Scale a bit higher the next time. What about a goal of saving $80 this month, since that would be $20 each week?

CSO: I like that, because then if I can't come up with the $20 for one week, I can make it up another week and still reach my $80 monthly goal.

THERAPIST: Exactly! But before I add it to the Goal Setting form, let's see if it satisfies the five guidelines. Go for it!

CSO: It's concise, stated in a positive way, and specific. And I think it's a reasonable amount and under my control. I do have a little extra cash each week that seems to mysteriously disappear. Yes, I can do it.

THERAPIST: Say no more! It's going on the goals form. What about a plan, a strategy, for reaching that goal? What can you do differently?

CSO: I'd like to track where my money, and my husband's money, is going first before I decide where I'm going to take it from.

THERAPIST: And when you say you're going to track it, what will that look like?

CSO: I know of a budget program online that shows you how to type in everything you spend in a week. It puts everything in categories. I've thought of doing that before but I never got around to it. I think it will be fun.

THERAPIST: Sounds like you're off to a good start. How about the guidelines for this strategy?

CSO: It's concise and clear, positive, specific, and reasonable. I'm not sure it's completely under my control though, because if my husband doesn't tell me everything *he* spends, I'll miss some things.

THERAPIST: How could you reword it so that it *is* under your control, and it still mostly accomplishes what you want it to?

Note: Given the CSO's high skill level in terms of goal setting, the therapist allows the CSO to lead the review of the guidelines and to make the first attempt at correcting any problems with the wording of the assignment. For CSOs with minimal goal-setting skills, you would play a more active role in reviewing the guidelines and developing new strategies (refer to Box 10.6 for samples of goals with problematic and improved strategies for other CSOs).

BOX 10.6

Goals with Problematic and Improved (Weekly) Strategies

Sample goals that adhere to the Goal and Strategy Guidelines are presented first, and examples of both problematic and improved strategies for achieving the goals follow. The problematic strategies violate the Goal and Strategy Guidelines—specific explanations as to why are provided. Several examples of improved strategies that adhere to the guidelines are offered next. The time frame for accomplishing each strategy is 1 week.

Goal (*social life category*): "Join an organization that specializes in outdoor activities and begin attending biweekly."

Problematic strategy: "Find an organization focused on outdoor activities; avoid ones that are probably geared toward seniors and ones that cost too much."

- Does not adhere to guidelines 2 (second half does not say what *will* be done) and 3 (not specific).

Improved strategies: (1) "Look up outdoor activity organizations using an Internet search and narrow it down to the top three most interesting ones," (2) "Narrow it down further to the ones that specialize in activities for 25- to 45-year-olds and that have a membership fee of $25 or less," and (3) "Contact the organization(s) that satisfy these requirements and see if I can attend one event in the next 2 weeks without officially joining."

Goal (*communication category*): "Compliment my teenage son during dinner at least four times a week."

Problematic strategy: "Think of something nice to say and don't get angry or annoyed if he doesn't respond."

- Does not adhere to guidelines 2 (second half does not say what *will* be done), 3 (not specific), 4 (second half not entirely reasonable), and 5 (second half not entirely under CSO's control).

Improved strategies: (1) "Make a list of potential compliments and select two for the first week," (2) "Rehearse the compliments using positive communication skills," (3) "Deliver two compliments during dinner the first week," and (4) "Remind myself that it's OK if my son doesn't respond positively."

CSO: I should say that I'm going to record what *I* spend, and that I'll ask my husband either to tell me what he spends, or to record it himself in the budget planner.

THERAPIST: Perfect. Since you'll be doing this assignment all week, I'll just put next session's date for the time frame for completing it. What about obstacles to getting this done? This is a much larger assignment than you contacting the Sociology Department.

CSO: Arthur will probably prefer to record it himself instead of telling me, so I'll need to show him how to use the program. I'll do that tonight. And I'd better leave myself a note the first few days until I get into the habit of recording the expenses.

Have CSO repeat back entire assignment.

One way to determine whether the CSO remembers and understands the assignment is to have him or her repeat it back to you. If the CSO has trouble with this step, you can offer assistance immediately. Furthermore, this tends to be the time when a CSO expresses any existing hesitation about doing an assignment. If this occurs, it can be addressed, such as through a CRA procedure called Systematic Encouragement (see Box 10.7).

THERAPIST: Once again—great job, Stella! I think you've now got plenty to work on this week. In fact, it's probably a good idea that we revisit everything you plan to do this week, just to make sure we're on the same page. And in case it helps, it's all written down on this Goal Setting form [Form 10.3; see Figure 10.2]. I'll send you home with a copy. Go ahead; tell me what your strategies are for the week!

COMMON PROBLEMS TO AVOID

The Happiness Scale is easy to administer, but clinicians sometimes do not take full advantage of the valuable information it contains. The Goal Setting exercise appears straightforward, and yet clinicians frequently have difficulty adhering to the recommended guidelines when formulating the goals and strategies. Suggestions for these and other problems follow.

Problem: As mentioned previously when discussing the use of other CRAFT forms, therapists sometimes refer to the procedure/exercise as "filling out a form." It is best to avoid referring to the Happiness Scale and Goal Setting exercise as "forms" since this minimizes the importance of the task at hand and reduces it to "paperwork."

Safeguards:

- Refer to CRAFT procedures as exercises, tasks, . . . or procedures.
- Do your best to convey enthusiasm when introducing all CRAFT procedures so that CSOs get a sense of their importance from the start.

Problem: New CRAFT clinicians occasionally administer the Happiness Scale as if it is just an item on a checklist of things to get done in a session, and as a result they miss the

BOX 10.7

Taking the First Step

At times, CSOs have a clear goal and the strategy for achieving it, but they experience great difficulty taking the first step. Usually this becomes apparent when they report in the next session that they were unsuccessful at even attempting their assignment, or when they raise many potential obstacles to completing the assignment during the in-session review of the strategy for the week. In these cases, "Systematic Encouragement" is used to help CSOs take that first step of their homework assignment *during* the session (see Chapter 12).

opportunity to follow up on details regarding the people or activities that play critical roles in the CSOs' lives.

Safeguards:

- Always assume that a CRAFT form is being administered for an important clinical reason, and that the information will be incorporated into the CSO's therapy in some manner.
- Remind yourself that the Happiness Scale is not a "one-and-done" instrument, but a tool that "keeps on giving" because it is built around CSOs' reinforcers: the rewards they need help working toward to make their lives happier.

Problem: Therapists have also been known to work on the Goal Setting exercise in one session and to file away the form upon completion, never returning to it again. The Goal Setting form is a treatment plan, and treatment plans need to be constantly reviewed and updated with new goals and new assignments.

Safeguards:

- Automatically have the Goal Setting form (Form 10.3) out and ready to go for each session. Since it contains the assignments from the previous week, they routinely should be reviewed at the beginning of a session. Even if new goals are not added, assignments should be updated weekly and added to the Goal Setting form.

Problem: Clinicians frequently use vague language when helping CSOs set goals and devise strategies. The use of specific wording reduces uncertainty about what CSOs are expected to accomplish and how. Given that it is unnatural for individuals to use highly specific language when speaking, it is no surprise that the first attempts at goal setting sound quite general.

Safeguards:

- Every time a goal/strategy is noted, ask yourself, "Can this be made more specific?" Also ask yourself, "If someone else (besides the CSO) were to read this, would she or he know exactly what it means and what to do?"

Problem: Sometimes clinicians do a beautiful job helping CSOs develop goals and assignments, but they end the exercise without asking about obstacles. Or, in other cases, the therapists ask about obstacles, but they do not inquire about potential solutions to the obstacles. Asking CSOs to anticipate barriers is an excellent way to get them to think about all the possible things that can go wrong, and to have the CSOs come up with reasonable methods for addressing these barriers should they present themselves during the week.

Safeguards:

- Get into the habit of always posing the question "Obstacles?" every time an assignment is given.
- Challenge CSOs to beat you to the punch to raise the question of obstacles when assignments are formulated.

Problem: At times, CRAFT therapists assume goal setting is a totally independent exercise that has no relationship to other CRAFT procedures. However, there are several procedures (e.g., Improving CSOs' Communication Skills) that provide CSOs with the skills needed to make progress toward the goals. And as noted previously, the Problem Solving procedure can be worthwhile when a CSO has trouble generating ideas for reaching a goal (e.g., coming up with new independent social activities that are inexpensive and fun).

Safeguards:

- When assisting a CSO in selecting strategies for obtaining goals as part of the Goal Setting exercise, get into the habit of asking yourself whether the CSO would have a better chance of successfully completing the strategy (homework) if another CRAFT procedure was introduced or reviewed first (e.g., Problem Solving, Improving CSOs' Communication Skills).

SUMMARY

This chapter deviates from the other chapters thus far, inasmuch as the focus is on the CSO's goals *aside from* getting the IP to reduce use and enter treatment. One noteworthy advantage of this focus is that CSOs can improve the quality of their lives regardless of whether their IP ever starts therapy. The Happiness Scale and Goal Setting exercise that dominate the chapter are borrowed from CRA, the treatment for IPs (see Chapter 12).

FORM 10.1

Helping CSOs Enrich Their Own Lives: Checklist

1. Give the rationale for focusing on the CSO's own happiness.

- ☐ a. State that CSOs' own happiness and health is an important part of CRAFT.
- ☐ b. Explain that CSOs often are isolated and suffering emotionally as a result of their IP's problem.
- ☐ c. Explain how CSOs are better able to take care of their IPs if the CSOs are taking better care of themselves, and as a result feel better (e.g., less anxious and depressed).

2. Introduce and provide the rationale for the Happiness Scale.

- ☐ a. State that the Happiness Scale is a tool that will allow the CSO to rate her or his happiness in different life areas.
- ☐ b. Explain that the information helps the CSO set goals for areas in which the CSO would like to see changes.
- ☐ c. Explain that the Happiness Scale will also be used to monitor progress in achieving goals over time.

3. Give instructions for the Happiness Scale.

- ☐ a. Explain that the CSO should rate her or his current happiness in each of the categories using the 1–10 scale.
- ☐ b. Ask the CSO to rate each category independent of the others, and to focus on how she or he is feeling today.
- ☐ c. Encourage the CSO to ask questions at any point.

4. Review some of the ratings on the Happiness Scale.

- ☐ a. Discuss the ratings of at least several categories by asking why a particular rating was given.
- ☐ b. Ask what would have to *change* in order for the rating to improve by a point or two.

5. Select a category from the Happiness Scale for setting a goal.

- ☐ a. Encourage the CSO to select a category on which she or he wants to work in the upcoming week, ideally one rated in the 4-7 range.

(continued)

6. Establish a goal and a strategy for attaining it.

- ☐ a. Set a goal that meets the goal and strategy guidelines.
- ☐ b. Create a strategy for achieving the goal that meets the goal and strategy guidelines.
- ☐ c. Discuss potential obstacles to completing the assignment, and generate solutions when necessary.
- ☐ d. Decide whether to add more strategies for the week to the current goal.

7. Set additional goal/strategies if indicated.

- ☐ a. Decide whether to add another goal (and strategies)—if so, follow guidelines.
- ☐ b. Have CSO repeat back entire assignment.

FORM 10.2

Happiness Scale

This scale is intended to estimate your *current* happiness with your life in each of the areas listed below. The blank box in the first column is for adding an area that is not already represented but is relevant to you. Ask yourself the following question as you rate each area:

How happy am I with this area of my life?

Circle one of the numbers (1–10) beside each area. Numbers toward the left (lower numbers, like 1) indicate various degrees of unhappiness, while numbers toward the right (higher numbers, like 10) reflect various levels of happiness.

In other words, state according to the numerical scale (1–10) exactly how you feel **today**. Also, try not to allow one category to influence the results of the other categories.

	Completely unhappy									**Completely happy**
Social life	1	2	3	4	5	6	7	8	9	10
Job or education	1	2	3	4	5	6	7	8	9	10
Money management	1	2	3	4	5	6	7	8	9	10
Substance use	1	2	3	4	5	6	7	8	9	10
Health and wellness	1	2	3	4	5	6	7	8	9	10
Family relationships	1	2	3	4	5	6	7	8	9	10
Legal issues	1	2	3	4	5	6	7	8	9	10
Emotional life	1	2	3	4	5	6	7	8	9	10
Communication	1	2	3	4	5	6	7	8	9	10
Spirituality	1	2	3	4	5	6	7	8	9	10
Other: ________________	1	2	3	4	5	6	7	8	9	10
General happiness	1	2	3	4	5	6	7	8	9	10

FORM 10.3

Goal Setting

Keep the goal and strategy guidelines in mind when filling out this form:

1. State goals/strategies that are concise and uncomplicated.
2. Use positive/action-oriented wording, indicating what *will* be done.
3. Use specific, measurable behaviors.
4. Design goals/strategies that are reasonable.
5. Select goals/strategies that are under the CSO's control.

Problem areas/goals	Step-by-step strategy (weekly assignment)	Time frame
1. In the area of **social life,** I will:		
2. In the area of **job or education,** I will:		
3. In the area of **money management,** I will:		

(continued)

Problem areas/goals	Step-by-step strategy (weekly assignment)	Time frame
4. In the area of **substance use,** I will:		
5. In the area of **health and wellness,** I will:		
6. In the area of **family relationships,** I will:		
7. In the area of **legal issues,** I will:		

(continued)

Problem areas/goals	Step-by-step strategy (weekly assignment)	Time frame
8. In the area of **emotional life,** I will:		
9. In the area of **communication,** I will:		
10. In the area of **spirituality,** I will:		
11. In the area of ________________________________, I will:		

Chapter 11

Inviting the Identified Patient to Enter Treatment

This chapter presents a procedure that teaches CSOs how to invite their IP to begin treatment by building a conversation that capitalizes on the factors that are most likely to influence the IP to agree. In addition to addressing the language and timing of the treatment invitation, this chapter outlines steps that should be taken to ensure that the IP is able to have a session with an appropriate therapist quickly. Finally, it prepares CSOs for handling a variety of possible IP responses to the treatment invitation.

Although CSOs are eager to learn this procedure, CRAFT therapists typically delay its introduction until the CSOs have learned other foundational procedures first, such as Improving CSOs' Communication Skills and Rewarding Non-Using Behavior. Not only does this equip CSOs with the skills to make the request and to deal with its consequences, but it often affords CSOs the opportunity to become more confident overall and to improve their relationship with their IP. Furthermore, the additional time and the CSOs' new skills can be instrumental in reducing the IP's substance use prior to extending the treatment invitation. The net result is that these IPs should be more open to sampling treatment.

THE BASICS

General Description

CRAFT's procedure for Inviting the IP to Enter Treatment consists of three distinct parts. As mentioned above, the procedure first focuses on crafting the conversation that increases the odds that the IP will agree to treatment. This process entails utilizing information that the CSO has already shared about the IP's reinforcers, and examining motivational hooks—additional potential rewards linked to treatment engagement that might entice the IP upon hearing about them. The composition of the treatment invitation is also influenced by whether the IP already knows that the CSO is in therapy. If the IPs *are* aware of their CSO's treatment, the CSOs typically refer to their own treatment in some manner as part of the treatment invitation. If the IPs are *un*aware of their CSO's ongoing therapy, then the CSOs commonly share that information with their IP at the start of the treatment engagement conversation. In terms of the timing of the delivery, CSOs learn how to use "windows of opportunity" as ideal times to invite their IPs to treatment.

Once CSOs are prepared to deliver the treatment invitation, they still must approach the issue of lining up a therapist who not only treats individuals with substance use problems, but also commits to seeing their IP *within a day or two* of when the IP agrees to treatment. The importance of finding a therapist who is similar in theoretical orientation to the CRAFT therapist is also discussed. The third part of Inviting the IP to Enter Treatment involves exploring how CSOs will handle the various reactions their IPs could have to the request, such as an IP agreeing to treatment but then never actually attending, or beginning treatment but terminating prematurely. The need for the CSO's continued emotional and behavioral support for the treatment-engaged IP is emphasized as well.

Procedure Timing

Although this is typically the last new procedure introduced in CRAFT, multiple factors still influence the decision regarding when it is time for CSOs to learn the specifics of extending a treatment invitation. As noted, at the very least, they will need to have had communication training, but usually they will have worked with you on most of the other procedures as well. Occasionally you might be convinced that the CSO is going to head home and prematurely extend a treatment invitation to the IP despite it not being the ideal time. In such cases you might opt to provide basic training in how to invite the IP to engage in treatment, regardless of whether other important CRAFT procedures have been taught.

Forms

- Inviting the IP to Enter Treatment: Checklist (Form 11.1)
- Using Motivational Hooks and Positive Communication to Invite Your Loved One to Attend Treatment (Handout 11.1)

CLINICIAN GUIDANCE AND SAMPLE DIALOGUE

The components for the CRAFT procedure Inviting the IP to Enter Treatment are presented below. Again, a sample case with clinician–CSO dialogue is included. The components for conducting this exercise are outlined in Form 11.1, Inviting the IP to Enter Treatment: Checklist, found at the end of this chapter.

Case Description

The CSO (Seri) is an unmarried 34-year-old Asian American female who lives in her own apartment. She has always had a close relationship with her half-brother, the 27-year-old IP (Ju Meok). Ju Meok lives with his (and Seri's) mother and a younger brother in the same apartment complex as Seri. The IP started to use substances while associating with a problematic group of friends after graduating from high school. At that time, Seri was influential in getting Ju Meok to stop using drugs and to begin college. The first 2 years of college went reasonably well, but Ju Meok became distraught after a breakup with a girlfriend. He reconnected with the friends who used substances, and quickly fell back into that lifestyle. Ju Meok's mother asked Seri to intervene again, which she willingly did. However, this time Ju Meok was unwilling to change his behavior. Consequently, Seri began CRAFT treatment. Although she does not live with Ju Meok, she has almost daily face-to-face contact with him. After several CRAFT sessions, Seri was influential in getting him to reduce his use and to increase his healthy social activities. Nonetheless, both Seri and her therapist believed it would be beneficial for Ju Meok to attend treatment so that his progress could continue.

1. Discuss motivational hooks for treatment invitations.

Motivational hooks are enticements presented by CSOs to their IP to make the idea of starting therapy more appealing (see Box 11.1). Since these hooks are built on the assumption that the CSOs already have revealed their own involvement in therapy to the IP, CSOs who have *not* done so yet would lead into the hooks discussion by informing their IP about their own treatment. Importantly, IPs tend to be more willing to listen to the message about their CSO's treatment (and to the treatment invitation that follows) if the CSOs do *not* directly state that they sought professional help exclusively or primarily to deal with the IP's substance use problem. Examples of CSOs revealing their therapy involvement at the start of their treatment invitation include:

- "You mentioned the other day that I've been in a better mood lately. I think you're right, and I'm guessing it's because I've been seeing a therapist. I've had lots of things on my mind that have been stressing me out, like work, the kids, and our frequent arguing. I think therapy is really helping."
- "I probably should have told you that I've been seeing a therapist for a few weeks now. My life felt like it was spiraling out of control. We've had our own troubles for a while now, as you know, some of them related to your drinking. Anyway, I've been feeling quite a bit better."

Present several motivational hooks.

THERAPIST: Seri, you've done a great job using the CRAFT procedures, and as a result Ju Meok has cut back his substance use considerably *and* has gotten back in touch with some of his old friends who don't use. How are you feeling about this progress?

CSO: I feel really good. But I still think he could benefit from getting into treatment. He still hangs out with his "troubled" friends and uses every now and then. I'm afraid his progress could fall apart at any minute.

THERAPIST: I agree that we shouldn't stop. It's a perfect time to move on to the CRAFT procedure that focuses on inviting a loved one into treatment. And you've already learned the basic skills to carry this off successfully. So let's go over some things you can tell him that might get him more interested in attending. We call these motivational hooks. I'll go over these hooks, and then we'll narrow it down to the ones you think might work with him. You can also add some of your own. And I know you've

BOX 11.1

Motivational Hooks to Bolster Treatment Entry Request

a. The IP can meet the CSO's therapist informally if desired:
- IPs are curious to find out about the individual who has been treating their loved one; the CRAFT therapist's warm and welcoming style then "seals the deal."

b. The IP can have his or her own therapist:
- IPs are reassured to learn that they would *not* be getting their CSO's therapist, as they assume the CSO's therapist would be biased against them.

c. The IP can sample a treatment session or two before making a decision regarding whether to attend regularly:
- IPs find this "no strings attached" offer less stressful and less overwhelming.
- IPs like the idea of having an easy way "out" if they do not like their therapist.

d. The IP can provide major input into the treatment goals and plan, including the extent to which the focus is on substance use:
- Some IPs respond to the idea that they will not necessarily have to "admit" they have a substance use problem that will need to be worked on right away.
- IPs may react favorably to the opportunity to receive assistance with depression or anxiety, job searches, relationship issues, and so on.

e. The IP can expect to be treated with respect and without confrontation or judgment:
- Many IPs assume they will be judged for their behavior, so this guarantee elicits curiosity and intrigue (and naturally some skepticism).

f. The IP can maximize therapy benefits (reduced use) now, in anticipation of a timely upcoming reward for substance-free behavior (e.g., the IP will be allowed to attend a child's school event in one month *if* abstinent for several weeks by then):
- IPs respond favorably to a short-term goal/challenge that seems manageable, especially if it is linked to a specific and highly valued reward.

already told him about being in therapy yourself, so we'll keep that in mind as we go through these.

Note: Since the IP already knows that the CSO is in her own treatment, the therapist does not need to cover this preliminary part of the conversation for the motivational hooks discussion. Case examples 2 and 3 in Handout 11.1, found at the end of this chapter, represent CSOs who have *not* yet told their IPs about being in treatment, and thus they include that information as part of the IP treatment invitation.

CSO: I'm eager to hear your suggestions.

THERAPIST: Great! I'm going to give you this handout so you can follow along (*gives CSO Handout 11.1*). The first one involves asking Ju Meok if he'd like to meet *your* therapist, me. This would be very informal. It could take place outside the office, such as at a coffee shop, if Ju Meok felt more comfortable there. This brief meeting would serve several purposes. Ju Meok might be curious about what you've been doing in therapy but be afraid to ask. This way he could hear directly from me what's been going on. And it would give me a chance to tell him what his own therapy would look like with his own therapist, which in turn would allow me to play a more central role in trying to get him into treatment.

Note: The therapist is uncertain which hook will be most appealing to the IP, and thus is simply going down the list and getting the CSO's reaction to each one. Prior to the session a new CRAFT therapist would have reviewed the list of hooks (see Box 11.1) and the reasons for using each one.

CSO: I think my brother *would* be curious about you, but somehow I can't imagine him agreeing to come meet you.

THERAPIST: Not a problem, we have others. The next hook, letter "b" on your handout, entails telling your brother that he could have his own therapist, that he wouldn't be getting yours. It's surprising what a difference this makes to individuals who are on the fence about coming in. I guess they automatically assume they'll be sharing the same therapist, and they're afraid the therapist will be biased against them.

CSO: That might be appealing to Ju Meok, but again, I'm not sure it would be enough to get him to come in.

THERAPIST: That's fine. You also might tell Ju Meok that he could simply "sample" treatment. In other words, he could go to a session or two and see if he likes it before deciding whether to make a bigger commitment. Lots of people are reluctant to start therapy because they're worried about whether they'll like their therapist. Sampling treatment lets them find out and offers an easy "escape" if they don't make a good connection. Also, the idea of starting therapy feels like a really big step to most people, and so sampling treatment is much more appealing. The funny thing is that they could do this anyway; just come in a few times and then stop. But somehow our straightforward invitation for them to do this is appreciated and seriously considered.

CSO: Now this one *would* probably appeal to Ju Meok. You've got some interesting ideas.

Note: Although the CSO announces that one of the hooks probably will appeal to her brother, the therapist continues to present them anyway in order to arm the CSO with several solid ones for her upcoming conversation.

THERAPIST: And there's more! This next hook, letter "d," would let your brother know that he'd play a major role in deciding what he'd be working on in therapy. In other words, his treatment would *not* have to be exclusively about his substance use, but could also address other problems of his choosing. You mentioned he'd been struggling over a breakup with his girlfriend—*that* could be a therapy topic. Or maybe he'd want to talk to someone about taking courses again. Naturally, the substance use problem would be brought up, too, given that he'd be seeing a therapist who regularly treats individuals with substance use problems, but it could be brought up in the context of the other things Ju Meok wanted to work on.

CSO: I'm not sure he'd believe this. Heck, I'm not even sure *I* believe it!

THERAPIST: That's understandable. But the reason we can claim this is because we're going to get a therapist lined up in advance for your brother that will allow this to happen. And in addition to having a therapist who lets Ju Meok be active in deciding the direction of therapy, we'll make sure this therapist shows him respect and isn't confrontational, which is letter "e" here on your handout. So you can tell your brother that, too: he won't be judged or confronted.

Note: The therapist is referring to the second part of the Inviting the IP to Enter Treatment procedure in which a therapist with specific characteristics is arranged in advance for the IP. This part of the procedure will be introduced later in the session.

CSO: Maybe if I explain all of that, he'll believe me.

THERAPIST: Well, remember that you won't be using *all* of these hooks, just the ones that seem best suited for your situation. And now the final hook, letter "f." For this one you'd be telling your brother that if he goes into therapy *now* and reduces his use, then he'd be more likely to get something important he's looking forward to a few weeks from now, something that's currently off limits due to his use. Common examples include a substance-using individual not being invited to a big family event, or being prohibited from attending a child's championship soccer game. Can you think of any upcoming event for which your brother would only be welcome if he's reduced his use? Maybe something associated with his younger brother?

CSO: I'd have to think about that. His little brother isn't involved in sports. I'm not sure. I can't think of anything right offhand.

THERAPIST: That's OK. We can add it later if something comes to you.

Note: It is not necessary for the therapist to spend considerable time on every motivational hook if it seems clear that some of them will not be suitable.

Help the CSO select the hook(s) that she or he will use with the IP.

THERAPIST: It sounded like some of these hooks might be worth trying, right?

CSO: Yes. I'd better use a couple. I liked the one about getting Ju Meok to agree to just trying out therapy without making a real commitment. He might be curious enough to do that. And he'll probably like hearing that he can use the sessions to work on other stuff, too.

THERAPIST: Good. What are the other things you think he'd want to work on?

CSO: I doubt he'll want to talk about his old girlfriend—well, maybe if he sticks with therapy for a while. He just seems kind of "lost" lately. He's definitely not happy.

THERAPIST: If you think he might be interested in therapy to work on his unhappiness, we could spend a few minutes now figuring out how you'd word that as part of the invitation to start treatment. And then we'll practice the entire conversation. Keep in mind that we want to make the idea of going into therapy to work on his mood *appealing* to him—we want it to serve as a hook.

CSO: He'll definitely know what I mean if I stick with lost, because I've said it to him before. Hopefully he'll be receptive to the invitation.

2. Conduct a role play of the treatment invitation and provide feedback.

Remind the CSO to use positive communication and motivational hooks.

As noted previously, since CSOs do not automatically include elements from their positive communication training (see Chapter 4) when they are developing new conversations, each role play is another opportunity for you to remind CSOs to do so. To assist CSOs with incorporating motivational hooks into the conversation, be sure they have Handout 11.1 in front of them to use as a reference.

THERAPIST: Let's go ahead and practice the conversation you'll have with your brother about inviting him to treatment, while remembering that you'll want to use the motivational hooks we just discussed. Feel free to refer to the handout (*refers to Handout 11.1*). And as always, it's important to use some of the positive communication phrases, too. Any idea as to which of those you'd like to incorporate into your invitation?

CSO: I think it would be easy to use an "understanding statement" because I could comment on how hard it might seem to start talking to a stranger about problems. I always use the "offer to help"; I'll keep it real general, so he can ask for anything he wants.

THERAPIST: Terrific choices. Any others?

CSO: I might need a quick reminder of what the others are.

THERAPIST: No problem. Here (*points to the Positive Communication Guidelines on Handout 11.1*).

CSO: Oh, right. I think I'd like to try the one for "accept partial responsibility." I could say that I should have had a specific plan, like to see a therapist, when I've mentioned being worried about him on other occasions.

THERAPIST: Good. I think we're set then. I'll start it off by playing Ju Meok. As always, make believe this is really happening right now.

Note: There is no correct number of positive communication elements for a CSO to consider using, so the therapist relies on personal judgment of the CSO's capabilities when deciding whether to encourage her to incorporate more of them into the conversation.

Engage in the role play.

As always, keep in mind the Role-Play ("Practicing") Guidelines (Chapter 4, Box 4.4).

THERAPIST (*as Ju Meok*): What did you want to talk to me about? Am I getting another lecture?

CSO (*in role play*): No, no lecture. Nobody likes those. I'll just get right to my point, because I want to be totally up front with you. I've noticed that you seem kind of "lost" lately. Maybe you're unhappy? I don't know.

THERAPIST (*as Ju Meok*): Maybe. But why? What are you getting at?

CSO (*in role play*): I'm thinking it might be helpful to talk to a professional, a therapist, about how you're feeling. I know it could be awkward talking to a stranger at first, but it gets comfortable fast. You remember that I'm in therapy, right?

THERAPIST (*as Ju Meok*): Yes, but why in the world are *you* in therapy? Oh, never mind. It's none of my business. Anyway, I don't think so.

CSO (*in role play*): You know I'm not going to give up that fast (*laughs*)!

THERAPIST (*as Ju Meok*): Are you sure this isn't your way of trying to get me into drug rehab?

CSO (*in role play*): I won't lie to you; I'm guessing your drug use *would* come up. But it wouldn't have to be the main focus. My own therapist said she'd help find a therapist who would let *you* be in charge of what you wanted to work on.

THERAPIST (*as Ju Meok*): I find that hard to believe.

CSO (*in role play*): I know what you mean; that's what I thought at first, too. But remember that my therapist will help find someone like that. Oh, and another thing to think about: You could decide to just give therapy a try. If you don't like it, or you don't get along with your therapist, after a session or two you could just stop going, with no questions asked. What do you think?

THERAPIST: Let's stop now and discuss how it went. For starters, what did you like about how you did?

CSO: I like how I tried to keep it upbeat even though it's a serious conversation.

THERAPIST: Yes, you definitely kept the conversation upbeat, and much of this was due to your positive communication skills. Let's talk about them first. Can you tell me which elements of positive communication you used? Feel free to refer to your handout with the Positive Communication Guidelines on it. I'll help if you get stuck.

Note: The therapist checks to make sure the *CSO* knows which parts of positive communication she used, as opposed to telling her. This allows the therapist to see the extent to which the CSO has learned the positive communication material.

CSO: I used an "understanding statement" when I said it could be awkward to start therapy with a stranger. Let's see. Looking at this list (*scans Positive Communication Guidelines section of Handout 11.1*), I think I did the first thing, too—be brief. I got right to the point about him seeing a therapist. Oh, and maybe the third one: I was specific about what I wanted him to do.

THERAPIST: Geez—listen to you! Not only was your conversation a very good one, but you even remember which parts of good communication you used! Oh, and I should add that I actually counted you making three understanding statements! In addition to the one you mentioned, you showed empathy or understanding when you reassured Ju Meok that nobody likes getting lectured, and when you agreed that it was hard to believe he'd be allowed to work on things of his own choosing in therapy.

CSO: I guess those *were* understanding comments, too. But as I think about it, I didn't make an offer to help.

THERAPIST: Not a problem. It went very smoothly without it. But since we're going to practice it again, you can add it this time. There was one other type of communication you initially said you were going to use that I didn't hear. Do you remember what it was? It had to do with specifically mentioning that he should see a therapist.

CSO: Oh, right. Yes. I was going to accept partial responsibility. I should be able to add that this time, too.

Discuss which motivational hooks were used (if any), and work to improve them within the conversation.

THERAPIST: Before we practice it again, let's review the motivational hooks you used. You did a really good job with those, too.

CSO: Thanks. They were easier to remember than I thought they'd be. Let's see. I think I did OK with pushing the idea of him starting therapy to work on feeling lost. At the same time, I was honest and didn't disagree when he said his drug use might come up. Oh, and I told him he could just sample treatment for a session or two.

THERAPIST: Yes, you presented both of the hooks you settled on: pointing out that he could be in charge of the treatment focus and therefore it wouldn't have to be about drugs all the time, and suggesting he sample a couple of sessions. Excellent. And you sort of presented another hook, the one about him getting his own therapist, because you said that I'd be helping find a therapist for him.

CSO: That's true. Maybe I should have made that more obvious.

THERAPIST: It wouldn't hurt, right? I'm guessing that we don't need any more hooks. But let's definitely incorporate some of those additional positive communication statements. Are you ready to try it again, or do you want to discuss it first?

CSO: I'm not sure I can remember all the pieces. Can we talk through it once more first?

THERAPIST: Absolutely! And once you feel comfortable, we'll practice it again.

Note: See Handout 11.1 (Example 1) for the final "polished" conversation for this CSO. In addition to encouraging the CSO to use the communication elements she had already mastered in the first role play (i.e., using an understanding statement, being brief, and naming a specific behavior), the final conversation shows that the therapist also worked with this CSO to:

- Accept partial responsibility (number 6 on the Positive Communication Guidelines list) by saying that she should have suggested seeing a therapist earlier.
- Make an offer to help (7 on the Positive Communication Guidelines list) by simply asking whether she could do anything to make the visit with a therapist happen.
- Add a feelings statement (4 on the Positive Communication Guidelines list), such as by expressing worry or concern.

3. Discuss "windows of opportunity" for inviting the IP to begin treatment.

As stressed throughout CRAFT, choosing the best *time* for a conversation with the IP is as important as choosing the best words. "Windows of opportunity" represent occasions associated with many IPs being more open to the idea of treatment. Thus, these windows typically are presented to CSOs (see examples in Box 11.2). The first window is specific to IPs who already are aware of their CSO being in treatment, whereas the other windows can be adapted to fit that situation or one in which the IP is *not* aware of the CSO being in therapy. Regardless, you do not need to review the entire list, particularly if another occasion already has been identified as being ideal for inviting the IP to attend treatment.

BOX 11.2

Common "Windows of Opportunity" for Inviting the IP to Begin Treatment

- The IP inquires about the CSO's (CRAFT) treatment (e.g., "What exactly goes on during those meetings you've had with a therapist?"; "What do you and your therapist talk about?").
- The IP asks why the CSO's behavior has changed lately; essentially when referring to the CSO's implementation of CRAFT procedures, such as Improving CSOs' Communication Skills, Rewarding Non-Using Behavior, and Withdrawing Rewards for Using Behavior (e.g., "Why are you being so nice all of a sudden? You must want something"; "You're acting really different lately. Why won't you hang out with me anymore?").
- The IP appears remorseful in the aftermath of a significant substance-related incident (e.g., driving while intoxicated [DWI], physical injury, arrest, job loss).
- The IP appears upset about a substance-related remark (e.g., overhears the daughter saying that she does not like having friends over because dad acts weird around them when he's drunk; the boss questions the IP about reports from coworkers that they smell marijuana on her clothing).

Present several common windows of opportunity.

THERAPIST: Seri, now that you have a good idea of *what* you want to say to Ju Meok, I'd like to talk about possible times for having this conversation. It turns out that certain "windows of opportunity," as we call them, are often associated with our loved ones being more receptive to hearing the invitation to begin treatment. I don't know if these will appeal to you, or will even be necessary, but shall I go over them briefly just in case?

CSO: Yes, absolutely.

THERAPIST: Great! I'll start with one that actually popped up in our practice conversation earlier. Do you remember reminding Ju Meok that you were already in treatment? My response, while playing him, was something along the lines of first asking *why* you were in therapy, but then quickly saying it was none of my business. And then the conversation switched to something else.

CSO: Yes, I remember that coming up.

THERAPIST: If you hadn't *already* been suggesting to your brother, as part of the role play, that he see a therapist, this would have been considered a window of opportunity because it would have been an opening to tell him that you were in treatment, at least partially due to your concern about him and your relationship with him. This could have then naturally led up to a treatment invitation.

CSO: I see how that could work. Hmm. You never know; maybe I'll end up using it.

Note: Although the CSO may not need this particular window of opportunity (at least initially), the therapist still describes it because it is such a clear illustration of the construct and is a reasonable backup plan for the CSO.

THERAPIST: Good. But there's no need to change your planned conversation right now, since you seem pretty comfortable bringing up the idea of treatment for him. Let's put this on the back burner in case you need it later. Now, another window of opportunity would be if Ju Meok asked you outright why you were acting differently at a time when you happened to be using one of the CRAFT procedures you'd learned. For example, this could occur when you were withdrawing a reward because he was using, or when you were using your positive communication skills to say something nice when he *wasn't* using. In other words, he might notice you behaving or talking differently and get curious about it.

Note: This window would be an excellent opportunity to inform an IP about a CSO's own treatment if it had not yet been revealed to the IP.

CSO: I like that one. I bet he *would* ask what was up if I used my communication skills to explain why I was rewarding his non-using behavior in some way.

THERAPIST: And then you could use a hook or two and see if he was interested in sampling treatment himself, with his own therapist, maybe so that he could learn some of the same communication skills to work on some problem of his choice.

CSO: Oh, OK. I see how the windows and hooks could work well together.

Note: The therapist mentions hooks b, c, and d from Box 11.1.

THERAPIST: Excellent. Another window would be if something really bad happened as a result of Ju Meok's use, and he was remorseful. This window usually follows something like a drug-related arrest for possession or assault. Or maybe the substance-using person spent their entire paycheck on drugs, or threatened a family member or friend while under the influence.

CSO: I guess I wouldn't rule that one out. I've worried about him getting into fights while high.

THERAPIST: Fair enough. The final common window would open if Ju Meok got very upset over an unexpected negative remark about his use. We'd have to explore what this might look like for him, but maybe it would be something along the lines of him overhearing his younger brother say he's too embarrassed to bring friends over after school because the whole apartment smells like marijuana. Although Ju Meok might be angry upon first hearing this comment, once he'd settled down he might agree it was time to work on his substance use.

Help the CSO decide which window of opportunity to use or help select a different specific time for the conversation.

THERAPIST: Seri, keep in mind that we don't *have* to rely on any of these four common windows for your conversation with your brother. I presented them just in case they might be helpful.

CSO: I know, but if it turns out to be hard to bring up the topic on my own, I could use the first one you mentioned, the one where I answer his question about why *I'm* in treatment by turning it into a treatment invitation for him. I'd definitely be able to ask him under those circumstances.

THERAPIST: That's fine. But there's a chance you might be waiting a long time if your therapy just doesn't happen to come up in any conversation. Is there anything you could do to help the topic come out?

CSO: I could make *sure* I mention something about my treatment. And if he doesn't ask me about it, I'll offer to tell him anyway.

THERAPIST: Very good. So for now we'll assume that you'll go ahead with the conversation we've been practicing. We just need to figure out exactly *when* you plan to have that conversation in terms of a day and time. And your backup plan will be to use a variation of our first window by mentioning your own therapy if he doesn't bring it up first, and telling him about it even if he doesn't ask. You'll link this up with an invitation for *him* to try out therapy. We can practice that part of the conversation, too, before you leave today.

Remind the CSO to have the conversation, if possible, when both the CSO and the IP are in good moods and the IP is substance-free.

THERAPIST: And keep in mind that this conversation is likely to go better if both you and your brother are in decent moods at the time. In other words, it's best not to invite him to treatment if either of you are really angry or upset; those conversations don't tend to turn out as planned. Also, he shouldn't be high or recovering from being high, if possible, since this would affect how he's thinking and feeling.

4. Discuss the selection of an appropriate treatment provider.

Discuss the need to identify an appropriate treatment provider for the IP, preferably one with a similar theoretical orientation that will likely honor the promises in the hooks.

It is not necessary for CSOs to know the type of treatment (i.e., behavioral or cognitive-behavioral) being sought for their IP if the CSOs are not identifying the therapist themselves. However, it is still useful for CSOs to know that you and their IP's therapist will have similar theoretical orientations (if possible), since this offers certain advantages (e.g., an understanding of each other's therapy language and procedures). Furthermore, since the motivational hooks that CSOs have been encouraged to use with their IP set up certain expectations regarding their IP's therapists (should they choose to begin treatment), it is important to be sure that the therapists fit the expectations. For example, these substance use therapists should be nonconfrontational/nonjudgmental, and should allow IPs to have considerable input into the goals of treatment (see Box 11.3 for these and additional desired qualifications for the IP's therapist).

THERAPIST: Seri, my plan is to help find your brother a substance use therapist who had behavioral or cognitive-behavioral training like I did. This way we'll know that Ju Meok will be getting what you promised: a therapist who isn't confrontational and doesn't judge, and who lets him have a say in what he works on in treatment. Also, Ju Meok will be learning some of the skills you've been taught, like positive

BOX 11.3

Desired Qualifications for the IP's Therapist

1. Has a behavioral or cognitive-behavioral theoretical orientation and training in the substance use field:
   - CSOs have been trained in a behavioral program (CRAFT), and thus would be better able to support the IP due to a common treatment conceptualization, "language," skills training (e.g., positive communication, problem solving) and exercises (e.g., Happiness Scale, Goal Setting).
   - Through the CSOs' use of motivational hooks, IPs have been "promised" several components of treatment that are part of behavioral and cognitive-behavioral treatments (e.g., ability to select main treatment goals).
2. Is nonconfrontational and nonjudgmental.
3. Is available to meet with the IP quickly, such as within 48 hours of the IP agreeing to begin treatment.
4. Can minimize the time spent on "paperwork" during the first session so that it can be devoted primarily to treatment engagement:
   - Ideally the IP's therapist would conduct the intake and assessment so that rapport building can start immediately, and the IP will not have to repeat the same information to several staff.
5. Is able to conduct couple therapy, too (if the CSO and IP are partners), in case the CSO eventually joins the IP for several sessions.

communication and problem solving. You'll have that in common, which might come in handy if you want to understand and support each other's treatment.

Explain the importance of the IP's therapist being available to meet with the IP quickly, such as within 48 hours of the IP agreeing to begin treatment.

THERAPIST: One major thing to keep in mind as we select this therapist is that he or she needs to commit to being available almost at a moment's notice, at least within 48 hours of your brother contacting her or him. Have you heard the saying, "Strike while the iron is hot"? It applies here, because once Ju Meok is willing to start treatment, it could be problematic to have him put on a wait list, since his motivation and interest could drop quickly in the meantime.

5. Arrange for a rapid intake.

One way to accomplish a fast turnaround time for an IP to be assigned to a therapist *and* begin treatment is to have therapists within an agency agree to pick up IPs for each other's CSOs without delay. Of course, practical considerations, such as the IP's health insurance (or the availability of free or sliding-fee clinics) and transportation to the agency or telehealth options, are always necessary considerations.

Help the CSO develop a rapid intake plan or discuss one that is already in place.

THERAPIST: Given how important it is to have a therapist ready to see your brother as soon as he agrees to begin treatment, let's figure out how to make that happen. One option would be for him to come to *this* agency, as I know that one of my colleagues would pick him up rather quickly, and the type of therapy that each of these colleagues offers is in line with what we want. What kinds of problems do you see with this? Regardless, we'll still come up with a few more options.

CSO: I'd love to have him come here, but it's not real close to public transportation, so it might be an excuse for him to miss sessions.

THERAPIST: We could do some problem solving to find possible solutions to his transportation problem in the event that he wanted to come here. For instance, we have telehealth options, too, if he'd be comfortable with that. Anyway, this place will be an option, but we definitely need more. Does Ju Meok have insurance for behavioral health services? If so, we'll look at my list of providers who have really come through for me in similar situations in the past. Also, we can look at the agencies that provide services on a sliding-fee or free basis. There are some excellent ones I can show you. We'll keep access to transportation in mind.

CSO: Yes, he has the same insurance as me. You mentioned telehealth. I don't think Ju Meok would want that. He's kind of joked about people who get their medical services over the phone or Internet.

THERAPIST: That's good to know. We'll steer clear of telehealth for now. Let's take a look at this list of potential therapists then so we can see where their offices are located. Together we should be able to figure out whether they are near public transportation. If you're OK with the idea, I'd like us to call our top choices while you're still here. If we can get through to a receptionist who does the scheduling for an agency, we could at least find out a therapist's upcoming availability. If we have to leave a phone message with a private therapist, we'll probably still hear back pretty quickly about availability. Either way, we should know in the next day or so what our options are in terms of who would be able to see your brother quickly if he agrees to treatment this week. Sound OK?

CSO: Let's go for it!

Note: If therapy time had been running short, the therapist probably would have asked the CSO to contact the short list of potential IP therapists as a homework assignment, and to call back with the outcome as far as who was tentatively lined up to be the IP's therapist. In this manner, the therapist would not need to wait until the next session (and waste precious time in the process) to find out whether the CSO had encountered difficulties in arranging for an IP therapist.

Develop a backup plan in case the initial rapid intake plan falls through.

THERAPIST: We should discuss a backup plan in case our original plan to get your brother a therapist tentatively lined up unravels at the last minute. For example, what if your brother agrees to treatment on a Friday night, and the therapist we've selected works at a clinic that isn't open until Monday? What's our plan? Should we get an emergency contact number? Should we try to get information about the people who would be on call there? Should we resort to a walk-in service for just the weekend? How much of a problem would it be to just wait until Monday? Lots to talk about.

6. Prepare for possible treatment refusal/dropout *or* ongoing treatment engagement.

Remind the CSO that it is fairly common for several treatment invitations to be extended before the IP agrees to treatment, and provide reassurance about having a plan for proceeding in such cases.

In discussing the possibility that the IP might refuse the treatment invitation (more than once), it is important to create a balance between being realistic *and* optimistic. In other words, CSOs should be prepared to view their own IP's treatment refusal (should it happen) in a broader context that allows them to refrain from judging themselves harshly. CSOs should also feel confident about successfully engaging their IP in treatment in the near future. In terms of the process, you should briefly explain how you would proceed *if* a treatment refusal occurred. The main considerations include determining whether the CSO delivered the treatment invitation as practiced (as far as how and when), and whether another invitation should be prepared and practiced immediately (if so, how and when) or delayed so that time can be devoted to the CSO's own personal goals instead. See Box 11.4 for detailed instructions for situations in which a treatment refusal *does* occur.

THERAPIST: Keep in mind that it's pretty common for loved ones to say "no" more than once before they finally agree to begin therapy. If your brother says "no," we'll examine the situation carefully to see if we can figure out what might have influenced his decision. For instance, we'll look at whether your invitation came across in the way we'd practiced and at the time you'd settled on. Regardless, we'll come up with a plan for moving forward.

CSO: I wouldn't want to give up right away, that's for sure.

THERAPIST: Good, I didn't think you would. Well, we might decide to make some changes in how you approach him or in what you say, but we also might decide to wait a bit before asking him again. Regardless, *if* this happens, I'll hang in there with you so we can figure out the next step together.

Discuss the CSO's anticipated reaction if the IP refuses the treatment invitation.

If you are concerned that the CSO would have considerable difficulty handling the rejection of a treatment refusal at this stage in the CRAFT program, your discussion might include conducting a role play in which the IP (played by you) refuses treatment. The role play would allow the CSO to experience any negative feelings associated with the refusal and for you to help process them.

THERAPIST: What do you make of the picture I've laid out for you here? Even if you do everything right in terms of how you invite your brother, he still could refuse treatment. What would that be like for you if he did? How do you think you'd feel?

CSO: I guess I wouldn't be that surprised, but I know I'd be disappointed.

BOX 11.4

Responding to a Treatment Refusal

1. Ask for a full description of the circumstances:
   - Did the invitation occur at the planned time?
   - Were the CSO and IP in good moods?
   - Did the CSO use motivational hooks and positive communication?
   - Were there extenuating circumstances?
2. Determine whether the CSO is interested in quickly making another request for the IP to enter treatment and whether it appears reasonable to do so:
   - If "yes":
     - Plan for the time and circumstances of the next treatment request.
     - Role-play the request, with an eye toward minimizing any problems identified from the last request.
     - Remind the CSO to continue with the other CRAFT procedures (e.g., Rewarding Non-Using Behavior, Withdrawing Rewards for Using Behavior) throughout.
   - If "no":
     - Help the CSO focus on personal goals with the procedure Helping CSOs Enrich Their Own Lives.
     - Encourage the CSO to continue with the other CRAFT procedures.
     - Agree on a time for revisiting the idea of inviting the IP to sample treatment.

THERAPIST: And what would you do with your disappointment? How would you deal with it?

CSO: I can picture myself avoiding him for a few days. In the meantime, I'd be trying to figure out what went wrong and how I can approach him again.

THERAPIST: Normally I might suggest that we practice a conversation in which you invite Ju Meok to treatment and he *refuses*, since these role plays are a good way to "try out" the hurt or angry feelings you might have. However, I'm convinced that you'd bounce back quickly regardless. And we'd definitely discuss it in here afterward anyway.

Plan for the possibility that the IP agrees to treatment but never actually attends or drops out prematurely.

As far as discussing what the plan would be *if* the IP failed to begin treatment despite promising to do so, you would inform CSOs that if they wanted to discuss the "no show" with their IP, a preparatory role play would be practiced. Additionally, various options for taking the next steps could be addressed through Problem Solving.

With regard to addressing IP treatment dropout (should it occur), you would explain that the strategy would begin with a discussion of the circumstances under which the IP dropout occurred. Depending on this information, you and the CSO together would decide whether it would be reasonable to (a) develop a plan to get the IP to reenter treatment (while utilizing CRAFT skills such as problem solving and positive communication), or (b) take a break from inviting the IP to sample treatment, and instead focus directly on the CSO's personal goals (via the Happiness Scale and Goal Setting exercise). Regardless, CSOs would be encouraged to continue using the procedures for Rewarding Non-Using Behavior and Withdrawing Rewards for Using Behavior. In general, responding to a treatment dropout is very similar to responding to a treatment refusal (see Box 11.4, number 2).

Although an overview of a basic plan can be presented to CSOs in anticipation of these possible IP "letdowns," the details cannot be solidified until the event occurs and the circumstances are reviewed. At that point, the primary issue is whether the CSO is still receiving CRAFT treatment. CSOs would be told that if they are in treatment, session time would be devoted to finalizing a strategy for responding to the IP's problematic behavior. You would also inform CSOs that if CRAFT treatment had ended for them, you might encourage them to resume treatment for a few sessions in order to develop a new plan for proceeding.

THERAPIST: Another thing we should plan for is the possibility that your brother agrees to start treatment . . . but then never shows, or he starts treatment but then drops out quickly.

CSO: Wow, that would be a drag. How would I even know if either of those things happened?

THERAPIST: Excellent question, since as you probably know, his therapist wouldn't be allowed to inform you without Ju Meok's permission. So how would you want to handle that?

CSO: I guess I'd check in with him a week or two after he supposedly had started therapy to see how it was going. I think he'd tell me if he never made it there or if he stopped going.

THERAPIST: Good. And we can practice that conversation once Ju Meok has agreed to start treatment, so you'll be ready. How do you think you'd feel in that situation?

CSO: To be honest, I feel annoyed just imagining it. I've been working really hard to get him into treatment. If he bails, I'd be upset. But I'm sure I'd settle down and eventually try again.

THERAPIST: It's perfectly understandable that you'd be annoyed and upset with him. Being the resilient person that you are, I'm not surprised that you'd be up for trying again to get him into treatment. We'd work on that together. But depending on what happened, we might also decide to take a break and focus back on *you* for a bit—to check on your progress toward your own goals. Again, we'd really need to review the circumstances and see what you wanted to do at that point. And we could always role-play any conversations you might want to have with your brother about what happened.

CSO: What if he drops out when I'm no longer coming to therapy?

THERAPIST: We'll talk a bit more about a plan before your treatment ends. But since we can only strategize so much without knowing the circumstances, you might decide at that point to come back into therapy for a session or two.

Discuss ways in which the CSO can support an IP who is in treatment.

A CSO's job is not done once the IP begins treatment. You should discuss the importance of the CSO:

- Continuing the standard CRAFT procedures (e.g., Rewarding Non-Using Behavior; Allowing for Natural, Negative Consequences of Use; Improving CSOs' Communication Skills).
- Attending some sessions with the IP if requested.
- Offering to help more generally (e.g., help plan pleasant non-using activities).
- Offering to discuss common exercises/procedures of the IP's and CSO's treatment if theoretical orientations are similar (e.g., Goal Setting, Problem Solving).

THERAPIST: And now, finally, we should discuss what to do when Ju Meok begins and *continues* in treatment, as your work isn't done! Any idea what I'm going to stress?

CSO: You're probably going to tell me to keep doing what I've been doing all along: Reward him when he's not using and allow for the negative consequences. That kind of stuff.

THERAPIST: You know me all too well! Yes, it would be important to keep doing the things that we think have helped him reduce his use and which we hope will help him decide to start treatment. I'm glad you recognize the importance of keeping that up, because some people assume they're done when their loved one enters therapy. OK. What else can you do? Since Ju Meok is your brother as opposed to being your partner, it's unlikely that his therapist would want you to attend any sessions with him. But if for some reason his therapist *did*, would you be OK with that?

CSO: I'll help in any way I can.

THERAPIST: Excellent answer. It also reminds me that it's always a good idea to simply use one of your favorite positive communication skill components: the one that offers to help. Even if Ju Meok isn't sure what he needs at the time, I'm guessing he'll appreciate the gesture. For example, since part of his treatment would probably focus on him finding non-using fun activities, and you've already worked on this for him in CRAFT, maybe you could continue this work. Of course, *this* time you could offer to do the selection and planning of the activities in conjunction with him.

CSO: I'd have no problem with that. I'd even enjoy it.

THERAPIST: You could let him know that you've probably learned some of the same skills in your own therapy that he's learning, like communication and problem solving. So if he ever wants to talk about them or things that are going on in therapy more generally, you'll know where he's coming from.

CSO: I'd be happy to compare notes!

THERAPIST: Excellent! As always, I'm here if you need me.

COMMON PROBLEMS TO AVOID

Inviting the IP to Enter Treatment is a highly anticipated procedure for CSOs, and one that most therapists enjoy. However, since the stakes are high for this treatment invitation, CSOs can be quite anxious as they prepare for it, and therapists can feel the pressure of the stressful situation as well. Therapist tips for conducting the procedure are outlined below.

Problem: It is common for clinicians to launch into the role plays for treatment invitations without reminding CSOs to incorporate their positive communication skills and without first reviewing them when necessary. Both the CSOs and therapists are focused on using the hooks, while forgetting the significant role of positive communication more generally.

Safeguards:

- You should get into the habit of reminding CSOs to use their positive communication skills before *every* new role play, regardless of the CRAFT procedure being practiced.
- Make an effort to routinely ask about which components of positive communication the CSOs used in a role play as part of your feedback (again, regardless of the CRAFT procedure), as it will serve as a cue for CSOs to remind *themselves* to think about using positive communication each time they start a role play.

Problem: Therapists who are teaching CSOs how to invite their IP to treatment have sometimes not done the groundwork for developing a list of appropriate and available therapists (with substance use expertise), or have not worked with CSOs to develop one. This runs the risk of CSOs going home and extending treatment invitations, but then either having no therapist available for the IP, or placing an IP with a therapist who has beliefs and practices that are not in line with what has been promised to the IP by the CSO.

Safeguards:

- Prior to accepting *any* CSOs for CRAFT sessions, you should spend time contacting potentially appropriate local substance use therapists to explore their treatment approach, and to determine their willingness to be part of a referral list of individuals who can respond quickly to treatment requests from IPs.

Problem: CRAFT therapists occasionally avoid the difficult discussions that are part of the Inviting the IP to Enter Treatment procedure—namely, that the CSO's treatment invitation might not "work" at first, or the IP's attempt at treatment might not "take" the first time. These conversations need to take place so that the CSO can be prepared both emotionally and in terms of having a backup plan.

Safeguards:

- You should carefully review each of the steps of Inviting the IP to Enter Treatment (see Form 11.1) prior to starting it with a CSO so that these last steps do not get overlooked and the session time does not run out before they can be addressed.
- Remind yourself that treatment engagement is often a process that starts and stops . . .

and then repeats. This understanding will allow you to prepare your CSOs (and yourself) for whatever path the treatment engagement takes.

SUMMARY

This chapter provides a structure for building CSOs' invitation for their IP to enter treatment. In addition to stressing the importance of relying on CSOs' positive communication skills more generally, motivational hooks and windows of opportunity are introduced to increase the likelihood of their IP accepting the invitation. The need to have a suitable therapist for their IP arranged in advance is addressed, and options for dealing with a variety of potential IP responses to the invitation are covered.

FORM 11.1

Inviting the IP to Enter Treatment: Checklist

1. Discuss motivational hooks for treatment invitations.

☐ a. Present several motivational hooks.

☐ b. Help the CSO select the hook(s) that she or he will use with the IP.

2. Conduct a role play of the treatment invitation and provide feedback.

☐ a. Remind the CSO to use positive communication and motivational hooks.

☐ b. Engage in the role play.

☐ c. Discuss which motivational hooks were used (if any), and work to improve them within the conversation.

3. Discuss "windows of opportunity" for inviting the IP to begin treatment.

☐ a. Present several common windows of opportunity.

☐ b. Help the CSO decide which window of opportunity to use or help select a different specific time for the conversation.

☐ c. Remind the CSO to have the conversation, if possible, when both the CSO and the IP are in good moods and the IP is substance-free.

4. Discuss the selection of an appropriate treatment provider.

☐ a. Discuss the need to identify an appropriate treatment provider for the IP, preferably one with a similar theoretical orientation that will likely honor the promises in the hooks.

☐ b. Explain the importance of the IP's therapist being available to meet with the IP quickly, such as within 48 hours of the IP agreeing to begin treatment.

5. Arrange for a rapid intake.

☐ a. Help the CSO develop a rapid intake plan or discuss one that is already in place.

☐ b. Develop a backup plan in case the initial rapid intake plan falls through.

6. Prepare for possible treatment refusal/dropout *or* ongoing treatment engagement.

☐ a. Remind the CSO that it is fairly common for several treatment invitations to be extended before the IP agrees to treatment, and provide reassurance about having a plan for proceeding in such cases.

☐ b. Discuss the CSO's anticipated reaction if the IP refuses the treatment invitation.

☐ c. Plan for the possibility that the IP agrees to treatment but never actually attends *or* drops out prematurely.

☐ d. Discuss ways in which the CSO can support an IP who is in treatment.

HANDOUT 11.1

Using Motivational Hooks and Positive Communication to Invite Your Loved One to Attend Treatment

Following the lists of Motivational Hooks and Positive Communication Guidelines are examples of conversations that use both of these techniques in treatment invitations. The precise hooks and positive communication elements used within the sentences are cited in brackets.

Motivational Hooks

a. Your loved one can meet your therapist informally if desired.
b. Your loved one can have his or her own therapist.
c. Your loved one can sample a treatment session or two before making a decision regarding whether to attend regularly.
d. Your loved one can provide major input into the treatment goals and plan, including the extent to which the focus is on substance use.
e. Your loved one can expect to be treated with respect and without confrontation/judgment.
f. Your loved one can maximize therapy benefits (reduced use) now, in anticipation of a timely upcoming reward for substance-free behavior.

Positive Communication Guidelines

1. Be brief (uncomplicated).
2. Use positive/action-oriented wording (indicating what you would like to see happen).
3. Mention specific behaviors.
4. Label your feelings.
5. Offer an understanding statement.
6. Accept partial responsibility (for something related to the problem situation, *not* for the substance use).
7. Offer to help.

Examples

The *letter* of the hook and the *number* of the positive communication guideline used are in brackets.

Example 1: The CSO is the 34-year-old half-sister of the IP (the person with the substance use problem who refuses treatment), a 27-year-old male.

CSO: "Hey, I was hoping you had a few minutes to talk. I'm worried about you [4].

(continued)

You seem really 'lost'; you never seem happy anymore [1]. I probably should have suggested this a while ago [6]: What do you think about getting some professional help? I imagine the idea of talking to a stranger may seem odd at first [5], but I promise you, it gets easier each time. My own therapist says he could help find somebody [b] who'd let you work on whatever *you* wanted to; it wouldn't all be left up to your therapist to decide [d]. And you wouldn't have to make a big commitment up front; you could just try a few sessions to see if you like it. If you don't, you can just stop going [c]. What do you think? Is there something I can do to help make this happen [7]?"

Example 2: The CSO is the wife of a 48-year-old man who drinks heavily (IP). The IP has been unhappy with his job for a long time.

CSO: "Maybe I should have told you this earlier [6]: I've been going to therapy for a few weeks now. I've been sad and upset about how our relationship has been lately [4], and it'll be no surprise to you that I think at least some of this is related to your drinking. But I think we can both get back to being happy again if we work at it [2]. I know you've been really stressed at your job [5], so maybe you'd be willing to see a therapist about that? What I'm trying to say is that although I hope you'd want to work on your drinking with a therapist, it wouldn't have to be the *only* thing you work on [d]. With my own therapist's assistance, I could help you find *your* own therapist [b, 7]; one who wouldn't be confrontational [e] and who would welcome your input as far as your goals for treatment [d]. Would you be willing to try it for a week or two for the sake of our marriage [c]? If you hate it, you can stop going. But if it does go well, I'd consider going with you to that big dinner coming up at your company in a few weeks, because I wouldn't be so worried about your behavior there [f]."

Example 3: The 30-year-old CSO had always had a solid relationship with his 26-year-old sister (IP), but this changed about 3 months ago when she started dating a small-time drug dealer and began using herself.

CSO: "Melody, I know you've wanted a serious boyfriend for a long time now. I get that [5]. It makes me happy to see *you* happy [4]. At the same time, I miss the old, crazy, friendly 'you' that was 'high' without the drugs [2, 4]. And I'm worried about you [4], precisely *because* of the drugs [1, 3]. I think it's partly my fault though, because I should have spoken up months ago when I saw the two of you starting to hang out [6]. Maybe I can help in some way now? [7]. Anyway, I've been meeting with a therapist to work on my own stuff *and* to talk about my concerns related to you. Would you be open to the idea of trying out therapy yourself, even if it's just for a few sessions [c]? We could find you a therapist who wouldn't judge your lifestyle [e, 7], and who'd let *you* decide what you wanted to work on in treatment [d]. For example, you said a while ago that you were wondering if you should finish college. A therapist could help you sort that out [d]. What do you think about the idea of meeting my therapist, like for a cup of coffee, so she can tell you more about the type of therapist she has in mind for you [a, b]?"

Chapter 12

Using the Community Reinforcement Approach with the Identified Patient

This chapter provides an introduction to the Community Reinforcement Approach (CRA), a behavioral treatment for individuals with substance use problems. The individual in the therapy room when receiving CRA is *not* a CSO but either a former treatment-refusing IP who ultimately has agreed to enter treatment, or a nonresistant client with a substance use problem. As in the rest of this book, to minimize confusion, this chapter refers to the client with the substance use problem (who is receiving CRA) as the IP.

As the name implies, CRA helps individuals find ways to rearrange or rebuild their "community" (i.e., home, family, work, church, social activities) such that it reinforces (rewards) a healthy lifestyle that does not rely on alcohol or drugs. In other words, the goal of CRA is to set up these environmental contingencies so that substance-free behavior is more rewarding than substance-using behavior. CRA accomplishes this, in part, by the IP and therapist examining the factors associated with the onset of substance-using episodes and the positive consequences that maintain them. Using CRA, IPs are taught the skills needed to change their lifestyle to one that is healthy, fulfilling, and importantly . . . enjoyable.

This CRA chapter is intended primarily to pique CRAFT therapists' interest in learning more about this scientifically supported treatment (Campos-Melady, Smith, Meyers, Godley, & Godley, 2017; Roozen et al., 2004; Roozen & Smith, 2021, in press; Smith, Gianini, Garner, Malek, & Godley, 2014; Smith, Meyers, & Delaney, 1998) that also has been used successfully with diverse populations (Venner, Serier, et al., 2016; Venner, Smith, et al., 2021) and adolescents (A-CRA; Garner et al., 2009; M. D. Godley et al., 2017; S. H. Godley et al., 2014; Smith, Davis, Ureche, & Dumas, 2016; Welsh et al., 2019). CRA overlaps significantly with CRAFT in terms of both the theory and procedures, and thus CRA would be relatively easy for CRAFT therapists to learn. In addition to having another empirically supported treatment with which to treat individuals with substance use problems, why might you want to learn CRA? CRA-trained therapists clearly would satisfy the desired qualifications for the IP's therapist (discussed in Chapter 11, Box 11.3) in terms of therapist style and theoretical orientation. Importantly, if you were trained in both CRAFT and CRA, you could enter into an arrangement with another similarly trained clinician to accept IPs for each other without any problematic delays (see Chapter 11).

Detailed information about how to implement CRA can be found in *Clinical Guide to Alcohol Treatment: The Community Reinforcement Approach* (Meyers & Smith, 1995; Roozen & Smith, 2021, in press). The treatment manual for the adolescent version of CRA (A-CRA) is *The Adolescent Community Reinforcement Approach: A Clinical Guide for Treating Substance Use Disorders* (Godley, Smith, Meyers, & Godley, 2016).

THE BASICS

General Description

As noted in Chapter 1, the CRAFT program is an outgrowth of CRA. Therefore, many of the CRA procedures presented in this chapter will look familiar, and the novel ones will be comprehendible due to the common theoretical foundation. The procedures that are shared across CRAFT and CRA are mentioned briefly with attention to their usage in CRA (including some examples). The procedures that are not contained within CRAFT are presented in more detail to provide a fuller picture of the CRA program.

Procedure Timing

Similar to CRAFT, the CRA procedures are not assigned to specific sessions, and yet several of the procedures commonly *are* conducted near the start of therapy. Specifically, the CRA Functional Analysis of Drinking or Using Behavior (see Form 12.1, found at the end of this chapter) is one of the first procedures, since it provides assessment information. The Happiness Scale and Goal Setting are two additional procedures that are conducted near the beginning of CRA treatment, as they form the foundation for the treatment plan. Finally, Sobriety Sampling is often one of the first CRA procedures introduced for those IPs who report an interest in working on their substance use early in treatment. In contrast, when CRA Relationship Therapy is included as part of the CRA program (i.e., when IPs are good candidates for having their partner involved in several sessions; see the "CRA Relationship Therapy" section below), it typically is scheduled well into the treatment process. This allows time for IPs to learn critical CRA skills (e.g., positive communication) and to demonstrate progress with their substance use. The remaining CRA procedures are introduced as clinically indicated.

Forms

- CRA Functional Analysis of Drinking or Using Behavior (Form 12.1)
- CRA Functional Analysis of a Fun, Healthy Behavior (Form 12.2)
- Social/Recreational Activities 2 × 2 (Form 12.3)
- CRA Functional Analysis for Relapse (Form 12.4)
- Relationship Happiness Scale (Romantic Partner Version) (Form 12.5)
- Relationship Goal Setting (Romantic Partner Version) (Form 12.6)
- Daily Reminder to Be Nice (Form 12.7)

PROCEDURES COMMON TO CRA AND CRAFT

Approximately half of CRA's procedures are contained within the CRAFT program, and thus they already have been described in detail in previous chapters. These procedures are (1) Functional Analysis of [a Loved One's] Drinking or Using Behavior; (2) Functional Analysis of a [Loved One's] Fun, Healthy Behavior; (3) [Improving CSOs'] Communication Skills; (4) Problem Solving; (5) Happiness Scale; and (6) Goal Setting. With the exception of the two FA procedures, the steps and forms for these overlapping procedures are the same across CRAFT and CRA; CRA items 5 and 6 are combined in the CRAFT procedure Helping CSOs Enrich Their Own Lives. Unique applications of these procedures within CRA treatment are explained below.

Functional Analysis of Drinking or Using Behavior

The CRA Functional Analysis of Drinking or Using Behavior (see Meyers & Smith, 1995, pp. 20–29; Roozen & Smith, 2021, in press) is somewhat easier to administer than the CRAFT Functional Analysis of a Loved One's Drinking or Using Behavior (see Chapter 3, Form 3.2), because the CRA version is administered directly to the individual with the substance use problem. Therefore, when administering the CRA FA (Form 12.1), an individual (the CSO) does *not* have to speculate about the thoughts, feelings, and behavior of the individual with the substance use problem (the IP), since the IP is responding to the questions directly him- or herself. Furthermore, the assignments that are outgrowths of the FA are focused on changing the behavior of an individual directly (the IP). In contrast, the CRAFT FA requires a plan in which the CSO will behave differently toward the IP in an effort to influence the IP's behavior.

Functional Analysis of a Fun, Healthy Behavior

Similar to the FA conducted for substance use, the FA that is done in an effort to increase *enjoyable* activities is somewhat easier to administer in its CRA version (see Meyers & Smith, 1995, pp. 29–33; Roozen & Smith, 2021, in press) as opposed to its CRAFT version (see Chapter 6, Form 6.2), and for the same reasons. Nonetheless, this particular CRA FA (Form 12.2) is not administered with IPs as often as the CRAFT version is administered with CSOs, given that the CRA program has several procedures available for working with IPs on their social/recreational life (see the "Social/Recreational Activities" section below).

With that said, if you genuinely enjoy administering FAs, it would be a natural choice for you to conduct one when working on an IP's social life (see Form 12.2). And some therapists specifically turn to the CRA Functional Analysis of a Fun, Healthy Behavior (instead of using other CRA Social/Recreational Activities procedures) when they want to scrutinize the IP's thoughts/feelings that are triggers for the decision to engage in a fun and healthy behavior as opposed to the decision to use alcohol or drugs.

Communication Skills

Positive communication skills training is virtually the same for both CRAFT and CRA. The CRA procedures that tend to rely heavily on positive communication skills include

Social/Recreational Activities, CRA Relationship Therapy, and some of the goals established as part of Goal Setting.

When communication skills are taught within CRAFT (see Chapter 4), the CSOs most commonly are preparing for conversations with their IPs. Within CRA (see Meyers & Smith, 1995, pp. 102–105; Roozen & Smith, 2021, in press), the IPs primarily prepare for conversations with their CSOs. However, IPs also might be rehearsing for conversations with friends with whom they have lost contact since starting to use heavily, bosses who have passed them over for raises despite recent significant improvements in work performance, family members who have banned them from get-togethers due to their past using behavior, and ex-partners (or judges) who play a role in reestablishing visitation rights for their children.

Problem Solving

The Problem Solving procedure is exactly the same in CRAFT (see Chapter 9) and CRA (see Meyers & Smith, 1995, pp. 105–111; Roozen & Smith, 2021, in press). Representative problems addressed with this procedure during CRA treatment include coping with cravings in the evening while watching television, having difficulty falling asleep when not using, finding new non-using friends, and getting transportation to meetings (e.g., AA/Narcotics Anonymous [NA], Smart Recovery).

Happiness Scale

The Happiness Scale's format, administration, and purpose is standard across CRAFT (see Chapter 10, Form 10.2) and CRA (see Meyers & Smith, 1995, pp. 80–84; Roozen, Bravo, Pilatti, Mezquita, & Vingerhoets, 2022). Within CRA, the Happiness Scale is given routinely to IPs in one of the first sessions, as it is viewed as a fundamental part of their treatment planning. For CRAFT, although the Happiness Scale often is administered to CSOs early in treatment as well, it is also acceptable to administer it somewhat later in CRAFT (see Chapter 10).

Goal Setting

Given that CRA's Goal Setting builds directly upon the Happiness Scale, it is not surprising that this procedure is the same in CRAFT (see Chapter 10) and CRA (see Meyers & Smith, 1995, pp. 84–94; Roozen & Smith, 2021, in press). One unique aspect is that therapists within CRA programs often wonder whether IPs will select the "Substance Use" category from the Happiness Scale and use it to set goals during Goal Setting. As noted earlier (Chapter 11), IPs are told by their CSOs that when they begin CRA treatment, *they* will determine the areas they want to address. Interestingly, even when IPs do *not* set explicit goals in the "Substance Use" category initially, their substance use typically emerges as a barrier to achieving their goals in other areas (e.g., job or education, family relationships, legal issues, health and wellness). When this occurs, you would bring the issue back to the *IP's own goals* and ask whether it is worth addressing the substance use in order to obtain those other goals.

PROCEDURES UNIQUE TO CRA

As mentioned, the overall goal of CRA is to help IPs rearrange their "community" (home, work, social activities, church, etc.) such that a *non-using* lifestyle is more rewarding (reinforcing) than one that revolves around alcohol or drugs (see Meyers & Smith, 1995; Roozen & Smith, 2021, in press; Smith, Crotwell, Simmons, & Meyers, 2015). During the introductory (first) CRA session, you should (1) describe the overall goal of CRA, (2) outline several procedures (e.g., Communication Skills, Problem Solving), (3) emphasize the importance of completing weekly assignments as part of the program, (4) establish positive expectations for change by mentioning the research support, (5) describe the typical duration of treatment (e.g., 12 weekly sessions), and (6) start to identify IP reinforcers (i.e., things of value to IPs that would influence their decision to stop/reduce their substance use). One should note that in addition to the standard CRA procedures described next, CRA also has an optional Job Counseling procedure that helps IPs obtain and keep jobs (see Meyers & Smith, 1995, pp. 121–126; Azrin & Besalel's, 1980, *Job Club Counselor's Manual*). Below we discuss each CRA-specific procedure, its purpose, and steps for implementation.

Sobriety Sampling

Sobriety Sampling is an alternative to the often intimidating message from many treatment programs that an individual can *never* drink/use again for the rest of his or her life. Although lifelong abstinence *may* be in some individuals' best interest, Sobriety Sampling allows IPs with all types of goals, including that of moderation, the opportunity to "sample" an initial time-limited period of sobriety. This inviting and nonjudgmental approach to treatment ultimately is associated with many IPs eventually deciding to pursue abstinence rather than moderate use. Yet, regardless of an IP's long-term goal and willingness to engage in Sobriety Sampling, CRA clinicians are encouraged to welcome all individuals into treatment. One basis of support for this inclusive approach is the recent research evidence for expanded definitions of alcohol recovery (e.g., Witkiewitz et al., 2020).

Sobriety Sampling can be adapted to a harm reduction interpretation (Marlatt, Larimer, & Witkiewitz, 2012; Marlatt & Witkiewitz, 2010) that supports the sampling of small periods of abstinence *within a day*. This typically is reserved for IPs who are unwilling to commit to abstinence for any length of time (e.g., several days). For example, you might reasonably negotiate with an IP to smoke marijuana only in the evenings as opposed to multiple times throughout the day.

Steps of the Procedure

1. ***Offer a rationale for sampling sobriety.***
   - Present the reasons that are most relevant to your IP and link them to your IP's unique situation. For example, a time-limited period of sobriety at the start of treatment:
     - Enables IPs to set reasonable and attainable goals.
     - Enhances self-efficacy when these attainable goals are reached.

- Disrupts old habits, thereby giving IPs the chance to develop new positive coping skills.
- Builds family support and trust.
- Provides a "time-out" from drinking/using so IPs can experience the sensation of being abstinent and thereby decide whether they want to continue it.

2. ***Negotiate the period of sobriety.***
   - Be prepared to suggest a lengthy period of sobriety (often based on the IP's longest past period), and negotiate downward:
     - Suggest a lengthy period of sobriety (e.g., 30 days? 90 days?).
     - Justify your selected period of time. Examples:
       - The first 90 days is a high relapse period.
       - Mutual help groups (AA, NA) strongly suggest 90 meetings in 90 days.
       - An upcoming important event (e.g., court date, notable family activity) for the IP aligns with the suggested period.
     - Expect that the IP will want to negotiate a shorter period of sobriety.
     - Agree on a reasonable period of time for sampling sobriety, making sure it extends at least to the time of your next session. (*Note:* If abstinence *within a day* is negotiated instead, specify the parameters.)

3. ***Plan for time-limited sobriety.***
   - Work with the IP to generate a plan for successfully reaching the sobriety goal:
     - Identify the biggest upcoming threats to sobriety.
     - Develop a plan for tackling those threats that does *not* simply rely on past unsuccessful methods.
     - Make sure the plan involves a specific behavior that is measurable, simple/straightforward, and under the IP's control.
     - Discuss obstacles and develop backup plans.
     - Offer additional sessions in the upcoming week if deemed necessary.
     - Remind the IP as to *why* he or she is working hard to sample sobriety.

Drink/Drug-Refusal Training

The three-step procedure of Drink/Drug–Refusal Training teaches skills for anticipating high-risk environments, increasing a supportive social network for those situations, and developing and practicing a repertoire of assertive refusal responses to use if faced with offers of alcohol or drugs.

Steps of the Procedure

1. ***Review upcoming high-risk situations.***
   - Discuss potential high-risk situations that may occur prior to the next session.
   - Identify the specific triggers in those situations.
   - Develop a plan (and a backup plan) for dealing with the triggers.

2. ***Enlist social support.***
   - State the need for individuals supportive of the IP's substance-free lifestyle.
   - Help identify at least one person who could be supportive at the high-risk time.
   - Discuss how to ask this individual in advance to support the IP's desire to remain substance-free during the high-risk situation.
   - Make the assignment for the IP to contact this individual explicit.

3. ***Review and practice assertive drink/drug–refusal response options.***
   - Present a standard list of assertive options with examples:
     - Show confident body language (stand up tall, look the person in the eye).
     - Say, "No, thanks" (without guilt!).
     - Suggest alternatives ("No thanks, but I'd really love an iced tea/coffee").
     - Change the subject ("Can you believe how crazy the weather has gotten?").
     - Address the aggressor assertively about the issue ("Please don't keep asking; I'm not going to drink").
     - Leave the situation.
     - Carry a "prop" (an alcohol-free beverage).
     - Other ideas?
   - Ask the IP to select several options and to put them into his or her own words.
   - Role-play the high-risk situation; offer specific feedback (praise *and* shape the behavior); repeat the entire role-play process (see Chapter 4, Box 4.4).

Social/Recreational Activities

Social/Recreational Activities is a "package" procedure that contains options for several other CRA and CRAFT procedures as well as new ones: Problem Solving and Functional Analysis of a Fun, Healthy Behavior (see Step 2 below). The overall goal is to help IPs improve their substance-free social and recreational lives (Roozen et al., 2008). Rich, healthy, social lives play a critical role in competing with the decision to use substances (Delmée, Roozen, & Steenhuis, 2018).

Steps of the Procedure

1. ***Discuss the importance of an enjoyable, healthy social/recreational life.***
   - Convey the need to have a social life that is healthy *and* rewarding so that it can compete with substance use.
   - Report that feeling bored and lonely are two common triggers for substance use.

2. ***Identify a reasonable social/recreational activity.***
   - Steer clear of activities that the IP regularly engaged in while using substances in the past.
   - Focus on activities that are neither too complex nor too expensive.
   - Settle on an activity that the IP can imagine doing in the next week or two.
   - If the IP needs additional help in identifying an activity, use one of the following procedures:
     - Problem Solving (see Chapter 9).
     - Functional Analysis of a Fun, Healthy Behavior (see Chapter 6 for instructions and the modified form to suit IPs, Form 12.2).
     - Social/Recreational Activities 2 × 2 (Form 12.3). Help the IP generate ideas within these categories and save for future use with this IP (and with other IPs).

3. ***Develop a precise plan for sampling the new activity.***
   - Refer to the Goal and Strategy Guidelines (see Chapter 10, Box 10.3).
   - Use the Homework Assignment Guidelines (see Chapter 3, Box 3.1).

Systematic Encouragement

Systematic Encouragement is recommended when an IP voices a commitment to carrying out an assignment, but you remain unconvinced that the IP will follow through with it in the upcoming week. Your belief is likely based on the IP's past behavior or the IP's hesitance to embrace the assignment. This brief procedure provides momentum by assisting the IP in taking that first difficult step during the therapy session, thereby making it more likely that the rest of the assignment will be completed for homework. The procedure also enables the IP to ascertain whether he or she is actually ready to tackle the task, and it gives you the opportunity to observe the IP's skills in the moment and to offer support afterward. Systematic Encouragement typically is used in conjunction with other procedures in which homework assignments are made (see Box 12.1 for examples). (Note that we mentioned this procedure in Chapter 10 in terms of its potential use with CSOs.)

Steps of the Procedure

1. ***Give a rationale for taking the first step of a difficult assignment during the session.***
   - The rationale may include:
     - This "gets the ball rolling" and thereby makes it more likely that the rest of the assignment will be completed during the week.
     - It makes the assignment "real" and thus lets the IP determine whether he or she is truly ready to attempt the task.
     - It affords you an opportunity to observe the IP's skills in action and to offer feedback.
     - It gives you the chance to lend support afterward.

BOX 12.1

Examples of Systematic Encouragement Used within CRA Procedures

- Social/Recreational Activities
  - An IP commits to calling an old friend to see whether she is willing to meet for coffee. The IP has not had any contact with this friend for over 6 months and is worried that the friend might refuse to meet. Since the IP has had difficulty making the first contact for similar past assignments, the therapist rehearses the phone call (using positive communication) with the IP in the session, and then asks the IP to make the actual call before the session ends.
- Sobriety Sampling
  - An IP agrees to sample sobriety for 1 month. Part of his plan for achieving this entails attending three AA meetings a week. The IP expresses concern about being able to find a suitable meeting, and reluctance about walking into an AA meeting alone the first time. The therapist helps the IP search for meeting options on the Internet and to select one. The therapist then has the IP leave a prepared and practiced phone message that asks an AA member to contact him prior to the meeting so that a plan can be in place to meet the IP when he arrives at his first meeting.
- Medication Monitoring
  - An IP agrees that it would be in his best interest to have his wife serve as his monitor for taking his antidepressant medication daily. The therapist helps rehearse the conversation (using positive communication) in which the IP asks his wife to serve in this role. The IP reports that although he definitely wants to ask his wife to be his monitor, he is afraid he might back out of making the request. After a brief discussion about the wording, the IP sends his wife a text during the session in which he asks if they can sit down to discuss an important issue after dinner that evening.

2. ***Help the IP prepare for taking the first step in the session.***
   - For first steps that involve contacting someone:
     - Plan and rehearse the conversation, or
     - Help write the note/text/email.
   - For first steps that involve removing barriers (e.g., helping IPs find days/times/locations/costs for specific activities):
     - Plan how to address the barriers.

3. ***Have the IP take the first step during the session.***
   - Observe the IP making the contact (phone, email, text, etc.) or addressing the barriers.
   - Discuss how the IP experienced the in-session activity and review the outcome.

4. ***Finalize the assignment.***
   - Make any necessary adjustments to the homework assignment.
   - Make the assignment explicit (see Homework Assignment Guidelines in Chapter 3, Box 3.1).
   - Remind the IP that the homework will be reviewed at the next session.

Medication Monitoring

The procedure enlists the assistance of a supportive loved one (a monitor) in an effort to increase the chance that IPs take their prescribed medications as directed. A monitor is used with IPs who are at risk for *not* taking their medication for a variety of reasons, such as forgetting, being ambivalent, or simply not making it a priority. The procedure originally was developed to help IPs take disulfiram (Antabuse), but now it is used for many different medications.

Steps of the Procedure

1. ***Discuss the pros and cons of taking the prescribed medication.***
   - Ask about several possible *dis*advantages to taking the medication, such as:
     - Uncomfortable side effects
     - An unwelcome feeling of reliance on medication
     - Stigma
   - Suggest several advantages to taking the medication, such as:
     - Less family worry
     - Fewer "slips"
     - An increase in self-confidence
     - More productive use of therapy time
     - A better chance of reaching treatment goals overall

2. ***Discuss the role of the monitor.***
   - Explain that the monitor is trained to offer words of encouragement while observing the IP taking the medication as prescribed (e.g., daily).
   - Emphasize the monitor's role in increasing medication adherence by:
     - Providing support
     - Allowing for accountability

3. ***Select an appropriate monitor.***
   - Explain that the monitor (e.g., the CSO) should be readily available and reliable.
   - Help the IP select a monitor.
   - Role-play the conversation for inviting the individual to be the IP's monitor.

- Discuss whether the monitor should be invited to attend the next session to learn the monitoring protocol (or whether the IP will teach the monitor at home; see Note below).
- Finalize the homework assignment for inviting the individual to be the monitor.

4. ***Set up the monitoring protocol (ideally with the monitor present).***
   - Determine *when* and *where* the medication will be given.
   - Discuss how the IP wishes the monitor to handle the situation if the IP refuses to take the medication. Options might include having the monitor:
     - Do nothing unless the IP refuses 2 days in a row.
     - Simply ask how she or he might be of help.
     - Call the IP's therapist.

5. ***Practice administration of the medication (ideally with the monitor present).***
   - Using positive communication, prepare the conversation for administering the medication.
   - Practice the conversation (see Chapter 4).
   - Emphasize the importance of this being a pleasurable and supportive event for both the IP and the monitor.

Note: Ideally the monitor will attend the session for Steps 4 and 5. Otherwise, the IP will consult with the monitor outside of the session and train her or him on the administration techniques that have been practiced in session using role plays.

CRA Relapse Prevention

CRA Relapse Prevention is a "package" that offers strategies for either preventing the occurrence of a relapse or intervening if a relapse has taken place. It consists of *three distinct procedures*: the CRA FA for Relapse, the Behavioral Chain Leading to Relapse (partially based on Marlatt, 1985), and the Early Warning System. These procedures can be introduced at almost any time, since relapse prevention technically starts the first day of CRA treatment. With that said, the first two procedures are built around a relapse. Thus, if it has been an extremely long time since the IP relapsed, you would need to decide whether it still would be worthwhile to have the IP work with one of those older relapse episodes. Another option would be to select the Early Warning System procedure instead. These three procedures that are part of the CRA Relapse Prevention package follow.

CRA FA for Relapse

- Focus specifically on a recent relapse episode instead of asking about a typical/common using episode (as is done for the initial FA).
- Use the CRA Functional Analysis for Relapse form (Form 12.4).

Behavioral Chain Leading to Relapse

- Discuss how a careful review of the chain of events that led to the relapse will help the IP "connect the dots" between the series of small decisions made earlier in the day and the eventual relapse.
- Start when the IP awoke on the relapse day and draw the chain of events that led up to the relapse (see Figure 12.1 example). The links in the chain (represented as ovals) can be behavior, thoughts, or feelings.
- Explain that it is much easier to make changes earlier in the chain of events as opposed to later when the relapse cues are stronger.
- Help the IP identify new ways to respond to a similar situation in the future in terms of:
  - Making different (small) decisions along the chain that lead to a healthy outcome as opposed to a relapse. Suggested places for starting a conversation about making different (healthier) decisions the next time the IP faces a similar situation are pointed out (see rectangles).
  - Relying on better coping strategies and being prepared to address obstacles associated with implementing them. Suitable places for discussing coping strategies different from the ones the IP used (and which ultimately led to relapse) are indicated (see hexagons).

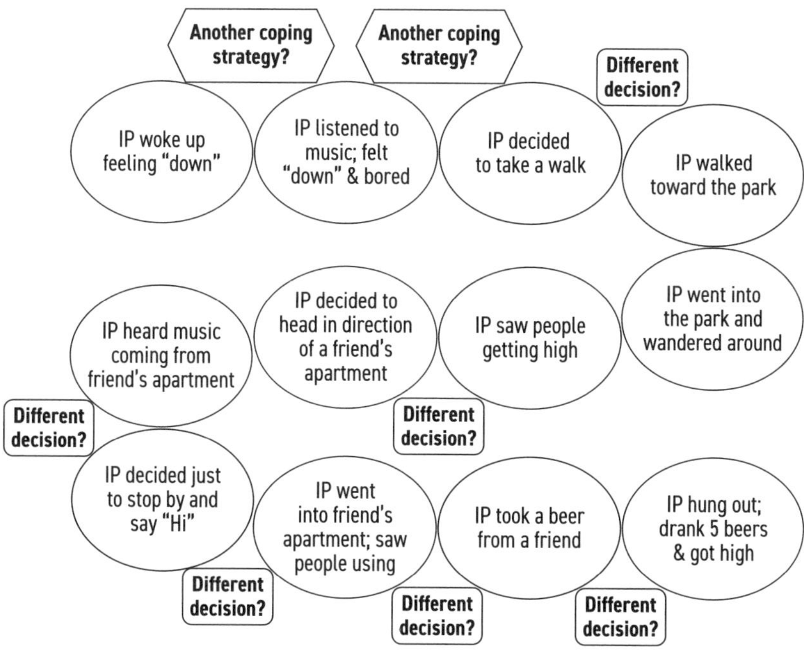

FIGURE 12.1. Example of a Behavioral Chain Leading to Relapse.

Early Warning System

- Explain that this system is a preplanned response by an IP and a monitor (e.g., a CSO) to a high-risk situation (based on the IP's known triggers).
- Refer to the section earlier in this chapter on the procedure Medication Monitoring for specific steps to select and train a monitor. The monitor's specific task would be different in this relapse prevention scenario, since medication would not be administered. Instead, the monitor would be watching for relapse triggers and responding to them in a manner preplanned by both the monitor and the IP.

CRA Relationship Therapy

CRA Relationship Therapy is also a package of procedures, comprising an overview and several procedures for working with romantic partners to address their present-day problems. Unlike CRA Relapse Prevention in which the three distinct procedures are intended to stand alone, the expectation when conducting CRA Relationship Therapy is that *all* of the procedures will be utilized. This structured approach primarily entails teaching skills in positive communication and goal setting, skills that are generalizable to a variety of interpersonal situations. If the IPs already have been trained in these skills as part of individual CRA treatment, they are asked to assist in teaching the skills to their partner. However, if the partners are CSOs who have received CRAFT, they will be familiar with the skills already. CRA Relationship Therapy is introduced for cases in which IPs would appear to benefit from having their partner attend several therapy sessions with them. It should be noted that with appropriate modifications, CRA Relationship Therapy can be used with nonromantic relationships as well, such as a parent and teen as part of A-CRA (see S. H. Godley et al., 2016).

Procedures in the Package

1. ***Overview of the Process.***
    - Describe how therapy is action oriented and focuses on the here-and-now.
    - Explain that attempts will be made to keep the sessions upbeat and positive.
    - State that the IP and partner will learn to use positive communication with each other and set agreed-upon goals.
    - Mention that the IP may be interested in helping teach the partner some of the basic skills if already trained in them.

2. ***Three Positive Things Exercise.***
    - Explain that a positive tone is established for the session by having the IP and partner start by taking turns looking directly at each other and saying three positive things about the other person.
    - Offer assistance if someone has trouble identifying three positive things, and praise any reasonable efforts.

- After hearing the three positive things, ask the person *about whom they were said* to report what he or she heard *and* what he or she is *feeling* in reaction to the words.
- If the person misheard or misunderstood what had been said about him or her, have the person who delivered the three positive things restate them.

3. ***Goal Setting.***
   - Relationship Happiness Scale (Romantic Partner Version; see Form 12.5):
     - Explain that the purpose of this scale is to allow the IP and partner to rate their current level of happiness *with each other* in several areas of their relationship.
     - State that these ratings will be used to identify goals for each partner to work toward, and to monitor progress toward the goals over time.
     - Give instructions for completing the scale, being sure to highlight the anchor points (1 = *completely unhappy*; 10 = *completely happy*).
     - Have each individual complete the scale independently.
     - Review several ratings for each individual by asking *why* the rating was given *or* asking what would need to change in order for the rating to improve.
     - Ask the partners to each select one category in which they would like their *partner* to work on a goal for the upcoming week.
   - Relationship Goal Setting (Romantic Partner Version; see Form 12.6):
     - Work with each individual so that his or her goal (for his or her partner) satisfies the Goal and Strategy Guidelines (see Chapter 10, Box 10.3).

4. ***Communication Skills Training and Practice.***
   - Discuss the importance of positive communication (see Chapter 4).
   - Define at least three of the seven Positive Communication Guidelines (see Chapter 4, Box 4.1) and give examples relevant to the case. For CRA Relationship Therapy, the following three guidelines (of the seven) are recommended:
     - Offer an understanding statement (Positive Communication Guideline 5).
     - Accept partial responsibility (6).
     - Offer to help (7).
   - Help each individual use positive communication to formulate a request for the partner to work on the goal already selected for him or her.
   - Have one individual present the request verbally to the partner.
   - While encouraging the use of positive communication, help the partners negotiate the terms of the request.
   - Add the negotiated goal to the Relationship Goal Setting (Romantic Partner Version) form (Form 12.6).
   - Repeat the process with the second individual, beginning with presenting the verbal request to the partner.
   - Make sure the partners know that these goals are the homework for the week (see Homework Assignment Guidelines, Chapter 3, Box 3.1).

5. ***Daily Reminder to Be Nice.***
   - Explain that the purpose of this exercise is to give their relationship a "jump start" by reintroducing some of the pleasant, small things that used to happen automatically in their relationship.
   - Mention that although the actions might not feel genuine at first, this will change with time and practice.
   - Ask the partners to complete at least one item from the Daily Reminder to Be Nice form (Form 12.7) each day even if they are not sure whether their partner is doing so.
   - Encourage each individual to discuss or demonstrate one of the items from the form in the session, and assist if necessary.
   - Suggest that they find a place to keep the forms at home so that they neither get lost nor forgotten.

SUMMARY

This chapter describes CRA, the treatment designed to use directly with the individual with the substance use problem (as opposed to with the CSO). As noted, many of the CRA procedures serve as the foundation for CRAFT procedures. Those CRA procedures that are *not* incorporated into CRAFT are presented in more detail. Overall, CRA is a program that would be ideally suited for an IP who decides to seek treatment, given that it "delivers" on the CSOs' promises contained within the motivational hooks (Chapter 11).

FORM 12.1

CRA Functional Analysis of Drinking or Using Behavior

External triggers	Internal triggers	Drinking/using behavior	Short-term positive consequences (rewards)	Long-term negative consequences
1. *Who* are you usually with when drinking/using? 2. *Where* do you usually drink/use? 3. *When* do you usually drink/use?	1. What are you usually *thinking* about right before drinking/using? 2. What are you usually *feeling* right before drinking/using?	1. *What* do you usually drink/use? 2. *How much* (or *how many times* during the episode) do you usually drink/use? 3. Over *how long* a period of time do you usually drink/use?	1. What do you like about drinking/using with (*who*)? 2. What do you like about drinking/using (*where*)? 3. What do you like about drinking/using (*when*)? 4. What pleasant *thoughts* do you have while drinking/using? 5. What pleasant *feelings* do you have while drinking/using?	1. What are the negative results of your drinking/using in these areas: a. Family b. Friends/partners c. Physical d. Emotional e. Legal f. Job g. Financial h. Other

FORM 12.2

CRA Functional Analysis of a Fun, Healthy Behavior

External triggers	Internal triggers	Fun, healthy behavior	Short-term negative consequences (barriers)	Long-term positive consequences
1. *Who* are you usually with when you (*behavior*)? 2. *Where* do you usually (*behavior*)? 3. *When* do you usually (*behavior*)?	1. What are you usually *thinking* about right before you (*behavior*)? 2. What are you usually *feeling* right before you (*behavior*)?	1. *What* is your fun, healthy behavior? 2. *How often* do you engage in it? 3. *How long* a period of time does it last?	1. What do you dislike about (*behavior*) with (*who*)? 2. What do you dislike about (*behavior*) (*where*)? 3. What do you dislike about (*behavior*) (*when*)? 4. What unpleasant *thoughts* do you have while (*behavior*)? 5. What unpleasant *feelings* do you have while (*behavior*)?	1. What are the positive results of (*behavior*) in each of these areas: a. Family b. Friends/partners c. Physical d. Emotional e. Legal f. Job g. Financial h. Other

FORM 12.3

Social/Recreational Activities 2 × 2

Fill in each of these boxes with as many ideas for fun activities as you can. Remember that the goal is to add fun social and recreational activities to your life.

Things to do:

With money/with others	**With money/alone**
Without money/with others	**Without money/alone**

FORM 12.4

CRA Functional Analysis for Relapse

External triggers	Internal triggers	Drinking/using behavior	Short-term positive consequences (rewards)	Long-term negative consequences
1. *Who* were you with when you drank/used? 2. *Where* did you drink/use? 3. *When* did you drink/use?	1. What were you *thinking* about right before you drank/used? 2. What were you *feeling* right before you drank/used?	1. *What* did you drink/use? 2. *How much* (or *how many times* during the episode) did you drink/use? 3. Over *how long* a period of time did you drink/use?	1. What did you like about drinking/using with (*who*)? 2. What did you like about drinking/using (*where*)? 3. What did you like about drinking/using (*when*)? 4. What pleasant *thoughts* did you have while drinking/using? 5. What pleasant *feelings* did you have while drinking/using?	1. What are the negative results of your drinking/using in each of these areas: a. Family b. Friends/partners c. Physical d. Emotional e. Legal f. Job g. Financial h. Other

FORM 12.5

Relationship Happiness Scale (Romantic Partner Version)

This scale is intended to estimate your *current* happiness with your *relationship* in each of the areas listed below. Ask yourself the following question as you rate each area:

How happy am I today with my loved one in this area?

Circle one of the numbers (1–10) beside each area. Numbers toward the left (lower numbers, like 1) indicate various degrees of unhappiness, while numbers toward the right (higher numbers, like 10) reflect various levels of happiness.

In other words, state according to the numerical scale (1–10) exactly how you feel **today** with that particular relationship area. Also, try not to allow one category to influence the results of the other categories.

	Completely unhappy									**Completely happy**
Household responsibilities	1	2	3	4	5	6	7	8	9	10
Raising the children	1	2	3	4	5	6	7	8	9	10
Extended family relations	1	2	3	4	5	6	7	8	9	10
Social activities	1	2	3	4	5	6	7	8	9	10
Money management	1	2	3	4	5	6	7	8	9	10
Communication	1	2	3	4	5	6	7	8	9	10
Affection	1	2	3	4	5	6	7	8	9	10
Sexual relationship	1	2	3	4	5	6	7	8	9	10
Job or school	1	2	3	4	5	6	7	8	9	10
Emotional support	1	2	3	4	5	6	7	8	9	10
Drinking/drug use	1	2	3	4	5	6	7	8	9	10
Spiritual life	1	2	3	4	5	6	7	8	9	10

FORM 12.6

Relationship Goal Setting (Romantic Partner Version)

Under each area listed below, write down the behaviors that would represent an ideal relationship. Be brief, be positive, and state in a specific and *measurable* way what you would like to see occur.

1. In **household responsibilities,** I would like my partner to:

   a. ______________________________

   b. ______________________________

   c. ______________________________

   d. ______________________________

2. In **raising the children,** I would like my partner to:

   a. ______________________________

   b. ______________________________

   c. ______________________________

   d. ______________________________

3. In **extended family relations,** I would like my partner to:

   a. ______________________________

   b. ______________________________

   c. ______________________________

   d. ______________________________

4. In **social activities,** I would like my partner to:

   a. ______________________________

   b. ______________________________

   c. ______________________________

   d. ______________________________

(continued)

5. In **money management,** I would like my partner to:

    a. ______________________________

    b. ______________________________

    c. ______________________________

    d. ______________________________

6. In **communication,** I would like my partner to:

    a. ______________________________

    b. ______________________________

    c. ______________________________

    d. ______________________________

7. In **affection,** I would like my partner to:

    a. ______________________________

    b. ______________________________

    c. ______________________________

    d. ______________________________

8. In **sexual relationship,** I would like my partner to:

    a. ______________________________

    b. ______________________________

    c. ______________________________

    d. ______________________________

(continued)

9. In **job or school,** I would like my partner to:

   a. ____________________

   b. ____________________

   c. ____________________

   d. ____________________

10. In **emotional support,** I would like my partner to:

   a. ____________________

   b. ____________________

   c. ____________________

   d. ____________________

11. In **drinking/drug use,** I would like my partner to:

   a. ____________________

   b. ____________________

   c. ____________________

   d. ____________________

12. In **spiritual life,** I would like my partner to:

   a. ____________________

   b. ____________________

   c. ____________________

   d. ____________________

FORM 12.7

Daily Reminder to Be Nice

Make every effort to complete at least one of the items below each day. Check the box for it under the day.

Day/date:							
Did you express appreciation to your partner today?							
Did you compliment your partner today?							
Did you give your partner any pleasant surprises today?							
Did you express visible affection to your partner today?							
Did you spend some time devoting your complete attention to pleasant conversation with your partner?							
Did you *initiate* a pleasant conversation today?							
Did you make any offer to help before being asked?							
Other: ________________ ________________							

Chapter 13

Scientific Support for CRAFT

This final chapter presents the scientific evidence for CRAFT. Two systematic reviews (one from 2010 and another from 2019) are described in some detail first, and these are followed by newer studies that were not published at the time of the 2019 review and thus could not be included in it. We then present the CRAFT studies that did *not* focus on IP treatment engagement (entry), as these also were not included in the two systematic reviews. Tables are provided that contain the most salient information for all of the studies.

SYSTEMATIC REVIEWS OF CRAFT

Roozen, de Waart, and van der Kroft (2010)

The first CRAFT systematic review (Roozen et al., 2010) specifically compared CRAFT with Al-Anon/Nar-Anon and the Johnson Institute Intervention (JII). Four randomized controlled trials were examined that included 264 CSOs (Kirby, Marlowe, Festinger, Garvey, & La Monaca, 1999; Meyers, Miller, Smith, & Tonigan, 2002; Miller, Meyers, & Tonigan, 1999; Sisson & Azrin, 1986). The primary outcome variable was IP treatment engagement. For the secondary outcome interest, CSO improvement in functioning, there were data available for three of the four studies.

IP Treatment Engagement Results

- CRAFT facilitated treatment engagement (entry) for approximately two-thirds of the IPs.
- IP treatment engagement typically occurred after four to six CRAFT (CSO) sessions.
- IP engagement success was found across various substances, ethnic/racial groups, and CSO–IP relationships.
- A meta-analysis on the four studies showed that CRAFT's overall IP engagement rate of 67% was more than three times as effective as Al-Anon/Nar-Anon's 18% rate.
- The one study that compared CRAFT with the JII found that CRAFT's 64% engagement rate was more than twice as effective as JII's 30% rate.

CSO Functioning Results

- CSOs showed significant improvements in psychosocial functioning (depression, anger, family cohesion, family conflict, and relationship happiness) during the 6-month treatment time frame.
- These improvements occurred across treatment conditions and regardless of whether the IP had engaged in treatment.

Summary

CRAFT's engagement rates were more than three times that of Al-Anon/Nar-Anon and twice as effective as the JII. Overall, CSO functioning improved irrespective of treatment type and whether the IP entered therapy.

Archer, Harwood, Stevelink, Rafferty, and Greenberg (2019)

A recent systematic review (Archer et al., 2019) examined 20 different CRAFT treatment conditions that occurred within 14 studies. In other words, if a study had more than one CRAFT condition, each condition was reported separately. A total of 691 CSOs participated. They ranged in age from 18 to 81 years. Across the studies, 72–100% of the CSOs were female. The main outcome of interest was the treatment engagement (entry) rate for the IPs as reported by the CSOs up to 1 year after a CSO had started treatment.

IP Treatment Engagement Results

OVERALL:

- CRAFT was twice as effective as controls or comparison conditions.

BASED ON THE IP'S PROBLEM:

- Most studies had engagement rates of at least 60%. These percentages varied significantly depending on the IP's problem:
    - For studies in which IPs had a substance use disorder (SUD), engagement rates ranged from 40 to 86%.
    - For studies in which IPs had a gambling disorder, engagement rates ranged from 12.5 to 23.0%.
    - Archer and colleagues (2019) suggested that the lower engagement rates associated with the gambling studies might have been due to the fact that the gambling studies:
        - Mostly relied on self-directed workbooks instead of therapists.
        - Had questionable training of the therapists in the one study that used therapists.
        - Had recruitment flyers that did not specify that one goal of CRAFT was to get the IP into treatment.
        - Were dealing with a problem IP behavior that was more difficult to detect than substance use, and therefore it was harder for CSOs to properly implement the CRAFT procedures that revolved around rewarding the desired behavior.

BASED ON TREATMENT DELIVERY FORMAT:

- IP engagement rates varied across CRAFT delivery formats as well:
  - CRAFT treatment that contained *both* an individual and a group aspect had the highest engagement rates: 86% (Sisson & Azrin, 1986) and 77% (Meyers et al., 2002):
    - Sisson and Azrin (1986) reported that in addition to the individual sessions, group sessions were *an option at times* for role playing with other CSOs who had already engaged their IPs. However, the study did not indicate how often this occurred.
    - Meyers et al. (2002) supplemented the individual CRAFT sessions with 6 months of group treatment in their CRAFT + Aftercare condition. Yet no new IPs were engaged in treatment as a function of their CSO attending the aftercare groups.
    - It is possible that simply the act of offering CSOs multiple CRAFT formats was instrumental in achieving elevated IP engagement rates.
  - CRAFT individual session engagement rates ranged from 12.5 to 71.0%.
  - CRAFT group session rates were 60%.
  - CRAFT self-directed workbook engagement rates ranged from 13.3 to 40.0%.

BASED ON THE CSO-IP RELATIONSHIP, CSO AGE OR SEX, OR NUMBER OF SESSIONS:

- Overall, the type of CSO–IP relationship did *not* affect IP engagement. The only exception was one study that found that parents were significantly more effective (83% engaged) than nonparents (31% engaged; Meyers, Miller, Hill, &Tonigan, 1999).
- IP engagement rates were *not* affected by:
  - CSOs' age or sex.
  - The number of CSO sessions attended (or offered).

BASED ON ACCESSIBILITY OF IP TREATMENT:

- "Integrated" IP treatment entailed offering treatment to the IP either by the same team of therapists that offered CRAFT to the CSO or by someone associated with that team. For the 14 (out of 20) CRAFT conditions in which this occurred, IP engagement rates ranged from 52 to 86%. Archer et al. (2019) concluded that this easy/efficient way to schedule IPs that involves the CSO's same service agency might have improved treatment engagement.

Summary

Overall, CRAFT was twice as effective as the control or comparison conditions in terms of IP treatment engagement. Although engagement was considerably lower for the studies dealing with IP gambling problems as opposed to IP substance use, the gambling findings were probably at least partially the result of treatment implementation issues. In terms of treatment modality, the self-directed workbook delivery of CRAFT generally achieved the lowest engagement rates. With one exception (Meyers et al., 1999), IP engagement rates were not affected by the CSO–IP relationship, the CSO's age or sex, or the number of sessions attended. The use of "integrated" IP treatment may have supported IP engagement (see also Roozen & Smith, 2021, in press).

MORE RECENT ONLINE CRAFT STUDIES ADDRESSING IP ENGAGEMENT

Tables 13.1 and 13.2 contain all of the studies summarized in the Archer et al. (2019) systematic review, plus three additional ones. These more recent studies, which were offered online, each covered a different IP problem area. These three studies are summarized below.

IP Substance (Alcohol) Use (Eék et al., 2020)

Interested CSOs were randomly assigned to either a web-based, abbreviated CRAFT program (iCRAFT) that was therapist guided (i.e., therapists provided individualized feedback for completed exercises and homework) or to a wait-list (WL) condition (i.e., participants received the assessment only until the completion of the study, at which point they received iCRAFT). The IP engagement rate for iCRAFT was relatively low (21%) but it was twice that of the WL (11%) at 6 weeks. Importantly, compared to the WL at 6 weeks, CSOs in the iCRAFT condition were significantly less depressed and had more relationship happiness and better life quality. Eék and colleagues (2020) speculated that the low engagement rates might have been due to the following: (1) iCRAFT comprised just five (complex) modules, (2) the program did not offer any role playing, (3) IP treatment access varied considerably throughout the country, and (4) there was preemptive study closure.

IP Gambling (Magnusson, Nilsson, Andersson, Hellner, & Carlbring, 2019)

CSOs were randomized to either a WL or to a cognitive-behavioral therapy (CBT) program. The latter, which was delivered via the Internet and was described as "CRAFT inspired," also offered therapist phone calls or emails for support. The CBT program had low IP engagement rates (16%) and did not differ from the WL (14%) but showed promise as far as improved CSO functioning. The authors offered several possible explanations for the CRAFT-inspired condition's low engagement rates: (1) it was common for CSOs *not* to read all of the modules, including the module for IP treatment entry; (2) there were limited treatment services available for IPs with gambling problems; and (3) the treatment was somewhat difficult for CSOs to implement with their gambling IPs, since the absence of physiological signs of gambling interfered with CSOs' ability to administer the rewards contingently.

IP Posttraumatic Stress Disorder (Erbes et al., 2020)

CSOs were the spouses/partners of veterans who had been diagnosed with posttraumatic stress disorder (PTSD) but had not sought treatment. The study was conducted within the U.S. Department of Veterans Affairs (VA). CSOs were randomized to "VA-CRAFT" online or a WL. The IP engagement rates (as reported by the CSOs) were relatively low for both

TABLE 13.1. CRAFT Studies: IP with a Substance Use Problem

Authors (year) (sample size)[a]	CSO gender (female)	CSO ethnicity/race[b]	CSO age (range, average)	CSO's relationship with IP (CSO was the IP's . . .)
Sisson & Azrin (1986) (12 CSOs)	100%	NR	28–62 NR	Spouse (75%) Sibling (17%) Child (8%)
Miller et al. (1999) (130 CSOs)	91%	53% White 39% Hispanic 6% Native American 2% other	21–81 47	Spouse/partner (67.0%) Parent (30.0%) Child (1.5%) Grandparent (1.5%)
Meyers et al. (1999) (62 CSOs)	97%	48% Hispanic 47% White 3% Native American 2% African American	18–73 45	Parent (56%) Spouse (34%) Sibling (6%) Child (4%)
Kirby et al. (1999) (32 CSOs)	94%	75% White 22% African American 3% other	20–70 40	Spouse/partner (56%) Parent (38%) Sibling (6%)
Meyers et al. (2002) (90 CSOs)	88%	49% Hispanic 49% White (approx.)	NR 47	Parents (53%) Spouse/partner (30%) Sibling (10%) Child, friend (7%)
Waldron et al. (2007) (42 CSOs)	83%	48% Hispanic 48% White 4% Native American	NR 46	Parents/parent surrogates (100%)
Dutcher et al. (2009) (99 CSOs)	90%	76% White 59% Hispanic 21% other 2% American Indian	NR 51	Spouse/partner (48%) Parent (28%) Other (12%) Child (6%) Other relative (6%)
Manuel et al. (2012) (40 CSOs)	85%	65% White 30% Hispanic 2.5% Native American 2.5% mixed	26–76 51	Parent (62.0%) Spouse/partner (20.0%) Sibling (8.0%) Other (5.0%) Child (2.5%) Friend (2.5%)
Bisetto Pons et al. (2016) (50 CSOs)	76%	Conducted in Spain	NR 52	Parent (100%)
Bischof et al. (2016) (94 CSOs)	92%	Conducted in Germany	NR 49	Spouse/partner (80%) Child (10%) Parents (6%) Sibling (3%) Third-degree relative (1%)
Kirby et al. (2017) (115 CSOs)	77%	56% White 39% Black 5% other	NR 50	Spouse/partner (52%) Parent (26%) Other (22%)
Eék et al. (2020) (94 CSOs)	98%	Conducted in Sweden	NR 47	Partner (86%) Child (7%) Other (4%) Parent (2%) Friend (1%)

Note: NR, not reported; CRT, Community Reinforcement Training; FT, facilitation therapy; Tx, treatment; WL, wait list; TEnT, Treatment Entry Training.

[a]CSO sample size was calculated in different ways across studies. Randomized controlled trials (RCTs) commonly reported the number of participants randomized. Uncontrolled studies reported their CSO sample size as the number of CSOs who were recruited or assessed, or who attended treatment or completed follow-ups.

Treatment conditions	Treatment engagement rates	CSO functioning that significantly improved	Engagement window (months)	IP drug of choice[c]
• CRAFT (CRT) • Supportive counseling + Al-Anon referral	• 86% • 0%	NR	3	100% alcohol
• CRAFT • Johnson Institute Intervention • Al-Anon FT	• 64% • 30% • 13%	Depression, anger, family conflict and cohesion, relationship with IP (regardless of Tx condition and IP engagement status)	6	100% alcohol
• CRAFT	• 74%	Depression, anger, anxiety, physical symptoms (regardless of IP engagement status)	6	39% cocaine 29% stimulant 18% marijuana 9% opiates 5% "other"
• CRAFT (CRT) • Nar-Anon groups	• 64% • 17%	Total number of problems, mood, health, social adjustment (leisure, family unit), financial (regardless of Tx condition)	2.5	56% cocaine 22% heroin 22% "other"
• CRAFT • CRAFT + Aftercare group • Al-Anon and Nar-Anon FT	• 59% • 77% (collapsed 67%) • 29%	Depression, family functioning, physical (at $p < .05$ but not with correction at $p < .0026$) (regardless of Tx condition)	6	67% marijuana 63% cocaine 30% stimulant 19% opiates
• CRAFT	• 71%	Depression, state/trait anxiety, family cohesion and conflict (regardless of IP engagement status)	6	Primary interest was marijuana use; high levels of marijuana use reported at baseline (low alcohol levels)
• CRAFT	• 55%	Depression, state anger, state/trait anxiety, relationship happiness (regardless of IP engagement status)	6	91% alcohol 7% cocaine 1% heroin 1% methamphetamine
• CRAFT group + CRAFT self-help book • CRAFT self-help book	• 60% • 40%	Family cohesion and conflict (regardless of Tx condition)	6	100% alcohol or drugs (*not* further specified)
• CRAFT group	• 60%	Depression, self-esteem, state anger	2.5	56% marijuana 28% cocaine 12% alcohol 4% heroin
• CRAFT • WL control	• 40% • 14%	Depression, overall mental health, relationship happiness; with CRAFT > WL	3	100% alcohol
• CRAFT • TEnT • Al-Anon/Nar-Anon FT	• 62% • 63% • 37%	Depression, anxiety, anger, and problems (emotional, family, relationship) (regardless of Tx condition)	9	59% alcohol 30% stimulant 8% opiates 3% "other"
• iCRAFT (abbreviated, web based, therapist guided) • WL	• 21% • 11%	No within-group pre–post scores reported; iCRAFT significantly better than WL on several measures (depression, life quality, relationship happiness) but only at 6 weeks	6	100% alcohol

[b]Percentages do not necessarily add up to 100% since some studies collected information about ethnicity and race that allowed for the endorsement of multiple options, and other studies reported only on the predominant ethnicity/races.

[c]Numbers may exceed 100% if participants selected more than one drug.

TABLE 13.2. CRAFT Studies: IP with a Gambling Problem or PTSD Diagnosis

Authors (year) (sample size)[a]	CSO gender (female)	CSO ethnicity/ race[b]	CSO age (range, average)	CSO's relationship with IP (CSO was the IP's . . .)	Treatment conditions	Treatment engagement rates	CSO functioning that significantly improved	Engagement window (months)	Significant decrease in gambling behaviors (per CSO)[c]
Makarchuk et al. (2002) (31 CSOs)	87%	77% Canadian	19–78 45	Spouse/partner (71%) Parent (13%) Child (13%) Sibling (3%)	• "CRAFT" self-help manual • Control resource package	• 23% • 20%	Overall symptomatology, relationship happiness (regardless of Tx condition)	3	Negative consequences (regardless of Tx condition). "CRAFT" better than control for days gambling
Hodgins et al. (2007) (186 CSOs)	82%	67% Canadian 27% other 6% Native/ Métis	20–77 45	Spouse/partner (62%) Child (18%) Sibling (7%) Parent (6%) Friend (5%) Extended family (3%) (Total >100% reflects rounding)	• "CRAFT" self-help workbook • "CRAFT" self-help workbook + phone support • Control resource package	• 15% • 14% • 17%	Overall symptomatology, relationship happiness (regardless of Tx condition)	6	Negative consequences, money spent (regardless of Tx condition)
Nayoski & Hodgins (2016) (31 CSOs)	90%	84% Canadian 6% Italian 3% German 3% Hungarian 3% Chinese	NR 46	Spouse/partner (68%) Child (16%) Parent (13%) Ex-spouse (3%)	• "CRAFT" • "CRAFT" self-help manual	• 12% • 13% (Paper reports 17% based on those at follow-up)	(Comparison of effect sizes due to small sample; more promising for "CRAFT" condition)	6	Money spent (regardless of Tx condition)
Magnusson et al. (2019) (100 CSOs)	89%	Conducted in Sweden	NR 45	Partner (43%) Parent (43%) Other (14%)	• Internet CBT ("CRAFT" inspired) with therapist support available (phone, email) • WL	• 16% • 14%	Emotional consequences, anxiety, depression, relationship satisfaction (Internet CBT moderately positive effect compared to WL)	Posttest	Small inconclusive effects
Erbes et al. (2020) (41 CSOs)	100%	NR	NR NR	Spouse/partner (100%)	• "VA-CRAFT" • WL	• 36% • 21% (Numbers different with EMR; 0%, 11%)	Decrease in caregiver burden scores (total and objective) ("VA-CRAFT" better than WL)	3	N/A (PTSD diagnoses)

Note: PTSD, posttraumatic stress disorder; Tx, treatment; NR, not reported; "CRAFT," substantially modified version of CRAFT; WL, wait list; CBT, cognitive-behavioral therapy; EMR, electronic medical record.

[a]CSO sample size was calculated in different ways across studies. Randomized controlled trials (RCTs) commonly reported the number of participants randomized (but there were exceptions). Uncontrolled studies reported their CSO sample size as the number of CSOs who were recruited or assessed, or who attended treatment or completed follow-ups.

[b]Percentages do not necessarily add up to 100% since some studies collected information about ethnicity and race that allowed for the endorsement of multiple options, and other studies reported only on the predominant ethnicity/races.

[c]Reductions in gambling behaviors were reported in addition to IP treatment engagement rates, given that treatment for gambling is often neither available nor a goal of CSOs.

VA-CRAFT (36%) and the WL (21%), with no statistical difference between them. When the VA electronic medical records were used instead (which detected treatment specifically at the VA), the rates changed to VA-CRAFT (0%) and WL (11%). CSOs in the VA-CRAFT condition showed significantly better improvements than the WL on caregiver burden scores. Follow-up interviews determined that only a small percentage of CSOs in VA-CRAFT even raised the issue of treatment with their IP. Furthermore, CSOs required persistent reminders to log into the VA-CRAFT website to work on the course.

Summary

It appears sensible to develop an online version of CRAFT for today's world, given that treatment then becomes widely accessible to CSOs who might be unable to seek in-person CRAFT treatment due to a lack of available therapists or insurance to cover them, or to transportation or work and child-care schedule challenges. Yet the modest IP treatment engagement rates detected thus far might suggest that many challenges remain in developing a highly effective online version of CRAFT. At the same time, one cannot assume that these relatively low engagement rates were solely attributable to the online format, given that one of the studies was in the gambling area, and engagement rates for gambling studies in general have been suppressed. Additionally, one of the studies was with CSOs who had IPs diagnosed with PTSD; a particular IP problem area that has not yet been studied in a CRAFT face-to-face format. Importantly, there *were* notable improvements in CSO functioning.

A major challenge in developing an online version of CRAFT is presenting a sufficient amount of high-quality CRAFT material such that CSOs are able to receive an adequate "dose" of treatment *and* doing it in an interesting (perhaps personalized) way that minimizes CSO dropout. Conceivably this entails making the online material more interactive, but it also might require the involvement of therapist guidance/support. Research is needed to address these questions.

CRAFT STUDIES WITHOUT A PRIMARY FOCUS ON IP TREATMENT ENGAGEMENT

The final table (Table 13.3) contains CRAFT studies that did not focus on IP engagement, and thus were not included in the Archer et al. (2019) review.

1. **Focus of the CRAFT-T program: IP treatment retention.** The IPs were residents of a buprenorphine treatment program for opiate problems. IPs were randomized to CRAFT for Treatment Retention (CRAFT-T; Brigham et al., 2014) or to treatment as usual (TAU; education and referral). CRAFT-T sessions primarily were conducted with the CSOs (who were selected by the IPs), but IPs attended two CRAFT sessions. The results showed a trend for CRAFT-T to improve treatment retention; it reached significance when only the CSOs who were parental family were examined. IPs assigned to CRAFT-T significantly reduced their use of opiates and other drugs.

2. **Focus of the CRAFT groups: increase IP motivation for change.** These IPs had been referred by a National Addiction Help Line to a methadone clinic in Tehran, Iran,

TABLE 13.3. CRAFT Studies: IP Engagement NOT a Focus of Treatment

Authors (year) (sample size)[a]	CSO gender (female)	CSO ethnicity/race[b]	CSO age (range, average)	CSO's relationship with IP (CSO was the IP's . . .)	Treatment conditions	Primary IP treatment outcomes of interest	CSO functioning that significantly improved	Assessment window (months)	IP drug of choice (or other identified problem)
Brigham et al. (2014) (52 CSOs)	83%	90% White 6% African American 4% other	NR 42	Parent/aunt/grandparent (50%) Spouse/partner (38%) Sibling (6%) Friend (6%)	• CRAFT-T • TAU (support group + referral to Al-Anon or Nar-Anon)	Increase IP Tx retention: • CRAFT-T significant when CSOs were all parental family Reduce opioid and other drug use: • Significantly favored CRAFT-T	NR	9	100% opiates
Assadbeigi et al. (2016, 2017) (75 CSOs)	100%	Conducted in Iran	NR NR	Family member (100%)	(Quasi-experimental) • CRAFT group • Nar-Anon group • No-Tx control	Move IPs to a more advanced motivational stage of change: • IPs of CRAFT CSOs moved to a more advanced motivational stage of change	Quality of life (regardless of experimental Tx condition)	3	100% "drug use disorder"
Miller et al. (2016) (66 CSOs)	NR	NR	NR NR	NR	(Non-random assignment) • CRAFT • No-Tx comparison	Decrease 1-year recidivism: • 28% recidivism • 75%	NR	12	100% "substance using offenders"
Osilla et al. (2017) (234 CSOs)	95%	71% White 9% multi racial 6% African American 4% Hispanic/Latino	22–68 32	Spouse/partner (100%)	(Not entirely random assignment) • Partners Connect; abbreviated CRAFT + MI (web based) • WL control	(Focused exclusively on CSO)	Partners Connect significantly better than WL (anxiety, emotional and tangible social support); Partners Connect alone improved (relationship quality, family conflict)	5	100% alcohol
Ameral et al. (2020) (545 CSOs)	60%	82% White	26–79 55	Parent/parental role (100%)	• CRAFT-informed group	(Focused exclusively on CSO)	Ability to manage and cope with child's SUD; feeling less bothered or stressed by child's SUD	2	100% SUD
Kubo et al. (2020) (21 CSOs)	67%	Conducted in Japan	49–76 62	Parent (100%)	• Mental Health First Aid + CRAFT	Improve IPs' mental health and adaptive behaviors: • IPs had decreased obsessive-compulsive behavior, and increased adaptive behaviors (value) and activity	Perceived skills for managing a child with *hikikomori* and asking about depression and suicide; reduced stigma for mental health problems	6	100% *hikikomori* sufferers (severe social withdrawal)

Note: NR, not reported; CRAFT-T, Community Reinforcement and Family Training for Treatment Retention; TAU, treatment as usual; Tx, treatment; MI, motivational interviewing; WL, wait list; SUD, substance use disorder.

[a]CSO sample size was calculated in different ways across studies. Randomized controlled trials (RCTs) commonly reported the number of participants randomized. Uncontrolled studies reported their CSO sample size as the number of CSOs who were recruited or assessed, or who attended treatment or completed follow-ups.

[b]Percentages do not necessarily add up to 100% since some studies collected information about ethnicity and race that allowed for the endorsement of multiple options, and other studies reported only on the predominant ethnicity/races.

but their CSOs were eligible regardless of the IP's type of drug use. The paper (Assadbeigi, Pourshabaz, Mohamadkhani, & Farhoudian, 2016, 2017) reported that some of the IPs may have been in detox already. Using a quasi-experimental design, CSOs were assigned to one of three conditions: CRAFT group, Nar-Anon group, or a no-treatment control. The results indicated that only the IPs with CSOs in the CRAFT group improved their motivational stage of change. For example, those IPs moved from "precontemplation" or "contemplation" stages to the "preparation" stage, and from "preparation" to the "action" stage.

3. **Focus of CRAFT: decrease IP 1-year recidivism rates.** These IPs were jail inmates (substance-use offenders) who were receiving CBT. CRAFT was conducted with the CSOs (who were selected by the IPs) when the IPs were nearing their release date. IPs joined the CSOs for family sessions upon release. IPs who were not interested in this program were assigned to the no-treatment comparison condition (i.e., nonrandom assignment). According to the results (Miller, Miller, & Barnes, 2016), the IPs who had CSOs in the CRAFT program had significantly lower 1-year recidivism rates (28%) when compared to the no-treatment condition (75%). However, the potential role of IP motivation should be considered when interpreting the findings of this nonrandomized design.

4. **Focus of Partners Connect (abbreviated web-based version of CRAFT plus motivational interviewing): improve the mental health of military CSOs.** CSOs reported that their IPs, who were in the military, had alcohol problems (Osilla, Trail, Pedersen, Gore, & Tolpadi, 2017). The CSOs were randomized to Partners Connect or a WL condition (but the randomization was compromised). The outcome was that Partners Connect CSOs showed significantly greater decreases in anxiety and increases in social support compared to the WL CSOs. Partners Connect CSOs also had significant increases in relationship quality and decreases in family conflict over time, but these did not differ significantly from the WL.

5. **Focus of CRAFT-informed groups: increase CSOs' efficacy and empowerment regarding their child's SUD.** Parents (CSOs) who had a child (ages 14–26; IP) with an SUD were eligible for an 8-week CRAFT-informed group, regardless of whether their child was in treatment already (Ameral et al., 2020). The results showed that CSOs reported significant improvement in their ability to manage and cope with their child's SUD, and with their perceived stress about it. Overall stress was not reduced, however, and retention was somewhat problematic.

6. **Focus of CRAFT plus Mental Health First Aid groups: improve the CSOs' skills in managing a child suffering from *hikikomori*.** CSOs were the Japanese parents of a child suffering from *hikikomori* (severe social anxiety; IP; Kubo et al., 2020). The CRAFT part of this program was primarily an FA and positive communication skills training. The findings were that CSOs reported significant improvements in their ability to intervene for their depressed child (e.g., asking about feelings and suicidality), and a decrease in their own perceived stigma about mental health problems. CSOs reported significant improvement in several adaptive IP behaviors and a decrease in maladaptive behaviors, as well (see also Nonaka, Sakai, & Ono, 2013; Sakai & Sakano, 2010).

It is not possible to draw firm conclusions from these studies about the use of CRAFT for a purpose other than IP treatment engagement, given that (1) only six studies have been published that specifically used CRAFT (or a CRAFT-related treatment) for a primary purpose other than IP treatment engagement, (2) the studies all focused on different objectives (e.g., IP treatment retention, reduced IP recidivism rates, CSO management of a child with a mental health problem), and (3) only one study used a completely randomized design. Nonetheless, the findings were highly promising, with improvements in the expected direction (if not already significant) in each case. Thus, future research will determine the extent to which adaptations of CRAFT can be implemented successfully across a wide domain of problem areas.

SAMPLE OF ONGOING CLINICAL RESEARCH TRIALS WITH CRAFT

Listed below are the titles of several ongoing grant-supported clinical trials that are investigating various aspects of CRAFT.

1. "Combining Online Community Reinforcement and Family Training (CRAFT) with a Parent-Training Programme for Parents with Partners Suffering from Alcohol Use Disorder: Study Protocol for a Randomised Controlled Trial" (Lindner et al., 2018).
2. "Community Reinforcement and Family Training (CRAFT): Design of a Cluster Randomized Controlled Trial Comparing Individual, Group, and Self-Help Interventions" (Hellum et al., 2019).
3. "Study Design to Evaluate a Group-Based Therapy for Support Persons of Adults on Buprenorphine/Naloxone" (Osilla et al., 2020).
4. "Randomized Controlled Trial of CRAFT with American Indians" (Venner, Smith, et al., 2021).
5. "Improving Treatment Engagement in Individuals with Co-Occurring Substance Use and Psychosis: A Telemedicine Family-Based Approach" (McCarthy, 2021).
6. "A Randomized Controlled Trial of Coaching into Care with VA-CRAFT to Promote Veteran Engagement in PTSD Care" (Kuhn & Sayers, 2021).
7. "Scalable Digital Delivery of Evidence-Based Training for Family to Maximize Treatment Admission Rates of Opioid Use Disorder in Loved Ones" (Macky, 2019).

CONCLUSION

It is apparent from the ongoing studies listed above that CRAFT is moving in multiple exciting directions all at once. Not only is it being culturally tailored for racial/ethnic IP populations (e.g., American Indians) but it is also being adapted for work with IPs with psychological problems outside of the substance use and gambling realms (e.g., PTSD, psychosis). A new pilot study tested the feasibility of offering CRAFT via telehealth (the Zoom platform) for the CSOs of IPs with comorbid substance use and a chronic mental illness such as bipolar I disorder (McCarthy et al., 2022). The promising findings showed that the CSOs were extremely receptive to receiving CRAFT in this format, as evidenced by their

100% session-completion rate and their high satisfaction ratings. Furthermore, reports regarding CRAFT's acceptability with underrepresented racial groups are appearing in the literature (e.g., Calabria et al., 2013; Hirchak et al., 2020) along with their manuals for implementation (Rose, Calabria, Allan, Clifford, & Shakeshaft, 2014). Finally, CRAFT variations are being used in combination with other empirically supported treatments. One such project involves training the parents of children with substance use problems to be telephone coaches for other parents in similar situations (Carpenter, Foote, Hedrick, Collins, & Clarkin, 2020).

Future research should (1) continue to explore ways to improve the online versions of CRAFT, (2) test adaptations of CRAFT to better serve the CSOs of IPs with psychological problems other than SUDs, (3) determine the contribution of external factors that might be contributing to lower IP engagement rates (e.g., lack of easily accessible IP services), (4) identify the active treatment ingredients of CRAFT, and (5) determine the mechanisms of change for CRAFT.

References

Ameral, V., Yule, A., McKowen, J., Bergman, B. G., Nargiso, J., & Kelly, J. F. (2020). A naturalistic evaluation of a group intervention for parents of youth with substance use disorders. *Alcoholism Treatment Quarterly, 38*, 379–394.

Archer, M., Harwood, H., Stevelink, S., Rafferty, L., & Greenberg, N. (2019). Community reinforcement and family training and rates of treatment entry: A systematic review. *Addiction, 115*, 1024–1037.

Assadbeigi, H., Pourshahbaz, A., Mohamadkhani, P., & Farhoudian, A. (2016). Effectiveness of community reinforcement and family training (CRAFT) on motivational stages of change of drug abusers to engage in treatment. *International Journal of Humanities and Cultural Studies, ISSN 2356–5926*, 685–694.

Assadbeigi, H., Pourshahbaz, A., Mohamadkhani, P., & Farhoudian, A. (2017). Effectiveness of community reinforcement and family training (CRAFT) on quality of life and depression in families with drug abuse. *Global Journal of Health Science, 9*(3), 167.

Azrin, N. H. (1976). Improvements in the community reinforcement approach to alcoholism. *Behaviour Research and Therapy, 14*, 339–348.

Azrin, N. H., & Besalel, V. A. (1980). *Job club counselor's manual: A behavioral approach to vocational counseling.* Austin, TX: PRO-ED.

Azrin, N. H., Naster, B. J., & Jones, R. (1973). Reciprocity counseling: A rapid learning-based procedure for marital counseling. *Behaviour Research and Therapy, 11*, 365–382.

Azrin, N. H., Sisson, R. W., Meyers, R. J., & Godley, M. (1982). Alcoholism treatment by disulfiram and community reinforcement therapy. *Journal of Behavior Therapy and Experimental Psychiatry, 13*, 105–112.

Beck, A. T., & Steer, R. A. (1993). *Beck Anxiety Inventory manual.* San Antonio, TX: Psychological Corporation.

Beck, A. T., Steer, R. A., & Brown, G. (1996). *Beck Depression Inventory–II (BDI-II)* [Database record]. APA PsycTests. Retrieved from *https://doi.org/10.1037/t00742-000.*

Benishek, L. A., Carter, M., Clements, N. T., Allen, C., Salber, K. E., Dugosh, K. L., & Kirby, K. C. (2012). Psychometric assessment of a self-administered version of the Significant Other Survey. *Psychology of Addictive Behaviors, 26*, 986–993.

Benishek, L. A., Kirby, K. C., & Dugosh, K. L. (2011). Prevalence and frequency of problems of concerned family members with a substance-using loved one. *American Journal of Drug and Alcohol Abuse, 37*, 82–88.

Birkeland, B., Foster, K., Selbekk, A. S., Hoie, M. M., Ruud, T., & Weimand, B. (2018). The quality of life when a partner has substance use problems: A scoping review. *Health and Quality of Life Outcomes, 16*(1), 219.

Bischof, G., Iwen, J., Freyer-Adam, J., & Rumpf, H. J. (2016). Efficacy of the community reinforcement and family training for concerned significant others of treatment-refusing individuals with alcohol dependence: A randomized controlled trial. *Drug and Alcohol Dependence, 163,* 179–185.

Bisetto Pons, D., González Barrón, R., & Botella Guijarro, A. (2016). Family-based intervention program for parents of substance-abusing youth and adolescents. *Journal of Addiction.* Retrieved from *https://downloads.hindawi.com/journals/jad/2016/4320720.pdf*

Brigham, G. S., Slesnick, N., Winhusen, T. M., Lewis, D. F., Guo, X., & Somoza, E. (2014). A randomized pilot clinical trial to evaluate the efficacy of community reinforcement and family training for treatment retention (CRAFT-T) for improving outcomes for patients completing opioid detoxification. *Drug and Alcohol Dependence, 138,* 240–243.

Busby, D. M., Crane, D. R., Larson, J. H., & Christensen, C. (1995). A revision of the Dyadic Adjustment Scale for use with distressed and nondistressed couples: Construct hierarchy and multidimensional scales. *Journal of Marital and Family Therapy, 21,* 289–308.

Cacciola, J. S., Alterman, A. I., Lynch, K. G., Martin, J. M., Beauchamp, M. L., & McLellan, A. T. (2008). Initial reliability and validity studies of the revised Treatment Services Review (TSR-6). *Drug and Alcohol Dependence, 92,* 37–47.

Cafferky, B. M., Mendez, M., Anderson, J. R., & Stith, S. M. (2018). Substance use and intimate partner violence: A meta-analytic review. *Psychology of Violence, 8,* 110–131.

Calabria, B., Clifford, A., Shakeshaft, A., Allan, J., Bliss, D., & Doran, C. (2013). The acceptability to Aboriginal Australians of a family-based intervention to reduce alcohol-related harms. *Drug and Alcohol Review, 32,* 328–332.

Campos-Melady, M., Smith, J. E., Meyers, R. J., Godley, S. H., & Godley, M. D. (2017). The effect of therapists' adherence and competence in delivering the adolescent community reinforcement approach on client outcomes. *Psychology of Addictive Behaviors, 31,* 117–129.

Carpenter, K. M., Foote, J., Hedrick, T., Collins, K., & Clarkin, S. (2020). Building on shared experiences: The evaluation of a phone-based parent-to-parent support program for helping parents with their child's substance misuse. *Addictive Behaviors, 100,* 106103.

Cunningham, J. A., Sobell, L. C., Sobell, M. B., & Kapur, G. (1995). Resolution from alcohol treatment problems with and without treatment: Reasons for change. *Journal of Substance Abuse, 7,* 365–372.

Dawson, D. A., Grant, B. F., Chou, S. P., & Stinson, F. S. (2007). The impact of partner alcohol problems on women's physical and mental health. *Journal of Studies on Alcohol and Drugs, 68,* 66–75.

Delmée, L., Roozen, H. G., & Steenhuis, I. (2018). The engagement of non-substance-related pleasant activities is associated with decreased levels of alcohol consumption in university students. *International Journal of Mental Health and Addiction, 16,* 1261–1269.

Dutcher, L. W., Anderson, R., Moore, M., Luna-Anderson, C., Meyers, R. J., Delaney, H. D., & Smith, J. E. (2009). Community reinforcement and family training (CRAFT): An effectiveness study. *Journal of Behavior Analysis in Health, Sports, Fitness, and Medicine, 2,* 80–90.

Eék, N., Romberg, K., Siljeholm, O., Johansson, M., Andreasson, S., Lundgren, T., . . . Hammarberg, A. (2020). Efficacy of an Internet-based community reinforcement and family training program for AUD and to improve psychiatric health for CSOs: A randomized controlled trial. *Alcohol and Alcoholism, 55,* 187–195.

Epstein, E. E., McCrady, B. S., Morgan, T. J., Cook, S. M., Kugler, G., & Ziedonis, D. (2007). Couples treatment for drug-dependent males: Preliminary efficacy of a stand alone outpatient model. *Addictive Disorders and Their Treatment, 6,* 21–37.

Erbes, C. R., Kuhn, E., Polusny, M. A., Ruzek, J. I., Spoont, M., Meis, L. A., . . . Taylor, B. C. (2020). A pilot trial of online training for family well-being and veteran treatment initiation for PTSD. *Military Medicine, 185*(3–4), 401–408.

Falkowski, C. L. (2003). *Dangerous drugs: An easy-to-use reference for parents and professionals* (2nd ed.). Center City, MN: Hazelden.

Garner, B. R., Godley, S. H., Funk, R. R., Dennis, M. L., Smith, J. E., & Godley, M. D. (2009). Exposure to adolescent community reinforcement approach (A-CRA) treatment procedures as a mediator of the relationship between adolescent substance abuse treatment retention and outcome. *Journal of Substance Abuse Treatment, 36*, 252–264.

Godley, M. D., Passetti, L. L., Subramaniam, G. A., Funk, R. R., Smith, J. E., & Meyers, R. J. (2017). Adolescent community reinforcement approach implementation and treatment outcomes for youth with opioid problem use. *Drug and Alcohol Dependence, 174*, 9–16.

Godley, S. H., Hunter, B. D., Fernández-Artamendi, S., Smith, J. E., Meyers, R. J., & Godley, M. D. (2014). A comparison of treatment outcomes for adolescent community reinforcement approach participants with and without co-occurring problems. *Journal of Substance Abuse Treatment, 46*, 463–471.

Godley, S. H., Smith, J. E., Meyers, R. J., & Godley, M. D. (2016). *The adolescent community reinforcement approach: A clinical guide for treating substance use disorders*. Normal, IL: Chestnut Health Systems.

Haugland, B. S. M. (2005). Recurrent disruptions of rituals and routines in families with paternal alcohol abuse. *Family Relations, 54*, 225–241.

Haverfield, M. C., Theiss, J. A., & Leustek, J. (2016). Characteristics of communication in families of alcoholics. *Journal of Family Communication, 16*(2), 111–127.

Hellum, R., Nielsen, A. S., Bischof, G., Andersen, K., Hesse, M., Ekstrom, C. T., & Bilberg, R. (2019). Community reinforcement and family training (CRAFT): Design of a cluster randomized controlled trial comparing individual, group, and self-help interventions. *BMC Public Health, 19*(1), 307.

Hirchak, K. A., Hernandez-Vallant, A., Herron, J., Cloud, V., Tonigan, J. S., McCrady, B., & Venner, K. (2020). Aligning three substance use disorder interventions among a tribe in the Southwest United States: Pilot feasibility for cultural re-centering, dissemination, and implementation. *Journal of Ethnicity in Substance Abuse*. [Epub ahead of print]

Hodgins, D. C., Toneatto, T., Makarchuk, K., Skinner, W., & Vincent, S. (2007). Minimal treatment approaches for concerned significant others of problem gamblers: A randomized controlled trial. *Journal of Gambling Studies, 23*, 215–230.

Hunt, G. M., & Azrin, N. H. (1973). A community-reinforcement approach to alcoholism. *Behaviour Research and Therapy, 11*, 91–104.

Hussaarts, P., Roozen, H. G., Meyers, R. J., van de Wetering, B. J. M., & McCrady, B. S. (2011). Problem areas reported by substance abusing individuals and their concerned significant others. *American Journal on Addictions, 21*, 38–46.

Kaur, A., Mahajan, S., Sunder Deepti, S., & Singh, T. (2018). Assessment of role of burden in caregivers of substance abusers: A study done at Swami Vivekananda Drug De-addiction Centre, Government Medical College, Amritsar. *International Journal of Community Medicine and Public Health, 5*, 2380–2383.

Kirby, K. C., Benishek, L. A., Kerwin, M. E., Dugosh, K. L., Carpenedo, C. M., Bresani, E., . . . Meyers, R. J. (2017). Analyzing components of community reinforcement and family training (CRAFT): Is treatment entry training sufficient? *Psychology of Addictive Behaviors, 31*, 818–827.

Kirby, K. C., Marlowe, D. B., Festinger, D. S., Garvey, K. A., & La Monaca, V. (1999). Community reinforcement training for family and significant others of drug abusers: A unilateral intervention to increase treatment entry of drug users. *Drug and Alcohol Dependence, 56*, 85–96.

Krause, N., & Borawski-Clark, E. (1995). Social class differences in social support among older adults. *The Gerontologist, 35*, 498–508.

Kubo, H., Urata, H., Sakai, M., Nonaka, S., Saito, K., Tateno, M., . . . Kato, T. (2020). Development of 5-day hikikomori intervention program for family members: A single-arm pilot trial. *Heliyon, 6*, e03011.

Kuhn, E. R., & Sayers, S. (2021, January). A randomized controlled trial of coaching into care with VA-CRAFT to promote veteran engagement in PTSD care. Retrieved from *http://report.NIH.gov*

Lambert, M. J., Morton, J. J., Hatfield, D. R., Harmon, C., Hamilton, S., Reid, R. C., & Burlingame, G. M. (2004). *Administration and scoring manual for the OQ-45.* Nashville, TN: American Professional Credentialing Services.

Lander, L., Howsare, J., & Byrne, M. (2013). The impact of substance use disorders on families and children: From theory to practice. *Social Work Public Health, 28*, 194–205.

Lindner, P., Siljeholm, O., Johansson, M., Forster, M., Andreasson, S., & Hammarberg, A. (2018). Combining online community reinforcement and family training (CRAFT) with a parent-training programme for parents with partners suffering from alcohol use disorder: Study protocol for a randomised controlled trial. *BMJ Open, 8*(8), e020879.

Macky, J. (2019, September). *Scalable digital delivery of evidence-based training for family to maximize treatment admission rates of opioid use disorder in loved ones.* National Institute on Drug Abuse. Retrieved from *https://reporter.nih.gov/project-details/10044474.*

Magnusson, K., Nilsson, A., Andersson, G., Hellner, C., & Carlbring, P. (2019). Internet-delivered cognitive-behavioral therapy for significant others of treatment-refusing probem gamblers: A randomized wait-list controlled trial. *Journal of Consulting and Clinical Psychology, 87*, 802–814.

Makarchuk, K., Hodgins, D. C., & Peden, N. (2002). Development of a brief intervention for concerned significant others of problem gamblers. *Addictive Disorders and Their Treatment, 1*, 126–134.

Mancheri, H., Alavi, M., Sabzi, Z., & Maghsoudi, J. (2019). Problems facing families with substance abusers: A review study. *Jorjani Biomedicine Journal, 7*, 31–38.

Manuel, J. K., Austin, J. L., Miller, W. R., McCrady, B. S., Tonigan, J. S., Meyers, R. J., . . . Bogenschutz, M. P. (2012). Community reinforcement and family training: A pilot comparison of group and self-directed delivery. *Journal of Substance Abuse Treatment, 43*, 129–136.

Margolin, G., Talovic, S., & Weinstein, C. D. (1983). Areas of Change Questionnaire: A practical approach to marital assessment. *Journal of Consulting and Clinical Psychology, 51*, 921–931.

Marlatt, G. A. (1985). Cognitive assessment and intervention procedures for relapse prevention. In G. A. Marlatt & J. R. Gordon (Eds.), *Relapse prevention: Maintenance strategies in the treatment of addictive behaviors* (pp. 201–279). New York: Guilford Press.

Marlatt, G. A., Larimer, M. E., & Witkiewitz, K. (Eds.). (2012). *Harm reduction: Pragmatic strategies for managing high-risk behaviors* (2nd ed.). New York: Guilford Press.

Marlatt, G. A., & Witkiewitz, K. (2010). Update on harm reduction policy and intervention research. *Annual Review of Clinical Psychology, 6*, 591–606.

McCarthy, J. (2021, January). Improving treatment engagement in individuals with co-occurring substance use and psychosis: A telemedicine family-based approach. Retrieved from *http://report.NIH.gov*

McCarthy, J. M., Wood, A. J., Shinners, M. G., Heinrich, H., Weiss, R. D., Mueser, K. T., Meyers, R. J., Carol, E. E., Hudson, J. I., & Öngür, D. (2022). Pilot development and feasibility of telehealth Community Reinforcement and Family Training (CRAFT) for early psychosis and substance use. *Psychiatry Research, 317*, 114804. Retrieved from *https://doi.org/10.1016/j.psychres.2022.114804.*

McCrady, B. S., Owens, M. D., & Brovko, J. M. (2013). Couples and family treatment methods. In B. S. McCrady & E. E. Epstein (Eds.), *Addictions: A comprehensive guidebook* (2nd ed., pp. 454–481). New York: Oxford University Press.

McCrady, B. S., Wilson, A. D., Munoz, R. E., Fink, B. C., Fokas, K., & Borders, A. (2016). Alcohol-focused behavioral couple therapy. *Family Process, 55*, 443–459.

McKetin, R., Voce, A., Burns, R. A., & Quinn, B. (2020). The Short Barriers Questionnaire (SBQ): Validity, factor structure and correlates in an out-of-treatment sample of people dependent on methamphetamine. *Journal of Substance Abuse Treatment, 116,* 108029.

Meyers, R. J., Miller, W. R., Hill, D. E., & Tonigan, J. S. (1999). Community reinforcement and family training (CRAFT): Engaging unmotivated drug users in treatment. *Journal of Substance Abuse, 10,* 291–308.

Meyers, R. J., Miller, W. R., Smith, J. E., & Tonigan, J. S. (2002). A randomized trial of two methods for engaging treatment-refusing drug users through concerned significant others. *Journal of Consulting and Clinical Psychology, 70,* 1182–1185.

Meyers, R. J., Roozen, H. G., Smith, J. E., & Evans, B. E. (2014). Reasons for entering treatment reported by initially treatment-resistant patients with substance use disorders. *Cognitive Behaviour Therapy, 43,* 299–309.

Meyers, R. J., & Smith, J. E. (1995). *Clinical guide to alcohol treatment: The community reinforcement approach.* New York: Guilford Press.

Miller, J. M., Miller, H. V., & Barnes, J. C. (2016). Outcome evaluation of a family-based jail reentry program for substance abusing offenders. *Prison Journal, 96*(1), 53–78.

Miller, W. R. (1996). Form 90: A structured assessment interview for drinking and related behaviors. In M. E. Mattson & L. A. Marshall (Eds.), *Project MATCH monograph series* (Vol. 5, pp. 95–97). Rockville, MD: National Institute on Alcohol Abuse and Alcoholism.

Miller, W. R., Meyers, R. J., & Tonigan, J. S. (1999). Engaging the unmotivated in treatment for alcohol problems: A comparison of three strategies for intervention through family members. *Journal of Consulting and Clinical Psychology, 67,* 688–697.

Miller, W. R., & Moyers, T. B. (2021). Teaching therapeutic skills. In *Effective psychotherapists: Clinical skills that improve client outcomes* (pp. 145–157). New York: Guilford Press.

Miller, W. R., & Rollnick, S. (2014). The effectiveness and ineffectiveness of complex behavioral interventions: Impact of treatment fidelity. *Contemporary Clinical Trials, 37,* 234–241.

Nadkarni, A., Bhatia, U., Velleman, R., Orford, J., Velleman, G., Church, S., . . . Pednekar, S. (2019). Supporting addictions affected families effectively (SAFE): A mixed methods exploratory study of the 5-step method delivered in Goa, India, by lay counselors. *Drugs: Education, Prevention and Policy, 26,* 195–204.

National Institute on Drug Abuse. (2018, June). Commonly abused drugs. Retrieved from *www.drugabuse.gov/drugs-abuse/commonly-abused-drugs-charts*

Nayoski, N., & Hodgins, D. C. (2016). The efficacy of individual community reinforcement and family training (CRAFT) for concerned significant others of problem gamblers. *Journal of Gambling Issues, 33,* 189–212.

Nonaka, S., Sakai, M., & Ono, A. (2013). Effects of cognitive behavior group therapy for mothers of individuals with hikikomori: A trial intervention of community reinforcement and family training. *Seishin Igaku, 55,* 283–291.

Orford, J. (2017). How does the common core to the harm experienced by affected family members vary by relationship, social and cultural factors? *Drugs: Education, Prevention and Policy, 24,* 9–16.

Orford, J., Templeton, L., Velleman, R., & Copello, A. (2005). Family members of relatives with alcohol, drug, and gambling problems: A set of standardized questionnaires for assessing stress, coping, and strain. *Addiction, 100,* 1611–1624.

Orford, J., Velleman, R., Copello, A., Templeton, L., & Ibanga, A. (2010). The experiences of affected family members: A summary of two decades of qualitative research. *Drugs: Education, Prevention and Policy, 17,* 44–62.

Osilla, K. C., Becker, K., Ecola, L., Hurley, B., Manuel, J. K., Ober, A., . . . Watkins, K. E. (2020). Study design to evaluate a group-based therapy for support persons of adults on buprenorphine/naloxone. *Addiction Science and Clinical Practice, 15*(1), 25.

Osilla, K. C., Trail, T. E., Pedersen, E. R., Gore, K. L., & Tolpadi, A. (2017). Efficacy of a web-based intervention for concerned spouses of service members and veterans with alcohol misuse. *Journal of Marital and Family Therapy, 44,* 292–306.

Perumbilly, S. A., Melendez-Rhodes, T., & Anderson, S. A. (2019). Facilitators and barriers in treatment seeking for substance use disorders: Indian clinical perspectives. *Alcoholism Treatment Quarterly, 37,* 240–256.

Roozen, H. G., Boulogne, J. J., van Tulder, M. W., van den Brink, W., De Jong, C. A., & Kerkhof, A. J. (2004). A systematic review of the effectiveness of the community reinforcement approach in alcohol, cocaine and opioid addiction. *Drug and Alcohol Dependence, 74,* 1–13.

Roozen, H. G., Bravo, A. J., Pilatti, A., Mezquita, L., & Vingerhoets, A. (2022). Cross-cultural examination of the community reinforcement approach Happiness Scale (CRA-HS): Testing measurement invariance in five countries. *Current Psychology, 41,* 3842–3852.

Roozen, H. G., de Waart, R., & van der Kroft, P. (2010). Community reinforcement and family training: An effective option to engage treatment-resistant substance-abusing individuals in treatment. *Addiction, 105,* 1729–1735.

Roozen, H. G., & Smith, J. E. (2021). CRA and CRAFT: Behavioral treatments for both motivated and unmotivated substance-abusing individuals and their family members. In N. el-Guebaly, G. Carrà, M. Galanter, & A. M. Baldacchino (Eds.), *Textbook of addiction treatment: International perspectives* (2nd ed., pp. 475–492). Cham, Switzerland: Springer Nature.

Roozen, H. G., & Smith, J. E. (in press). Substance-related and addictive disorders: First-wave case conceptualization. In W. O'Donohue & A. Masuda (Eds.), *Behavior therapy: First, second, and third waves.* Cham, Switzerland: Springer International.

Roozen, H. G., Wiersema, H., Strietman, M., Feij, J. A., Lewinsohn, P. M., Meyers, R. J., . . . Vingerhoets. J. J. (2008). Development and psychometric evaluation of the Pleasant Activities List. *American Journal on Addictions, 17,* 422–435.

Rose, M., Calabria, B., Allan, J., Clifford, A., & Shakeshaft, A. P. (2014). *Aboriginal-specific community reinforcement and family training (CRAFT) manual.* Kensington, Australia: National Drug and Alcohol Research Centre, University of New South Wales.

Rosenberg, M. (1965). *Society and adolescent self-image.* Princeton, NJ: Princeton University Press.

Rotunda, R. J., West, L., & O'Farrell, T. J. (2004). Enabling behavior in a clinical sample of alcohol-dependent clients and their partners. *Journal of Substance Abuse Treatment, 26,* 269–276.

Sakai, M., & Sakano, Y. (2010). Behavioral group psychoeducation for parents whose adult children have withdrawn from social life (hikikomori). *Japanese Journal of Behavior Therapy, 36,* 223–232.

Sanchez-Samper, X., & Knight, J. R. (2009). Drug abuse by adolescents. *Pediatrics in Review, 30,* 83–93.

Sarason, I. G., Sarason, B. R., Shearin, E. N., & Pierce, G. R. (1987). A brief measure of social support: Practical and theoretical implications. *Journal of Social and Personality Relationships, 4,* 497–510.

Sisson, R. W., & Azrin, N. H. (1986). Family-member involvement to initiate and promote treatment of problem drinkers. *Journal of Behavior Therapy and Experimental Psychiatry, 17,* 15–21.

Smith, D. C., Davis, J. P., Ureche, D. J., & Dumas, T. M. (2016). Six month outcomes of a peer-enhanced community reinforcement approach for emerging adults with substance misuse: A preliminary study. *Journal of Substance Abuse Treatment, 61,* 66–73.

Smith, J. E., Crotwell, S. M., Simmons, J. D., & Meyers, R. J. (2015). CRA and CRAFT: Behavioural treatments for both motivated and unmotivated substance abusing individuals. In N. el-Guebaly, G. Carrà, & M. Galanter (Eds.), *Textbook of addiction treatment: International perspectives* (pp. 941–959). Milano, Italy: Springer Milano.

Smith, J. E., Gianini, L. M., Garner, B. R., Malek, K. L., & Godley, S. H. (2014). A behaviorally-anchored rating system to monitor treatment integrity for community clinicians using the adolescent community reinforcement approach. *Journal of Child and Adolescent Substance Abuse, 23,* 185–199.

Smith, J. E., & Meyers, R. J. (2004). *Motivating substance abusers to enter treatment: Working with family members.* New York: Guilford Press.

Smith, J. E., & Meyers, R. J. (2010). *Community reinforcement and family training (CRAFT) therapist coding manual.* Bloomington, IL: Lighthouse Institute.

Smith, J. E., Meyers, R. J., & Delaney, H. (1998). The community reinforcement approach with homeless alcohol-dependent individuals. *Journal of Consulting and Clinical Psychology, 66,* 541–548.

Spielberger, C. D. (1999). *Staxi–2: State–Trait Anger Expression Inventory–2.* Odessa, FL: Psychological Assessment Resources.

Spielberger, C. D., Gorsuch, R. L., Lushene, R., Vagg, P., & Jacobs, G. A. (1983). *Manual for the State–Trait Anxiety Inventory (STAI Form Y).* Palo Alto, CA: Consulting Psychologists Press.

Straus, M. A., & Douglas, E. M. (2004). *Conflict Tactics Scale—Short Form.* APA PsycTests. Retrieved from *https://doi-org.libproxy.unm.edu/10.1037/t43278–000.*

Straus, M., Hamby, S. L., Boney-McCoy, S., & Sugarman, D. B. (1996). *Revised Conflict Tactics Scales.* APA PsycTests.

Substance Abuse and Mental Health Services Administration. (2006). *Detoxification and substance abuse treatment: A treatment improvement protocol TIP 45.* Rockville, MD: Author. Retrieved from *https://store.samhsa.gov/sites/default/files/d7/priv/sma15-4131.pdf*

Substance Abuse and Mental Health Services Administration. (2019). Key substance use and mental health indicators in the United States: Results from the 2018 National Survey on Drug Use and Health (HHS Publication No. PEP19-5068, NSDUH Series H-54). Rockville, MD: Center for Behavioral Health Statistics and Quality, Substance Abuse and Mental Health Services Administration. Retrieved from *www.samhsa.gov/data*

Tsuji, Y., Aoki, S., Irie, T., & Sakano, Y. (2020). Dysfunctional cognition and the mental health of substance abusers' family members. *American Journal of Family Therapy, 49*(2), 170–184.

Venner, K. L., Greenfield, B. L., Hagler, K. J., Simmons, J., Lupee, D., Homer, E., . . . Smith, J. E. (2016). Pilot outcome results of culturally adapted evidence-based substance use disorder treatment with a Southwest tribe. *Addictive Behaviors Reports, 3,* 21–27.

Venner, K. L., Serier, K., Sarafin, R., Greenfield, B., Hirchak, K., Smith, J. E., & Witkiewitz, K. (2021). Culturally tailored evidence-based substance use disorder treatments are efficacious with an American Indian Southwest tribe: An open-label pilot-feasibility randomized controlled trial. *Addiction, 116,* 949–960.

Venner, K. L., Smith, J. E., & Meyers, R. J. (2021, January). Randomized controlled trial of CRAFT with American Indians. Retrieved from *http://report.NIH.gov*

Waldron, H. B., Kern-Jones, S., Turner, C. W., Peterson, T. R., & Ozechowski, T. J. (2007). Engaging resistant adolescents in drug abuse treatment. *Journal of Substance Abuse Treatment, 32,* 133–142.

Welsh, J. W., Passetti, L. L., Funk, R. R., Smith, J. E., Meyers, R. J., & Godley, M. D. (2019). Treatment retention and outcomes with the adolescent community reinforcement approach in emerging adults with opioid use. *Journal of Psychoactive Drugs, 51,* 431–440.

Witkiewitz, K., Pearson, M. R., Wilson, A. D., Stein, E. R., Votaw, V. R., Hallgren, K. A., . . . Tucker, J. A. (2020). Can alcohol use disorder recovery include some heavy drinking? A replication and extension up to 9 years following treatment. *Alcoholism: Clinical and Experimental Research, 44,* 1862–1874.

Yoshioka, M. R., Thomas, E. D., & Ager, R. D. (1992). Nagging and other drinking control efforts of spouses of uncooperative alcohol abusers: Assessment and modification. *Journal of Substance Abuse, 4,* 309–318.

Zimet, G. D., Dahlem, N. W., Zimet, S. G., & Farley, G. K. (1988). The Multidimensional Scale of Perceived Social Support. *Journal of Personality Assessment, 52,* 30–41.

Index

Note. f or *t* following a page number indicates a figure or table.